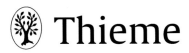

The Practice of Breast Ultrasound

Techniques—Findings—Differential Diagnosis

Helmut Madjar, MD
Professor of Gynecology
German Diagnostic Clinic
Director of the Department of Gynecology
Wiesbaden, Germany

Ellen B. Mendelson, MD, FACR
Professor of Radiology
Feinberg School of Medicine, Northwestern University
Chief, Breast and Women's Imaging Section
Northwestern Memorial Hospital
Chicago, IL, USA

With the collaboration of
Jack Jellins, PhD, Hon MD, FAIUM, FACPSEM
Sydney, Australia
Founding President of the
International Breast Ultrasound School

2nd edition

797 illustrations

Thieme
Stuttgart · New York

Library of Congress Cataloging-in-Publication Data is available from the publisher.

The following images in Chapter 3 are taken from: American College of Radiology (ACR). Breast Imaging Reporting and Data System Atlas (BI-RADS®Atlas). 4th ed. Reston, VA: American College of Radiology; 2003. They are reprinted with permission of the American College of Radiology. No other representation of this material is authorized without expressed, written permission from the American College of Radiology.

Figures 1, 2, 3, 4a and b, 5a and b, 6a and b, 7a and b, 8a and b, 9a, 10, 11a and b, 12, 13a and b, 14 a and b, 15a and b, 16a and b, 17a and b, 18a and b, 3.19a and b, 20, 21a and b, 3.22a and b, 23, 24a and b, 25, 26a and b, 27a and b, 29a–c, 32a and b, 3.37a and b, 38, 44, 46a and b.

Figure 11.2 is reproduced with permission of Elsevier Limited. The article was published in Radiologic Clinics of North America, Vol. 30(1), Mendelson Ellen B, Evaluation of the Postoperative Breast, pp. 107–138, Copyright Elsevier (1992).

Foreword to the Second Edition

This book comes at an opportune time when breast ultrasound examinations are increasing on a worldwide basis due to the availability of high-resolution imaging systems and the realization that ultrasound provides valuable information by differentiating between early cancers and benign lesions with a high degree of accuracy. Ultrasound is also the method of choice for interventional procedures, and plays an important role in patient management. In addition, the concept that ultrasound may have a role in "screening" for breast cancers in selected women will lead to an increase in examination numbers and require a better understanding of the potential of ultrasound imaging systems.

The text of this second edition has been completely revised to bring it up to date with current ACR BI-RADS ultrasound terminology, and, where required, images have been replaced to better illustrate the features described by the ultrasound lexicon. This makes the book suitable for clinicians in all countries and ensures that all descriptors are in accordance with the standard terminology.

Dr. Helmut Madjar and Dr. Ellen B. Mendelson are recognized international breast disease experts. They bring with them the clinical acumen and teaching experience to guarantee that the book not only meets the requirements for advanced breast imagers to optimize their skills in breast ultrasound but also fulfills the needs of beginners with little knowledge of the modality.

Dr. Madjar's ultrasonic skills in breast disease diagnosis, together with his long-term surgical experience, provide a distinctive insight into breast anatomy and pathology, which results in a clear understanding of the correlation between the disease processes and the associated feature descriptors.

Dr. Mendelson has made significant contributions to the book by introducing her knowledge and experience gained in chairing the ACR BI-RADS Ultrasound Expert Working Group responsible for the development of the ultrasound lexicon. Dr. Mendelson's devotion and commitment to high-quality breast imaging is reflected by her international reputation, and by bringing her experience to the book, its value as a comprehensive text has been greatly enhanced.

This book contains the material required to achieve high standards of examination and reporting, and is essential reading to ensure that the best results are obtained for all patients.

Jack Jellins   *Founding President—IBUS*

Foreword to the First Edition

The use of ultrasound for examining individuals presenting with breast problems has increased significantly in recent years. Attempts to delineate changes in breast tissue prior to intervention have become an essential part of modern clinical management. The goal is to avoid breast operations in women with benign lesions while also avoiding the dissemination of malignant cells that would compromise the chance for a cure. Recent advances in technology have facilitated the production of high-quality studies. High-resolution ultrasound images can be obtained in a specific area of interest within the breast volume, and if desired the whole breast can be quickly assessed by following a suitable scanning protocol.

Dr. Helmut Madjar has worked in the field of breast disease diagnosis and treatment since the early 1980s. By developing a systematic scanning protocol, he has contributed significantly to breast ultrasound by extending the capabilities of two-dimensional image interpretation. More recently, Dr. Madjar has further extended the capabilities of ultrasound techniques by evaluating the role of blood flow in the breast and analyzing pathologic features with a view to expanding the traditional criteria for ultrasound interpretation. Dr. Madjar's surgical experience, his expertise in mammography and pathology, and his years of work in various professional societies qualify him to produce a textbook on breast ultrasound which meets the guidelines of the German Society for Ultrasound in Medicine (DEGUM), the International Breast Ultrasound School (IBUS), and the German Union of Health Care Fund Physicians.

This book is structured to comply with the requirements of a three-tiered course of instruction in breast ultrasound covering material at the "basic," "intermediate," and "advanced" levels. It presents a range of diverse breast pathologies that will train the reader to recognize the critical features necessary for making a diagnosis. The inclusion of a standardized reporting format at the intermediate level facilitates the documentation of critical ultrasonic features and ensures that all essential features are included in the description of the area under investigation. This book will significantly improve the reader's ability to interpret breast ultrasound images, and it will provide a basis for the more effective utilization of the ultrasound modality.

Dr. Madjar's extensive experience in continuing education at national and international levels has established his reputation as a leading authority in breast ultrasound. His position as Seminar Director of DEGUM, President of the International Association for Breast Ultrasound (IABU), and Vice-President of IBUS make this clear.

The scientific and clinical results that Dr. Madjar has accumulated in his own research activities also help to make this book a valuable tool for all clinicians and sonologists interested in expanding the clinical capabilities of ultrasonic breast imaging.

Sydney, Australia
Fall 1999

Jack Jellins
President—IBUS

Preface

Ultrasound imaging of the breast has changed dramatically in recent years owing to advances in technology. In the 1970s and early 1980s, the indications for breast ultrasound were limited to palpable nodules and the differentiation of cystic and solid masses. Contrast resolution and spatial resolution at that time were relatively poor, consequently there was a limited capacity for soft-tissue discrimination and the detection of small lesions. Ultrasound technology has advanced significantly in recent years. In the late 1980s, 5-MHz transducers were considered state of the art. Today it is suggested that broad bandwidth linear transducers up to 17–5 MHz or 15–8 MHz with center frequencies of 7–8 MHz or higher be used. Considerable research has been conducted to develop spatial compounding, a speckle-reducing method that improves image quality, currently available in many high-end systems with high-resolution transducers used for breast imaging. Volume acquisitions, multiplanar reconstructions, and 3D/4D technology are available for existing and future applications.

Worldwide randomized controlled trial studies have shown that early detection of breast cancer is important and that mammography screening can reduce breast cancer mortality by 20–40%. These and other studies have also confirmed that high fibroglandular density can limit mammography's sensitivity and that adjunctive screening techniques can help to surmount this problem. Advances in handheld ultrasound have promoted confidence in differentiating between benign and malignant solid masses. Alongside this, there has been increased research interest in the potential of ultrasound for use in evaluating the breasts of women with newly diagnosed breast cancer for extent of the malignant process, as well as for additional screening of women whose risk of breast cancer is high and whose breasts are of high fibroglandular density on mammograms.

With the exception of skin cancers, breast cancer is the most common malignant disease in women of North America and Europe. The risk increases with aging and, as is currently thought, also with breast density, which is higher in younger women. Around 20–30% of breast cancers will develop prior to menopause. A positive family history, especially in first-degree premenopausal relatives, increases the breast cancer risk, and women with genetic mutations such as BRCA-1 and BRCA-2 have an estimated 70–80% risk of developing the disease. Many of these women develop breast cancer at an early age, underscoring the need for an intensive and technically optimal screening program that minimizes the effect of breast density.

In 2007, the American Cancer Society announced its new screening recommendations for contrast-enhanced breast MRI to be performed on an annual basis, in addition to (not replacing) mammography, for women with genetic mutations. Although research is being conducted in newer modalities that might be unaffected by breast density, such as positron emission and 99Tc sestamibi scanning using high-resolution cameras tailored for breast imaging, ultrasound is a leading contender for adjunctive screening of women of high risk (but not as high as that conferred by genetic mutation, previous mantle radiation to the chest for Hodgkin disease, or biopsy with histology of lobular carcinoma in situ) and with radiographically dense breast tissue. Technologic advances, including work on automated scanners, the development of standardized equipment specifications, improved education and training, an optimized examination technique, and data from multicenter studies such as ACRIN (American College of Radiology Imaging Network) 6666 are necessary to support the use of ultrasound for the detection of clinically and mammographically occult disease. Although its efficacy and cost-effectiveness in screening await confirmation from multicenter trial data, breast ultrasound has had a long, well-established history as a diagnostic modality. Use of ultrasound in evaluating palpable masses and breast thickening as well as lesions identified or suspected on mammograms has become the standard of care, helping to increase diagnostic specificity.

Owing to its superficial position, the breast is excellently suited for ultrasound evaluation. Nevertheless, the heterogeneous nature of the component breast tissues requires an examiner who has a basic understanding of ultrasound physics and acoustic artifacts, outlined in the first chapter. Also important for optimizing the power of ultrasound in both detection and diagnosis of breast abnormalities is recognition of breast anatomy and physiologic changes, which are addressed in the opening chapters of this text.

The German Federal Union of Health Insurance Fund Physicians (KBV) established guidelines for accreditation in breast ultrasound based either on in-clinic training or a specialized course of instruction. The latter involves a three-tiered program consisting of a basic, intermediate, and advanced course. This program also requires 200 examinations to be conducted under qualified supervision. The accreditation program represents a minimum requirement, and experienced examiners have realized that their proficiency would grow if they performed the examinations with attention to proper technique.

The format of this book, which was first published in German in 1999 and in English in 2000 with the second German edition appearing in 2005, is based on the progressive course levels of the KBV program and the training guidelines of the German Society for Ultrasound in Medicine (DEGUM) and is in accordance with all published international standards. It starts with basic technical principles, examination technique, the sonographic anatomy of the normal breast, and an outline of the examination protocol. Next, the intermediate course presents a systematic approach to the interpretation of specific benign and malignant breast lesions. Finally, the advanced course deals with specialized or evolving areas such as screening, surgical planning, the evaluation of microcalcifications, and interventional ultrasound, which covers ultrasound-guided fine-needle aspiration and core and vacuum-assisted biopsy techniques, the ultrasound-guided preoperative localization of nonpalpable lesions, and specimen ultrasonography for confirming the complete removal of small focal lesions. The book concludes with a review of innovative techniques that have made significant strides in recent years: 2D image reconstruction, 3D ultrasound imaging, and Doppler ultrasound techniques with and without contrast agents.

The second English edition has been revised to include North American practice patterns, similar in large measure but different in some respects from those of Germany presented in the first edition. Throughout the world, within the past 15 years and even longer, ultrasound has become an integral part of diagnostic breast evaluations, imaging-guided interventions, and patient management plans. The indications for breast sonography as well as the technical standards outlined in this text are in accord with those of

the American College of Radiology (ACR), which also has accreditation programs for breast sonography and ultrasound-guided interventions similar to those of European organizations such as the German Society for Ultrasound in Medicine (Deutsche Gesellschaft für Ultraschall in der Medizin: DEGUM). Added to this edition, helping to strengthen the role of ultrasound in the management of breast disease and offering the basis for self-audit of breast sonologists, is the presentation of the ACR's BI-RADS (Breast Imaging Reporting and Data System) for ultrasound, one of three multimodality lexicons based on a feature analytic approach used in standardizing description, reporting, and lesion assessment. The existence of these programs attests to the importance of ultrasound in managing breast lesions as well as to the commitment of breast imagers worldwide to do their very best in early detection and diagnosis of breast cancer.

Our format is intended to make it easy for the novice to learn about breast ultrasound, but it is also designed to provide a quick and practical reference for the experienced, practicing sonologist. The goal of the book is to help standardize the examination technique and the interpretation of findings, and thus to elevate the status of breast ultrasound as a diagnostic modality. We hope you will find this text useful, reach for it often, and enjoy reading it.

Helmut Madjar
Ellen B. Mendelson

Acknowledgements

We wish to express our great gratitude and profound appreciation to Annie Hollins and Elisabeth Kurz for their superb editorial expertise, meticulous attention to every word and illustration, and graciousness in communicating with two authors separated by the Atlantic Ocean and many time zones. Our special thanks also to the entire Thieme team involved in producing this text, which we hope will be useful to breast imagers everywhere.

Table of Contents

BASIC COURSE

1 Basic Principles   3

Physics 3
    Wavelength 3
    Speed of Sound 3
    Acoustic Impedance 3
    Attenuation 3
    Acoustic Enhancement 4
Technical Aspects of Ultrasound Equipment 6
    Pulsed Sound Waves 6
    Display Modes 6
    Focusing 6
    Transducers 7
    Current System Options Suitable for Breast Imaging:
    Spatial Compounding and Tissue Harmonic Imaging. 9
    Doppler Ultrasound 9
Equipment Operation 12
    Monitor Settings 12
    Documentation Unit 12
    Gain Settings 12
    Focusing 13
    Image Scale 13
    Demographic Documentation and Image Labeling .. 13
    Transducer Selection 14
    Transducer Frequencies 14
    Field of View 14
Quality Control and Test Phantoms 15
    General Considerations 15
    Characteristics of Test Phantoms 15
    Test Protocol 16
    Test Results 17
    Clinical Relevance 19

2 Examination Technique: Historical and Current   23

Water-Path Scanning 23
    Water-Bag Technique 23
    Immersion Technique 24
Real-Time Examination 28
    Patient Positioning 28
    Holding the Transducer 29

    Transducer Selection 31
    Coupling the Transducer 31
    Scanning Technique 32
Dynamic Examination 39
    Evaluating Spatial Extent 39
    Compression 40
Summary 41

3 BI-RADS For Ultrasound   43

Development of the BI-RADS–US System 43
Basis of the BI-RADS–US System: Feature Analysis 43
Classification Categories in the BI-RADS–US System ... 44
    Background Echotexture 44
    Masses 45
    Calcifications 55
    Special Cases 55
    Vascularity 58
Assessment Categories in the BI-RADS–US System 59
Quality Assurance 59
    American College of Radiology Accreditation 59
    American Institute of Ultrasound in Medicine
    Accreditation 59
    European Group for Breast Cancer Screening 60
    International Breast Ultrasound School 60
Summary and Conclusions 60

4 Sonographic Anatomy of the Breast and Axilla   61

Gross Anatomy 61
    Breast 61
    Parasternal Region 62
    Axilla 62
Sonographic Morphology 62
    Breast 62
    Parasternal Region 67
    Axilla 67

5 Standard Protocol for Breast Ultrasound Examinations   71

Patient History 71
Clinical Examination 71
Prior Mammograms 72

Other Studies... 72
Ultrasound Findings 72
Benign–Malignant Differentiation 75
Final Evaluation and Recommendation 76
Documentation 77

INTERMEDIATE COURSE

6 Fibrocystic Change   81

Clinical Significance.................................... 81
Diagnosis with Ultrasound........................... 82
    Common Findings................................... 82
    Less Common Findings 86
Diagnosis and Management, Pitfalls,
and When to Biopsy.................................... 92
Further Diagnostic Procedures 96
    MRI and Color Doppler 96
    Aspiration and Core Biopsy 97
    Ductography.. 97
Role of Ultrasound 98
Documentation 98

7 Cysts and Intracystic Tumors   99

Clinical Significance.................................... 99
Diagnostic Criteria...................................... 99
    Simple Cysts 99
    Complicated Cysts 100
Differential Diagnosis, Pitfalls 108
    Echogenic Cysts Versus Solid Tumors 108
    Fluid Levels 108
    Reverberations 109
    Malignant Tumors 109
Interventional Procedures........................... 114
    Aspiration 114
    Pneumocystography............................... 114
Role of Ultrasound 115
Documentation 115

8 Breast Implants   117

Clinical Significance................................... 117
Sonographic Findings 119
    Testing Ultrasound Properties of Different
    Implant Types 121

Implant Abnormalities: Fibrous Encapsulation,
Capsular Contracture, Extra- and Intracapsular
Implant Rupture.. 122
    Extra- and Intracapsular Implant Rupture,
    Silicone Migration, Granulomas, Siliconomas 123
    Primary and Recurrent Tumors............... 126
Differential Diagnosis, Pitfalls 128
Further Diagnostic Procedures 128
Role of Ultrasound 128
Documentation 129

9 Abscesses   131

Clinical Significance................................... 131
    Lactational Abscesses............................ 131
    Nonpuerperal Abscesses......................... 131
Diagnostic Criteria..................................... 132
    Edema 132
    Mass 132
    Additional Diagnostic Considerations...... 135
Management Procedures............................. 138
Role of Imaging 138
Documentation 139

10 Benign Solid Tumors   141

Clinical Significance................................... 141
Diagnostic Criteria..................................... 141
    Typical Findings of Fibroadenomas 141
    Less Common Findings of Fibroadenomas 145
    Other Benign Tumors............................. 145
Differential Diagnosis, Considerations, and Pitfalls 150
Further Diagnostic Procedures 153
    Ultrasound 153
    Mammography 153
    MRI.. 153
Documentation 156

11 Scars—The Treated Breast   157

Clinical Significance, Diagnostic Problems................. 157
Diagnostic Criteria, Postoperative Follow-Up 159
 Typical Findings.. 159
 Less Common Findings 160
Differential Diagnosis 164
Diagnostic Procedures.. 164
Role of Ultrasound 166
Documentation 166

12 Carcinoma   167

Clinical Significance.. 167
Diagnostic Criteria.. 168
 Typical Findings.. 168
 Less Common Findings 175

Differential Diagnosis 176
Further Diagnostic Procedures 188
Role of Ultrasound 189
Documentation 190

13 Lymph Nodes   191

Clinical Significance.. 191
Diagnostic Criteria.. 191
 Findings for Normal and Benign Lymph Nodes 191
 Findings for Malignant Lymph Nodes 192
Differential Diagnosis 196
Further Diagnostic Procedures 197
Role of Ultrasound 197
Documentation 198

ADVANCED COURSE

14 Interventional Ultrasound   201

Clinical Significance.. 201
Needle Insertion Technique 201
Fine-Needle Aspiration Cytology 205
 Solid Lesions 205
 Fluid-filled Lesions 207
Large Needle Biopsy:
Core, Vacuum-assisted, and Other Technologies 208
Ultrasound-Guided Localization.............................. 210
Specimen Ultrasonography..................................... 212
Summary 213

15 Preoperative Staging   215

Clinical Significance.. 215
Tumor Size... 215
Intraductal Carcinomas and
Intraductal Components.. 216
Multifocality and Multicentricity 218
Surgical Planning.. 220

16 Screening   223

Clinical Significance.. 223
Target Group for Extended Screening...................... 223

Prerequisites for Extended Screening...................... 223
Studies on Ultrasound Screening............................. 226
 Results of the Freiburg Screening Study 226
 Conclusions of the Freiburg Screening Study.......... 227

17 Follow-Up and Recurrence   229

Clinical Significance.. 229
Detection of Locoregional Recurrences 229
 Role of Ultrasound Compared with
 Other Modalities 234

18 Three-dimensional, Extended Field-of-View Ultrasound, and Real-time Compound Scanning   235

Clinical Significance.. 235
 Extended Field-of-View Ultrasound 235
 Real-time Compound Scanning............................. 235
Technical Principles 235
 Extended Field-of-View-Ultrasound...................... 236
 Real-time Compound Scanning............................. 237
Sample Applications of Three-dimensional
Ultrasound 238
Sample Applications of Extended
Field-of-View Imaging.. 239

Sample Applications of Compound Scanning............. 241
Discussion and Outlook............................... 243

19 Doppler Ultrasound   245

Clinical Principles 245
Historical Development............................... 245
Examination Technique 246
Interpretive Criteria.................................... 247
   Vascularity and Hemodynamic Parameters............. 248
Possible Applications.................................. 250
   Smoothly Marginated Carcinomas.......... 250
   Proliferative Fibroadenomas 250
   Multifocal and Multicentric Tumors 250

Scars.. 250
Lymph Node Evaluation........................... 251
Prognostic Evaluation.............................. 251
Chemotherapy and Follow-Up.................. 252
Use of Ultrasound Contrast Agents to Increase
Doppler Signal 252
   Practical Application.............................. 253

20 Breast Ultrasound Review Questions   255

Appendix: IBUS Guidelines 259
Further Reading 261
Index 264

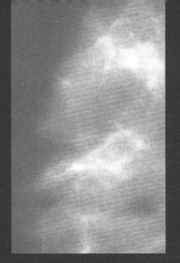

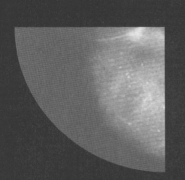

BASIC COURSE

1 Basic Principles   3

2 Examination Technique:
Historical and Current   23

3 BI-RADS For Ultrasound   43

4 Sonographic Anatomy
of the Breast and Axilla   61

5 Standard Protocol for
Breast Ultrasound Examinations   71

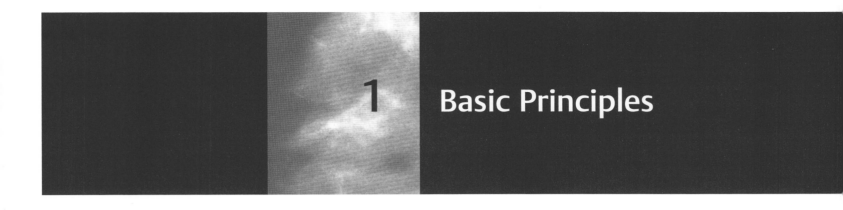

Basic Principles

Physics

Sound waves are mechanical waves that require a medium through which to propagate. Sound cannot travel through a vacuum. Different materials have different acoustic properties and therefore vary in their ability to transmit sound waves and reflect them at interfaces. The human ear is unable to hear sounds at frequencies higher than approximately 20,000 Hz (20 kHz). Frequencies beyond this range are known as *ultrasound*. Diagnostic ultrasound instruments generally operate at frequencies of 3–10-million Hz (3–10 MHz). High frequencies have shorter wavelengths, providing better spatial resolution and visualization of small tissue structures. To understand how images are produced with ultrasound, it is necessary to know something about the physics and technology of ultrasound. The most important basic concepts in ultrasound physics involve sound waves, the speed of sound, and acoustic impedance.

Wavelength

The following formula is used to calculate wavelength, λ:

$\lambda = c/f$, where c is the propagation velocity of sound in m/sec and f is the frequency or number of complete cycles in a unit of time (sec^{-1} or 1/sec).

Here are some examples of how wavelengths are calculated: Let us assume that a pure tone has a frequency of 262 Hz. The speed of sound in air is 330 m/s. The wavelength, λ, of the tone is calculated as follows:

$\lambda c = 330/262 = 1.3$ m

In soft tissue, the propagation velocity averages 1540 m/s. Using an ultrasound frequency of 5 million Hz (5 MHz), and taking into consideration that sound travels at greater speed through soft tissue than through air, in soft tissue $\lambda = 0.308$ mm.

Speed of Sound

The propagation speed of sound in air is very low. It is intermediate in water and soft tissues and relatively high in bone (**Table 1.1**).

Acoustic Impedance

In addition to propagation speed, tissue density has a major influence on the transmission and reflection of sound, and both propagation speed and physical properties of tissues are determinants of acoustic impedance (**Table 1.2**). As acoustic impedance increases, more of the sound energy is reflected and less is transmitted.

Because different soft tissues have similar impedances, most of the energy is transmitted at soft-tissue interfaces and a relatively small proportion of it is reflected. In diagnostic ultrasound, this permits the clear visualization of different tissues located at different depths within the body. If the sound encounters air or bone, however, the impedance mismatch is so great that almost all of the acoustic energy is reflected and nearly none is transmitted. This creates an *acoustic shadow* that obscures structures located deep to the air or bone.

Attenuation

As sound propagates through tissue, its amplitude and intensity are gradually decreased (attenuated) due to interactions between the sound waves and the medium. Causes of attenuation include sound absorption due to mechanical energy losses and the conversion of mechanical energy to heat. Reflections at interfaces also decrease the sound amplitude in proportion to increasing distance of travel. Sound is scattered when it bounces off small objects and is further attenuated by refraction when encountered by structures obliquely situated with respect to the direction of the beam

Table 1.1 Speed of sound in various media (m/s)

Air	330
Water	1520
Fatty tissue	1450
Muscle tissue	1580
Liver tissue	1560
Bone	3800

Table 1.2 Acoustic impedance of various media

Air	0.04
Water	152
Fat	138
Muscle	170
Liver	164
Bone	722

such as the curved interfaces of fat lobules. These components do not return to the transducer, so that their energy is lost and no echo signal is detected. The higher the frequency of the sound beam, the more it is attenuated. Thus, while high frequencies are theoretically desirable in imaging to optimize spatial resolution, attenuation limits the use of high frequencies in the deeper portions of the field of view. As a result, lower frequencies are needed for penetration to greater imaging depths, with the higher frequencies used in examining superficial structures. Broad bandwidth linear transducers offer the frequency ranges appropriate for breast imaging, up to 17 MHz in the near field and decreasing to 5 MHz for penetration of deeper areas.

Propagation of sound waves is optimal when the acoustic beam encounters tissue interfaces at 90°. Because of the impedance difference at interfaces, some of the energy is reflected back to the transducer and some continues to travel through the tissues in a straight line. If the sound meets a structure with an oblique angle of incidence, then part of the energy is reflected away from the interface at the same angle. The sound that enters the second medium undergoes refraction. The angle of refraction depends on the angle of incidence as well as the speed of sound in the adjacent medium. The more oblique the interface, the greater the deflection of the sound wave.

The critical angle between skin and connective tissue and between fat and parenchymal structures is approximately 50°. The refraction occurring at this angle is so great that the sound wave cannot penetrate the tissue interface. As a result, an acoustic shadow is formed, and the underlying structure is not visualized. Ultrasound examination technique can be modified to compensate for this effect (Chapter 2).

The various causes of attenuation explain why an acoustic shadow is frequently seen deep to carcinomas that have a heterogeneous internal structure (**Fig. 1.1**). Acoustic shadowing is an important feature to be applied in lesion analysis. The many fibrous elements present in scars lead to diffuse sound refraction, causing the tissue to appear hypoechoic and cast an acoustic shadow (**Fig. 1.2**). It is important to understand the cause of this phenomenon, because external compression can be applied to the breast with the transducer to flatten out the fibrous structures and decrease the refraction artifacts, bringing out the internal structural details of the scar tissue and diminishing acoustic shadowing (**Fig. 1.3**). This is a useful technique for helping to differentiate scar tissue from a malignant tumor.

Acoustic Enhancement

The structures located behind fluid and homogeneous tissues generally appear brighter (whiter) than other structures, creating an impression that the echoes have been amplified (**Figs. 1.4, 1.5**). In reality, however, the amplitude of the sound has not changed. When sound traverses a structure that absorbs less acoustic en-

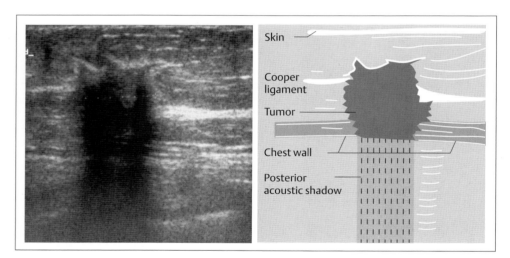

Fig. 1.1 Heterogeneous breast carcinoma with posterior acoustic shadowing. Sound is diffusely scattered within the heterogeneous internal structure of the tumor. The scattering, along with sound absorption in the tissue, creates a posterior acoustic shadow, associated with approximately 60% of primary breast carcinomas.

Skin

Cooper ligament

Tumor

Chest wall

Posterior acoustic shadow

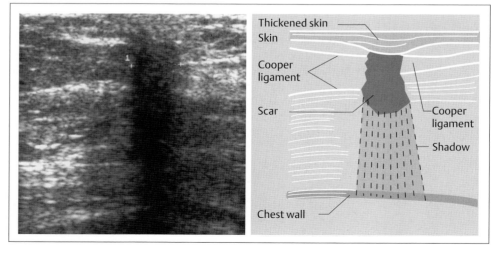

Fig. 1.2 Surgical scar with shadowing. The numerous connective tissue elements in this scar scatter the sound. Because of the refraction and attenuation, the scar appears hypoechoic and casts an acoustic shadow.

Thickened skin
Skin

Cooper ligament

Scar

Cooper ligament

Shadow

Chest wall

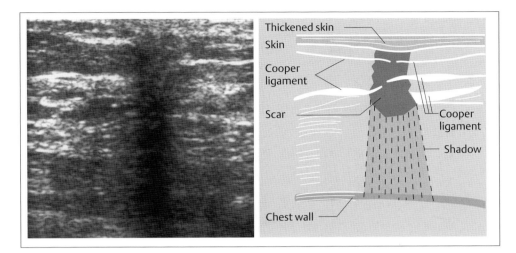

Fig. 1.3 Effect of compression. The same scar as in Fig. 1.2, but with slight pressure applied with the transducer. The external pressure flattens the connective tissue structures, improving sound penetration and reflection. This reduces acoustic shadowing and improves delineation of the internal structures. Scars also may change shape in orthogonal projections.

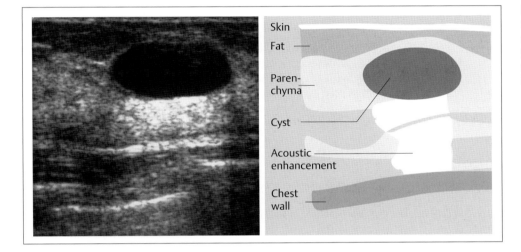

Fig. 1.4 Simple cyst with acoustic enhancement. Sound absorption in the surrounding parenchyma is higher than in the cyst. TGC (time gain compensation) corrects for the absorption, causing an apparent enhancement of echoes behind the cyst, where less attenuation occurs.

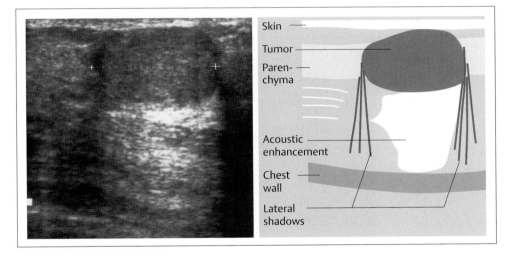

Fig. 1.5 Typical fibroadenoma. This solid, circumscribed homogeneous mass oriented parallel to the skin is less attenuating than the breast tissue, producing an acoustic enhancement effect similar to that in Fig. 1.4. Some complicated cysts with low-level internal echoes have a similar appearance.

ergy than surrounding tissues, the area located behind that structure will appear relatively brighter than its surroundings. This *acoustic enhancement* phenomenon is a typical feature of cysts and homogeneous solid masses, such as lymphomas.

Sound is attenuated as it travels through tissue, and ultrasound scanners (p. 12) can correct this effect with *time gain compensation* (TGC), which boosts the amplitude of echoes that are returned from more distant sources and can decrease overly bright echoes from superficial structures. A uniform brightness level is created over the full depth of the image, helping to improve the diagnostic quality of the image.

Technical Aspects
of Ultrasound Equipment

Pulsed Sound Waves

When a continuous sound wave (constant tone) is emitted, there is no way to calculate the travel time of the sound. To generate an image, it is necessary to transmit the sound in pulses of brief duration. The piezoelectric crystal in an ultrasound transducer is caused to vibrate by electronic impulses. A damping material at the back of the crystal limits the duration of the vibration, causing a short ultrasound pulse to be emitted. This pulse travels through the tissue, and sound waves are reflected back to the transducer from various depths. The reflected sound waves *(echoes)* that return to the transducer set up new vibrations in the piezoelectric crystal, which are converted to electrical signals. Given the relatively constant speed of sound in tissues, the time interval between the transmission and reception of the signal is proportional to the distance of the reflector from the transducer.

Display Modes

An ultrasound pulse can be used to interrogate a series of reflectors situated along a straight line. The different amplitudes that are received from various depths correspond to the impedance differences that are encountered in the tissues. The echoes registered along the path of the ultrasound pulse can be plotted on the x-axis of a monitor and their amplitudes on the y-axis to generate a one-dimensional sectional image. This display mode, in which distance is represented on the horizontal axis and amplitudes on the vertical axis, is called *A-mode* or *amplitude modulation* (**Fig. 1.6**). In the early years of ultrasound development, this was the only mode available for echo signal display. The disadvantage of the A-mode

trace is that it makes spatial and anatomic orientation difficult. Its advantage is that it allows the precise measurement of echo amplitudes. The sharp amplitude peaks provide accurate reference points for measuring transducer-to-reflector distances, and therefore A-mode is still used today for various applications.

Instead of displaying the different amplitudes of a one-dimensional image along the vertical axis, the amplitudes can be represented as spots of varying brightness: lower amplitudes appear darker, and higher amplitudes appear brighter. In this brightness-modulated mode, the one-dimensional display can be swept across the screen to depict changes along a temporal axis. This *M-mode* or *motion mode* is commonly used in echocardiography. The two-dimensional display represents the motion of the different tissue structures along a temporal axis (**Fig. 1.7**).

In the *B-mode (brightness modulation)* technique, multiple brightness-modulated lines of ultrasonic beams are displayed adjacent to one another on the monitor. This creates a two-dimensional sectional image in which different echo amplitudes are represented as different shades of gray, optimized by a broad dynamic range that offers the opportunity to perceive subtle differences in tissue echogenicity.

Real-time, gray-scale, B-mode display is currently the mainstay of diagnostic sonography. The impression of motion is obtained by rapid production of numerous individual two-dimensional images viewed in rapid sequence at rates of 15–60 frames per second.

Focusing

Various transducer design principles are employed in two-dimensional ultrasound imaging. The selection of a transducer for a particular imaging application is guided by its characteristic field of view and the way in which the sound beam can be steered. If the beam were not focused, the sound waves would diverge in a conical pattern and it would not be possible to accurately locate adjacent reflectors and portray them as separate structures. Beam

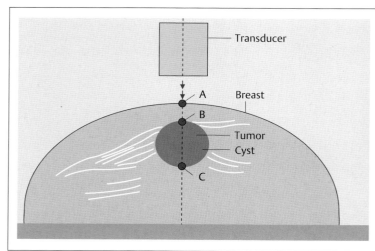
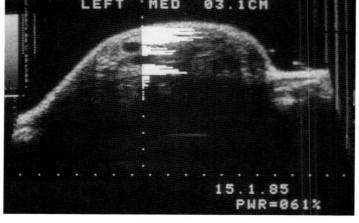

Fig. 1.6 Schematic diagram and monitor display of the A-mode (amplitude modulation) technique. This mode registers the echo amplitudes that are detected along one image line, producing a one-dimensional display of the sound amplitudes. Because the A-mode image does not provide anatomic orientation, it has been superimposed over a two-dimensional B-mode image of the breast. The image demonstrates a cyst.

The one-dimensional display of echo amplitudes in the A-mode image shows a circumscribed anechoic area, representing the cyst, flanked by high-amplitude echoes from the adjacent parenchyma. Acoustic enhancement accounts for the slightly higher amplitudes registered behind the cyst. High amplitudes appear bright in the B-mode image, and low amplitudes appear dark.

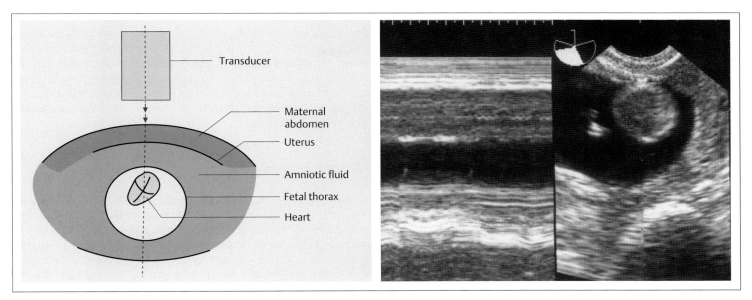

Fig. 1.7 Schematic diagram and monitor display (left) of the M-mode (time–motion) technique, illustrated here for a fetal heart. The motion of brightness-modulated spots is registered along a temporal (horizontal) axis. The echo amplitudes are represented as different levels of gray. Corresponding B-mode image is also shown (far right).

focusing is critical for achieving acceptable lateral resolution. Different transducers employ a variety of focusing methods, such as mechanical rotation, oscillation of the transducer, or electronic steering.

Transducers

Several types of transducers are available for two-dimensional B-mode imaging, the mode used for most clinical imaging studies (**Figs. 1.8–1.11 a–c**, **Table 1.3**). These transducers, along with their advantages and disadvantages in various applications, are discussed below.

Mechanical Sector Transducer

This type incorporates the simplest design principle (**Fig. 1.8**). A piezoelectric crystal is mounted on a rotation axis and driven by an electric motor that moves the crystal in a short circular or sector-shaped pattern. With each slight change in the crystal angle, a sound pulse is transmitted and received. The pattern of adjacent scan lines results in a sectional image of triangular shape, its apex at the top of the image. The advantage of this transducer is its relatively simple design. Disadvantages are the limited focusing options, the nonuniform field of view, and mechanical wear of the moving parts. The transducer is focused by using a curved piezoelectric crystal or interposing an acoustic lens to narrow the beam. This design results in a fixed focal zone located at a specific depth. One problem is the change in beam width at the near and far sides of the focal zone; variable focusing often cannot be achieved. Some transducers contain two or three crystals with different radii of curvature, providing a limited capacity for focusing at different depths.

Another disadvantage of the sector transducer is that the tissue directly beneath the probe is compressed during scanning. This unequal pressure distribution may displace mobile lesions out of the scan plane. Moreover, the small acoustic window of sector transducers provides more restricted near-field coverage than linear transducers, making sector transducers less useful for systematically surveying the entire breast. When a sector transducer is used for breast imaging, it should be used with a standoff pad to improve the visualization of more superficial structures as well as to obtain a broader and more linear coupling surface. Also, the standoff pad should be of appropriate thickness to place the focal zone of the transducer within the superficial breast layer.

These fixed-focus mechanical sector transducers are no longer commonly used for breast imaging.

Electronic Linear-Array Transducer

This transducer incorporates a different design principle. The transducer is elongated and contains many small piezoelectric crystals arranged side by side (**Fig. 1.9**). Each of these crystals (or small subgroup of crystals) is electronically fired in sequence, and each of the pulsed units transmits and receives one scan line. The parallel arrangement of the scan lines produces a two-dimensional, rectangular image. The time delay between successive crystal firing pulses can be varied as a means of directing and focusing the beam (**Fig. 1.10**). Pulsing the outer crystals first and then pulsing the inner crystals with a specified time delay results in a convergent sound wave with a variable focal distance. Increasing the pulsing delay between the outer and inner crystals short-

Table 1.3 Principal types of ultrasound transducer

▸ Mechanical sector transducer
▸ Electronic linear-array transducer
▸ Electronic convex-array transducer
▸ Electronic sector transducer
▸ Annular-array sector transducer

ens the focal distance and moves the focal point more into the near field. Decreasing the delay moves the focal point deeper in the field. A two-dimensional image is produced not by exciting individual crystals but by pulsing small groups of neighboring crystals in succession, each time shifting the pulsing sequence laterally by one crystal so that an image is built up line by line. The advantages are that the focal distance can be varied electronically, and that multiple focal zones can be produced simultaneously at various depths.

Variable focusing is an important advantage of linear-array transducers. Additionally, the parallel scan lines provide a uniform image field that is as broad in the near field as it is at greater depths. The flat transducer face is also advantageous for evaluating superficial structures, as it provides a relatively uniform coupling pressure at the skin surface. This avoids excessive deformation of the breast that would hamper the evaluation of anatomic structures. Electronic linear-array transducers used for breast imaging generally do not require a standoff pad except for the skin and most superficial tissues, and currently available transducers can focus to depths of less than 1 cm in the near field. With older or low-frequency transducers that do not provide acceptable near-field focusing, a standoff pad or thick mound of coupling gel should be used for examining superficial structures.

One disadvantage of linear transducers is that variable focusing is possible only in the image plane, resulting in a greater "image thickness" or slice thickness in the plane perpendicular to it. This adversely affects spatial resolution, although the effect may be difficult to appreciate in two-dimensional sectional images. Sector transducers focus the beam not just in the image plane but also in a circumferential pattern, but the focal zone of these probes is confined to a narrow region.

Electronic Convex-Array Transducer

Convex (curved) arrays are frequently used for abdominal imaging. The crystals are arranged side by side, as in the linear array, but the surface of the transducer is curved. This causes the beams to fan out, producing a trapezoidal image. The advantage over sector transducers is that the image can be electronically modified. As in the linear array, individual crystal groups can be pulsed with different time delays to modify the focal distance. The larger coupling surface provides a broader acoustic window in the near field, which is advantageous for evaluating superficial structures. Also, the scan lines are less divergent than in a sector transducer, resulting in a more uniform image field.

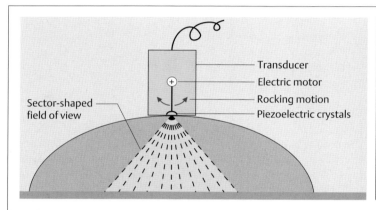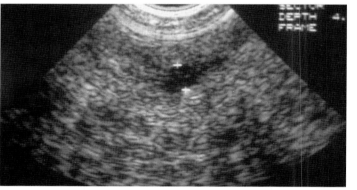

Fig. 1.8 Schematic diagram and monitor display of a mechanical sector transducer. As the motor-driven crystal transmits and receives ultrasound pulses, the constantly changing angle of the crystal produces a sector-shaped field of view. Disadvantages are the strong divergence of the scan lines and the limited focusing options. Mechanical sector transducers should no longer be used for breast imaging.

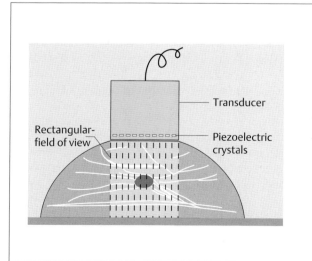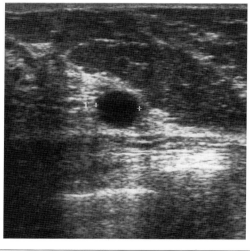

Fig. 1.9 Schematic diagram and monitor display of a linear-array transducer. This electronic multiple-element transducer contains an array of up to several hundred closely spaced piezoelectric crystals. Its advantages are a relatively uniform coupling pressure in the examination of superficial structures, the uniform field of view in the near and far fields, and the parallel arrangement of the image lines.

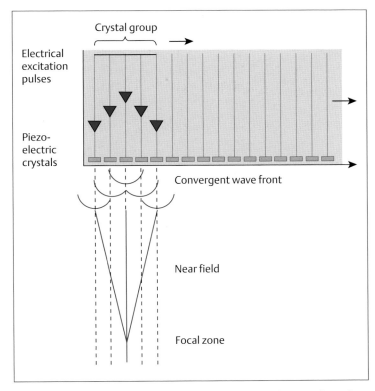

Fig. 1.10 Focusing in a linear-array transducer. The diagram shows how the crystal groups are pulsed in part of a linear array, which usually consists of 100–200 individual crystals. Shifting the pulsing pattern by one crystal with an appropriate time delay produces a convergent, electronically focused beam.

Labels in figure: Crystal group; Electrical excitation pulses; Piezo-electric crystals; Convergent wave front; Near field; Focal zone

Electronic Sector Transducer

These transducers have a smaller coupling surface than convex probes. They contain multiple crystals which are electronically pulsed to produce a sector-shaped image with variable focusing. As in mechanical sector probes, the image field is nonuniform due to convergence of the scan lines in the near field and divergence of the lines in the far field, and near-field coverage is limited.

Two-Dimensional Annular-Array Sector Transducer

This is an interesting design that employs multiple ring-shaped crystals in a concentric array (**Fig. 1.11 a–c**). As in electronic linear arrays, the crystals can be pulsed in a time-delayed sequence to shape and focus the beam. The whole array is mounted on a mechanically driven rotating axis that follows the principle of an ordinary sector transducer. This results in a sector-shaped sectional image. As in linear arrays, the crystal rings can be pulsed to position the focal zone or focus the beam synchronously at various depths. The advantages of this transducer are the spatial extent of the image (slice thickness) and the concentric focusing, which provides uniform image quality within the image plane. These probes should be used with a standoff pad to improve near-field coverage. Annular-array transducers are still relatively costly but increasingly available, and they provide a true alternative to electronic linear arrays. An advantage is that they can be focused in lateral as well as elevation planes. Additionally, they can collect

volumetric data needed for three-dimensional processing. One disadvantage, besides their high cost, is their large size and weight, which makes them relatively difficult to handle and maneuver. Another problem is the complexity of signal processing, resulting in a relatively slow frame rate.

Current System Options Suitable for Breast Imaging: Spatial Compounding and Tissue Harmonic Imaging

Research in transducer development continues, and in the future we will most likely see transducer designs offering three-dimensional and four-dimensional technology, the latter allowing for three-dimensional scanning in real time. Probes that enable elasticity measurements of tumors to be made are also approaching readiness for clinical use.

Spatial compounding is an important technical advance that has been available for some years. The scattering of ultrasound from small reflectors in breast tissue contributes to *speckle*, which can diminish contrast resolution. Speckle can obscure the margins of a mass, making it difficult to tell whether a mass is circumscribed or its margins are indistinct. With spatial compounding, between three and nine scanning angles are averaged, reducing the noise created by random scattering of sound in tissue. The resultant image is much smoother, and the margins of a mass can be analyzed more confidently for diagnosis. Posterior features (shadowing, enhancement) are less conspicuous but still recognizable.

Tissue harmonic imaging, important for reducing clutter and noise in deeper tissues and ineffective in superficial tissues, has been adapted to breast imaging. At 2–5 cm deep to the skin, it increases contrast and "cleans out" cysts. In the authors' view it diminishes the gray scale and subtlety of tissue differentiation obtainable with high-resolution transducers, giving the image an older style, high-contrast, more black-and-white image. The physics of harmonic imaging includes signal filtration or coded pulses to cancel artifacts occurring as a result of phase aberration (differential wave propagation speed through tissue, the high-pressure component moving more rapidly than the rarefactional component), thus distorting the wave.

Doppler Ultrasound

When a sound wave encounters a moving structure, the frequency of the reflected signal is altered. This phenomenon, called the Doppler effect, provides a means of detecting and recording blood flow. Structures (blood cells) moving toward the transducer increase the frequency of the reflected sound waves, while structures moving away from the transducer decrease their frequency. The difference between the two frequencies, called the Doppler shift, ΔF, is proportional to the velocity of the moving reflector ($\Delta F \sim F_R - F_T) = 2F_T v/c$). F_R represents the frequency of sound reflected from the moving structures while F_T is the frequency of sound transmission from the transducer; v is velocity of the structures moving toward the transducer and c, the frequency of sound in the particular medium.

The magnitude of the recorded frequency shift also depends on the cosine of the angle between the sound beam and the direction of blood flow (the course of the vessel) as defined by the equation: $\Delta F (F_R - F_T) = (2F_T)v \times \cos\Theta$.

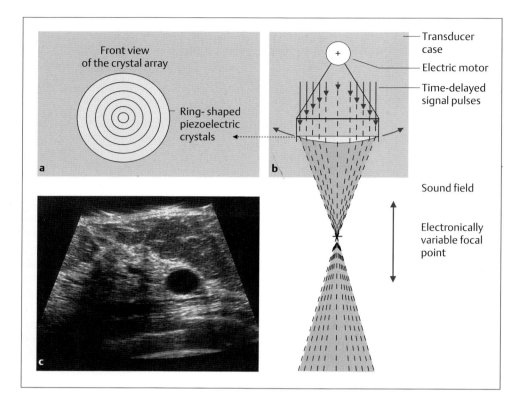

Front view
of the crystal array

Ring- shaped
piezoelectric
crystals

Transducer
case

Electric motor

Time-delayed
signal pulses

Sound field

Electronically
variable focal
point

a

b

c

Fig. 1.11 a–c Annular-array transducer. The basic design principle is like that of a sector transducer. But instead of one crystal, the transducer contains several ring-shaped crystals arranged in a concentric pattern. The array can be electronically pulsed to emit a focused beam. The diagram in panel **a** shows a front view of the annular crystal array. Panel **b** shows a side view of the transducer, and **c** illustrates the monitor view of a small breast cyst. This image was obtained with a fluid standoff pad, which widens the image to several centimeters in the near field.

The blood flow velocity can be calculated from the Doppler shift using the following equation:

$$v = \Delta F \cdot C/2F_T \cdot \cos\Theta.$$

This physical principle can be applied in various ways to record blood flow. Pulsed ultrasound systems (see below) can combine ultrasound imaging with Doppler flow analysis.

Various Doppler techniques have been developed. The simplest is *continuous-wave Doppler* (CW Doppler), which employs a pencil-shaped probe containing two crystals. The transmitting crystal emits sound continuously, and the receiving crystal receives the returning signal (**Fig. 1.12**) continuously. This technique is useful for detecting blood flow in the direction of the beam, but it cannot provide depth information or generate an image. The crystals do not have to be damped as in a pulsed system, making CW Doppler a highly sensitive technique for detecting low-velocity flows. Because the angle of the blood vessel cannot be determined, only the frequency shift can be measured with this technique. The frequency shift is proportional to the flow velocity, but angle correction is necessary to make a precise calculation.

Duplex Scanning

This technique employs a combination of B-mode imaging and Doppler flow sampling to simultaneously display a two-dimensional sectional image and the Doppler frequency spectrum from a selected sample volume (**Fig. 1.13**). As a general rule, duplex scanning is used only when the vessel of interest can be identified in the B-mode image. When the angle between the beam and vessel is known (angle correction), the flow velocity can be calculated. The advantage of duplex is the capacity for the selective interrogation of vessels that are visible in the image. One disadvantage is that ultrasound scanners in duplex mode usually operate at a lower frequency than the nominal frequency of the transducer.

Another disadvantage is that the Doppler signal and imaging beam are pulsed. This requires damping, and the lower frequency reduces sensitivity.

Color-Flow Doppler

This technique permits the two-dimensional imaging of blood flow within a real-time B-mode image. The measured frequency shifts are color-coded and displayed as color pixels (**Fig. 1.14 a–c**). The shade and brightness of the colors encode the direction and velocity of the flow. A spectral waveform can be generated by activating the duplex mode. The advantage is that a system with sufficient sensitivity can detect small vessels that are not visible in the B-mode image. This can be helpful in the evaluation of tumors and characterization of hypoechoic and nearly anechoic masses as cystic or solid. One limitation of color-flow Doppler is noise, represented by color, increasing as the gain is turned up, and ultimately intrusive.

Power Doppler

This technique, which also uses color coding, is based on amplitude rather than frequency as in color-flow Doppler. Its advantages over color-flow Doppler are less angle dependence, representation of noise by a homogeneous background color, and no aliasing. Artifactual noise is less of a problem, thus allowing higher gain settings to be used for heightened sensitivity to presence of flow. Power Doppler has also been used with vocal fremitus: for example, by having the patient hum or vocalize the vowel "e" over a long enough time to observe that a lesion, possibly benign or malignant, does not fill in with color while the surrounding isoechoic fat lobules reflect the vibration caused by the humming.

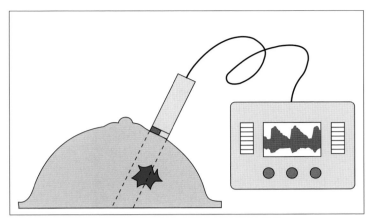

Fig. 1.12 Schematic diagram of a CW Doppler examination with a pencil-shaped probe. The Doppler frequency spectrum is displayed on the monitor.

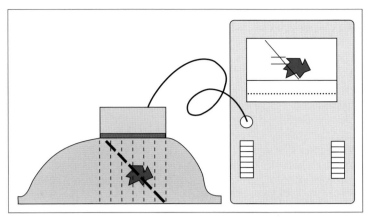

Fig. 1.13 The duplex examination combines B-mode imaging with Doppler flow sampling. Doppler frequencies can be measured within a selected sample volume in the B-mode image. Duplex scanning is feasible only when the vessel of interest can be identified in the B-mode image.

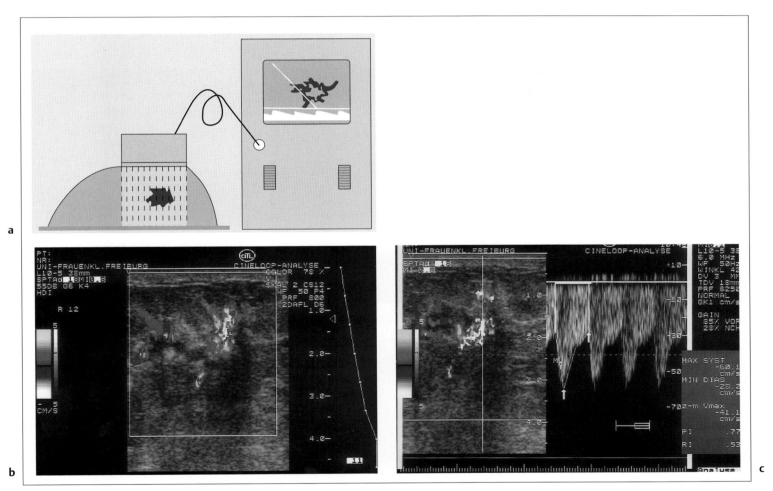

Fig. 1.14 a–c Color Doppler imaging. **a** As the diagram shows, frequency shifts are recorded throughout the image field and are displayed as color-coded pixels. Blue generally represents a negative frequency shift, indicating blood flow away from the transducer. Red indicates a positive frequency shift. The brightness of the color is a semiquantitative indicator of flow velocity. **b** Color Doppler display of invasive breast carcinoma. The color flow image shows a hypoechoic mass with irregular, ill-defined margins supplied by multiple blood vessels. **c** When the duplex mode is activated, selective flow analysis can be carried out in vessels demonstrated by color Doppler. The example shows a systolic flow velocity of 60.1 cm/s. The relationship of systole and diastole provides indices for describing the frequency profiles.

Equipment Operation

Monitor Settings

In B-mode imaging, the different echo amplitudes are displayed on the monitor in shades of gray. For many ultrasound systems, a gray-level scale with at least 16 different shades of gray is displayed at the edge of the screen. This aids the operator in adjusting the brightness and contrast of the monitor optimally so that different gray levels are distinguishable. If the contrast or brightness is set too low or too high, a portion of the gray-scale information will be lost (**Figs. 1.15 a–c, 1.16 a–c**).

Documentation Unit

There are many options for documenting ultrasound images. As the use of digital mammography becomes more widespread, mammograms, sonograms, and MRI images are now stored on picture archiving and communication systems (PACS) and mini-PACS systems. Also available is storage on film using laser systems, thermal printers, video clips and other systems. These systems, like the monitor, require brightness and contrast adjustments (**Figs. 1.15 a–c, 1.16 a–c**). The settings should be checked before every examination and calibrated to match the image on the monitors. If settings are faulty, the quality of the documentation may be insufficient to permit subsequent review of the images. Thus, the settings on the documentation unit are just as important as the monitor settings.

Gain Settings

Image brightness is affected by the power setting (amplitude of the transmitted signal), the gain setting (amplification of the received signals), and the *time gain compensation* (TGC). As the power setting is increased, a greater amount of sound energy is reflected back to the receiver, and the image appears brighter (**Fig. 1.17 a–c**). The same applies to the gain setting. It is also important to adjust the TGC, which compensates for energy losses by selectively amplifying the received signals in proportion to their depth (based on travel time). A knob or slide switch is used to adjust the TGC. If deep signals are not sufficiently amplified, the deeper portions of the image will appear too dark. If the gain is set too high, the image will appear washed out (too white).

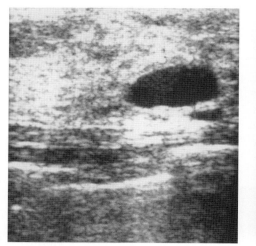 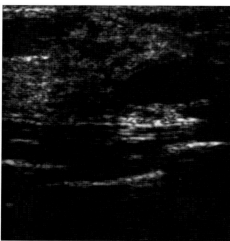 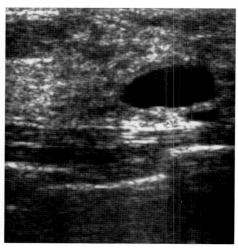

a, b   c

Fig. 1.15 a–c Brightness settings on the monitor or printer. **a** Background both too light and too bright, **b** too dark, **c** appropriate.

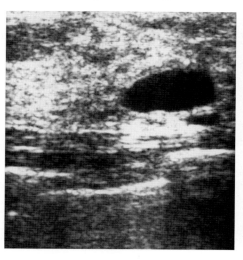 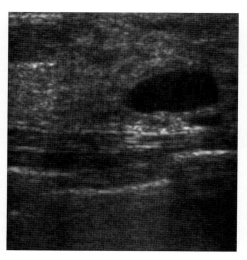 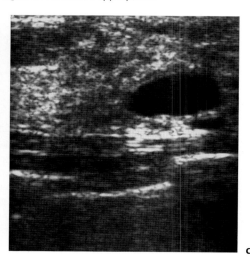

a, b   c

Fig. 1.16 a–c Contrast settings on the monitor or printer. **a** Too high, **b** too low, **c** appropriate.

The basic instrument settings should be adjusted at the center of the breast, as that region contains the greatest amount of parenchyma. With the power setting at an intermediate level, the operator should adjust the TGC so that the breast appears uniformly bright in the near and far fields (**Fig. 1.18 a–d**), bearing in mind that the subcutaneous fat in the near zone is of variable thickness. The subcutaneous fat should appear gray, not black, and should not be too bright. The parenchyma, which is more echogenic than fat, should be light gray, not white, and the darker gray ducts, some of them less than a millimeter in diameter, should be distinguishable as thin lines winding their way through the fibroglandular tissue. The connective tissue fibers are a convenient brightness gauge, as they can be seen both in the subcutaneous tissue and in deeper layers. If the sound output is insufficient to yield an image of acceptable brightness down to the chest wall despite maximum TGC, or if the highest TGC setting results in a noisy image, the power setting of the unit should be increased to deliver more sound energy to deeper tissues and the TGC should be simultaneously lowered in the near field.

Focusing

Variable focusing is available in linear probes, in convex and annular arrays, and in some sector probes. It should be adjusted to place the focal zone in the anterior to middle third of the region of interest between the skin and chest wall. Because the breast tissue is generally 2–4 cm thick beneath the acoustically coupled transducer in the supine patient, a focal depth between 1 and 2 cm is usually optimal. It is better to use a transducer that provides two or three focal zones, or one focal range, which will cover a depth from 0.5 to 3–4 cm. Having more than three focal zones slows the frame rate so that the image generation lags behind scanning, which is no longer in real time.

Image Scale

The size of the image should be adjusted to the individual breast size. It should be large enough to use as much of the screen as possible while also displaying the chest wall. Any additional depth,

ordinarily beyond 4–5 cm, would result in the lower portion of the image appearing black and devoid of information, with the minified breast tissue crowded into the upper part of the field. Too shallow a field of view amplifies the speckle pattern creating a noisy image. For the selective scrutiny of small focal lesions using the zoom function is a better choice than reducing the depth of the image, where noisy pseudomagnification of a mass hinders rather than helps in its characterization, particularly the analysis of its marginal characteristics.

Demographic Documentation and Image Labeling

Before every examination, the name of the patient should be entered. The patient may also be identified by an abbreviation or medical record number, birth date, or other unique identifier. Privacy regulations, such as HIPAA (Health Insurance Portability and Accountability Act, enacted by the United States Congress in 1996), must be observed.

The name of the facility and its location (city, state, zip code) should appear on the image, as should the initials or name of the sonologist or sonographer doing the scan.

As suggested in the *Practice Guideline for the Performance of the Breast Ultrasound Examination* (American College of Radiology, 2007), the location of the scan should be indicated by laterality (right or left), clockface notation, and distance from the nipple in cm. Because the nipple is a fixed point, distance from it is easily approximated by the length of the transducer face, e.g., 50 mm. The scan plane—radial, antiradial or transverse and sagittal (longitudinal)—should also be indicated. Another option is to use a body marker diagram to indicate scan plane, laterality, and clockface notation. Without this information, it would be virtually impossible to reproduce the examination at a later date and compare the image document with the written report. Image documentation is carried out after the real-time image has been captured and any focal lesions have been measured. Many currently available systems are equipped with a memory function and cine loop. These units can store in memory a series of ultrasound images acquired over a designated time interval. A trackball can then be used to review the prior successive images and select the image that is best for documentation.

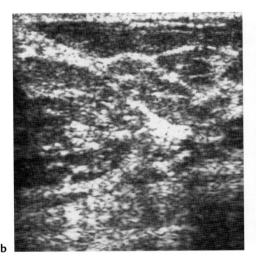 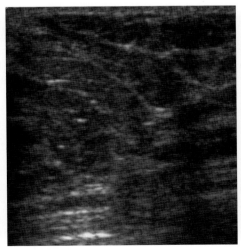 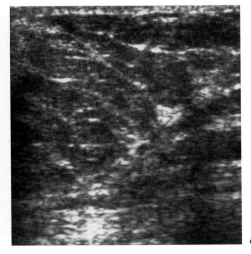

a, b   c

Fig. 1.17 a–c   Adjusting the power or gain setting on the ultrasound instrument. **a** Too high, **b** too low, **c** appropriate.

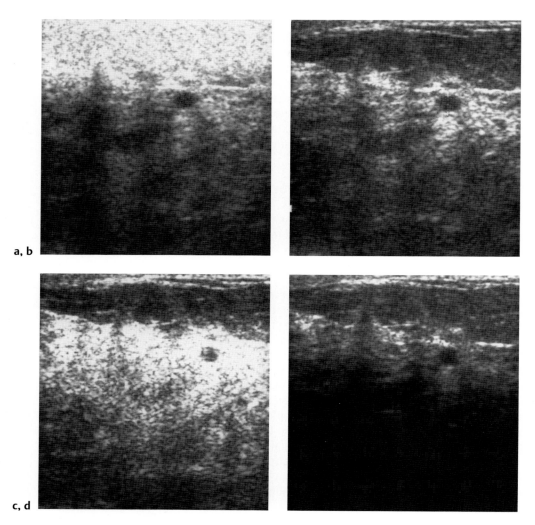

a, b

c, d

Fig. 1.18 a–d TGC settings.
a Near field too high.
b Appropriate.
c Far field too high.
d Too low throughout.

Transducer Selection

The advantages and disadvantages of sector, linear, and convex transducers are described above. The major differences relate to field of view, transducer coupling, focusing, and the pressure distribution in the tissue. Sector probes with a small coupling surface have an unequal pressure distribution that can displace mobile lesions out of the image plane. Other drawbacks are the "pie-shaped" field of view, the nonuniform image quality, and the unfavorable focusing properties.

Professional societies have emphasized the importance of using transducers with center frequencies of at least 7.5 MHz for breast examinations to obtain sufficient resolution. A 7.5-MHz transducer will provide adequate penetration depth even in a large breast. Because electronic linear-array transducers offer distinct advantages with regard to field of view, coupling, and focusing a high resolution linear-array transducer is currently considered best for most breast examinations. An annular-array sector transducer with a built-in standoff pad and a 7.5-MHz operating frequency would provide an acceptable alternative. Simple fixed-focus sector probes are not recommended for ultrasound examination of the breast.

Transducer Frequencies

Although 7.5 MHz has become standard, higher-frequency broad bandwidth linear probes can be used effectively for breast examinations and are now preferred. With their wide frequency ranges, these transducers can depict fine structures in the near field, enabled by transducers operating at 10, 12, 15, and 17 MHz yet able to penetrate to 5 cm at the low end of their frequency ranges, commonly 5 MHz. These transducers are used in most dedicated breast imaging facilities in the United States, and they are available for most ultrasound systems used for breast examinations.

Field of View

Many high-resolution transducers with footprints ranging from 38–50 mm provide only about a 3.5–7 cm field of view. Multichannel technology is used to focus these transducers, rather than the pulsing of small groups of crystals. This requires considerably higher computer capacity, since a great deal more signal information must be processed compared with simpler devices. This accounts for the higher cost of these high-resolution instruments. The computing requirements and necessary high line density limit the width of the image field to approximately 4 cm. The disadvantage is the small window for anatomic display. The advantage is substantially higher image quality. However, many manufacturers have expanded the field width of these probes to 5–6 cm, thus combining the advantages of high image quality and improved coverage of breast anatomy which is especially useful in efficient survey scanning and for large breasts. If the footprint becomes much greater than 6 cm, it will be difficult to maintain contact with the skin along the full length of the transducer. Such large footprints are impractical, especially in examinations of small breasts and the axilla.

Quality Control and Test Phantoms

General Considerations

Specifications of image geometry and transducer frequency issued by professional societies are helpful but are not sufficient for effective quality control. A better approach is to test whether an instrument is suitable for use in a particular body region. Experienced examiners can determine this by comparing the performance of different instruments under practical conditions in a large number of examinations. This is time-consuming, however, and it would not be possible to evaluate all available instruments. In addition, this type of evaluation is subjective.

Test phantoms are available for the simple, objective, and reproducible quality control of ultrasound imaging systems. Their relatively high cost, approximately $2500 at the time of writing, may discourage their use but they provide an objective means of evaluating image contrast, lateral and axial resolution, image geometry, focusing, and image field. Their use is encouraged and quality control is emphasized in the breast ultrasound accreditation programs of the American College of Radiology and the American Institute of Ultrasound in Medicine.

Characteristics of Test Phantoms

Several companies manufacture ultrasound phantoms. For comparison with actual examination conditions, it is important that the materials in the phantom simulate breast tissue in having physical properties similar to the acoustic properties of body tissue. We use the Model 550 Multipurpose Breast Scanning and Small Parts Phantom (ATS Laboratories, Bridgeport, CT) (**Fig. 1.19**). Other manufacturers also offer tissue-mimicking phantoms, including CIRS (Norfolk, VA), Gammex rmi (Madison, WI). For breast imaging, phantoms developed for high-resolution scanners should be used, since the particle size and target arrangement in many phantoms for testing general purpose ultrasound systems are suitable only for lower-resolution probes. Phantoms for high-resolution testing can be used to test transducers operating at frequencies of 7.5 MHz or higher. The ATS phantom is distinguished by its tissue-mimicking acoustic properties and the special arrangement of the target structures used to test imaging performance (**Table 1.4**). Its sound propagation speed is relatively low (1450 m/s), but the small difference compared with sound velocity in tissue is compensated for by geometrical corrections.

Table 1.4 Technical specifications of the ultrasound test phantom

General	
Material	Polyurethane
Ultrasound attenuation	0.504 dB/cm/MHz
Speed of sound	1450 m/s*
Line targets for image field evaluation	
Material	Nylon monofilament 0.05 mm diameter
Vertical	10 targets Spaced 0.5 cm apart Depth 0.5–5 cm
Horizontal	9 targets in 2 groups Spaced 0.5 cm apart Depth 2–4.5 cm
Axial-lateral resolution	
Material	Nylon monofilament 0.05 mm diameter
3 groups	10 targets per group Depth 2, 4, and 6 cm Axial offset 1 mm Distance 0.5, 1, 2, and 3 mm
Cysts	
Material	Anechoic tubes 1, 2, 3, and 4 mm diameter
4 target groups	6 target structures per group Depth 1–6 cm Spaced 1 cm apart
Gray-level contrast	
Material	Echogenic tubes 6 mm diameter
6 target structures	Depth 2.5 cm Spaced 1 cm apart
Contrast	-15, -6, -3, +3, +6, +15 (dB) (relative to background)

* Ultrasound instruments are usually calibrated to a sound velocity of 1540 m/s. To ensure accurate measurements, the test targets are positioned to correct for variations in sound velocity.

Phantoms from the other manufacturers listed above utilize the sound propagation speed of tissue (1540 m/s).

The phantom permits testing of the following characteristics:
- Image field (vertical and horizontal calibration, focal zone)
- Axial resolution
- Lateral resolution
- Sensitivity
- Functional resolution
- Dynamic range.

Image Field

The known distances between the targets provide a means of testing instrument calibration by measuring the phantom distances with the digital calipers of the scanner. The known spacing is

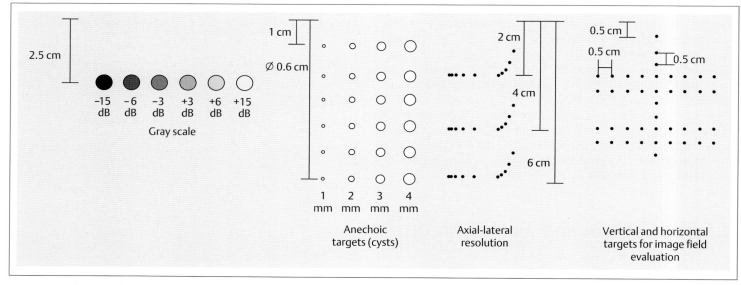

Fig. 1.19 Schematic diagram of the target structures in the test phantom used to make the illustrative images in this section (with permission of ATS Laboratories, Bridgeport, CT, USA).

compared with the caliper measurements to check for accurate calibration. This test is performed using the crossed pattern of vertical and horizontal line targets, which permits the entire focal region to be evaluated. If the wire appears as a dot, the resolution is optimal. If it appears as a horizontal line, the length of the line indicates the approximate width of the ultrasound beam.

Spatial Resolution: Axial, Lateral, and Elevation Plane

Axial and lateral resolution are tested on the monofilament thread targets. Axial resolution is the resolution along the axis of the ultrasound beam. It depends on the frequency and pulse length of the transducer, which are inversely proportional, the pulse length decreasing as the frequency increases. Lateral resolution depends on the width of the ultrasound beam, its frequency and focusing, and it is measured in the plane perpendicular to the beam, parallel to the transducer face. Because the beam diverges proximal and distal to the focal zone, the resolution outside the focal zone also affects image quality. This is tested on target structures located at various depths. The focal zone of the scanner can be moved into the near field or to deeper levels. Resolution in the elevation plane (azimuth) is related to slice thickness in the plane perpendicular to the beam and to the transducer

Sensitivity

The sensitivity of an ultrasound scanner refers to its ability to receive weak echoes from small, deeply situated structures. Depth sensitivity is influenced by the attenuation of the surrounding tissue. Breast imaging requires penetration depths of up to 5 cm in the supine patient. Imaging depths up to 6 cm can be tested in the phantom using the anechoic "cyst" targets.

Functional Resolution (Cysts)

Functional resolution is the ability of a system to detect anechoic structures within the test phantom and correctly portray their size and shape. A deficiency in performance is indicated if cystic structures are not sharply imaged, if they contain internal echoes, or if the structures are not visualized due to superimposed echoes from surrounding tissues.

Gray-Level Reproduction and Dynamic Range (Contrast)

The gray-level reproduction of a scanner refers to its ability to assign different brightness levels to echoes of different amplitudes. The dynamic range is the range from the faintest gray that can be registered to the brightest level, and higher dynamic ranges (measured in dB) are important in maximizing the number of shades of gray depicted in the image. These features are important in displaying echoes of varying amplitudes. They are tested in the ATS phantom by imaging a horizontal row of six gray-level tubes 6 mm in diameter.

Test Protocol

As a general rule, you get what you pay for: more expensive instruments provide better image quality than bargain scanners. In recognition of this fact, we assigned the ultrasound scanners to four different price classes and scored each quality criterion on a six-point rating scale (**Tables 1.5, 1.6**).

This scale provided a means of rating instrument quality independent of the subjective impressions of the examiners. The ratings were done independently by four radiologists, and the results were averaged (the scores differed from the average value by a maximum of ± 1 point).

Table 1.5 Price classification of ultrasound imaging systems

Price class 1	<$ 25 000
Price class 2	$ 25 000–50 000
Price class 3	$ 50 000–100 000
Price class 4	>$ 100 000

Table 1.6 Point scale for rating the quality of ultrasound scanners

6	Excellent
5	Good
4	Satisfactory
3	Adequate
2	Poor
1	Unsatisfactory

Table 1.7 Test results in all scanners for the four test criteria

Price class	Transducer MHz		Contrast In/out of focal zone		Resolution In/out of focal zone		Cysts In/out of focal zone		Image field
1	5	S	1	–	1	–	1	–	1*
	5	L	4	3.5	2.3	2	2.8	2.5	3
	5	L	4.5	4	2	2	2	2	4
	7.5	L	3.5	3.5	2	2	2	1.5	3.3
2	7.5	L	4	4	3	3	3	3	4.3
	7.5	L	5	1.8	4	1	4	1.5	2
	7.5	L	3.5	3.3	3	2.8	3.5	3.3	4
	7.5	L	4.3	4	4	3	4	4	4.3
	10	S	1.5	–	3.8	1	3.5	1	4.3**
3	7.5	L	5.5	1	4.5	1	5.5	1.8	1.8
	7.5	L	5	4	3	3	3.8	3.3	4
	7.5	L	5	5	5	4	4.3	4	5
	7	L	3.5	2	3.8	3.3	3.8	3.5	4.8
4	5	L	4	3	3.5	3.5	3	3	3.8
	7.5	L	4.8	3.5	3.8	3.5	5	4	4.5***
	10	L	4.5	4.5	5	4	6	4.3	5.3

Rating scale: excellent (6), good (5), satisfactory (4), adequate (3), poor (2), unsatisfactory (1). S = sector probe, L = linear array
* Focusing unsatisfactory (Fig. 1.**21**).
** Adequate sound penetration only to a depth of 2 cm.
*** Reverberations at a depth of 2.5 cm.

Test Results

The results are summarized in **Table 1.7** and **Fig. 1.20 a, b**. Scanners in *price class 1* (less than $ 25 000) are, for the most part, unsatisfactory. None can be recommended for breast imaging. The

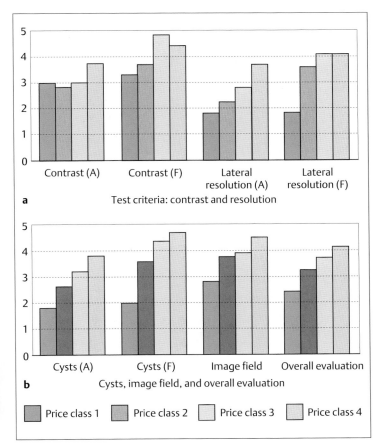

Fig. 1.20 a, b Average scores (1–6) assigned to class 1–4 instruments for various test criteria.
a Contrast 1 cm outside the focal zone (A) and in the focal zone (F), and lateral resolution 1 cm outside (A) and inside (F) the focal zone.
b Visualization of cysts (1–4 mm in diameter) 1 cm outside (A) and inside (F) the focal zone, image field evaluation, and overall evaluation.

poorest in this category is a scanner with a 5-MHz sector probe (**Fig. 1.21 a–d**). The six gray-scale tubes cannot be distinguished from the background or from one another. Cysts 1 mm and 2 mm in size are not detected, while 3-mm and 4-mm cysts are barely visible within the focal zone but are too blurry to be recognized as cysts. On resolution testing, the vertical nylon wires are well separated, but the horizontal wires blend together into a long streak-like echo, including the thread spaced farthest (3 mm) from the others. The poor lateral resolution is also apparent in the image field evaluation, where all the vertical and horizontal wires are blended together.

As **Table 1.7** indicates, electronic linear-array transducers perform somewhat better than the sector probe, and these instruments are just adequate for the simple, basic evaluation of a palpable breast mass. However, the poor lateral resolution would not permit the further investigation of subclinical masses.

Five scanners in *price class 2* were tested. A 10-MHz sector probe failed because of inadequate penetration depth. Lateral resolution in the focal zone is very good to a depth of 2 cm, but the strong divergence of the beam prevents image evaluation just 1 cm outside the maximum focal zone. The poor imaging depth of this probe would preclude a useful evaluation even with adequate sound penetration.

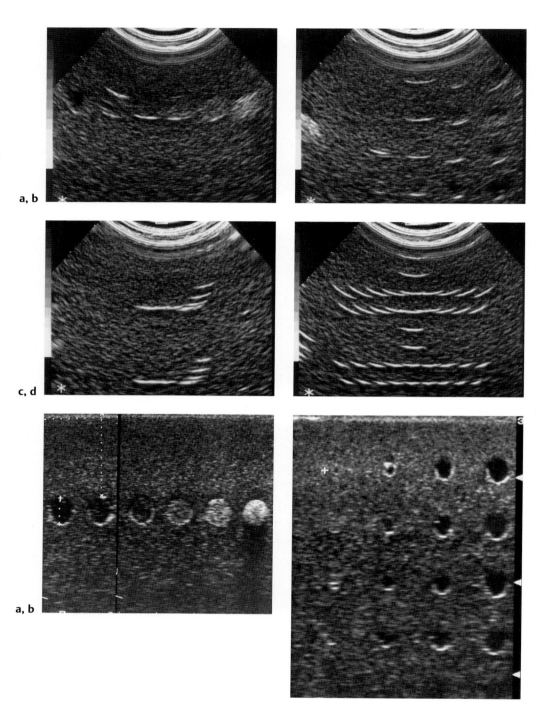

a, b

c, d

a, b

Fig. 1.21 a–d Example of unacceptable image quality from a class 1 scanner with a 5-MHz sector transducer.

a The six tubes for testing gray-level contrast are poorly demarcated.

b The cysts with diameters of 1, 2, and 3 mm are poorly visualized at depths of 1–4 cm. The 4-mm cyst is visible but is not clearly distinguishable as a cyst.

c All the horizontal wires for testing lateral resolution at depths of 2 cm and 4 cm are blended together. This means that the lateral resolution exceeds 3 mm.

d In the image field test, the scanner does not portray the target threads as dots anywhere in the depth range of 0.5–5 cm, indicating unacceptable lateral resolution throughout the image field.

Fig. 1.22 a–d Example of a good scanner in price class 2.

a Good contrast resolution of the gray-scale tubes.

b Good visualization of the anechoic tubes. The 1-mm cyst is just visible.

Fig. 1.22 c, d ▷

All the linear arrays show acceptable results. **Fig. 1.22 a, b** shows an example of a good scanner. Image contrast, resolution, and image field are good to satisfactory. A notable feature is the uniform beam outside the focal zone. As **Table 1.7** indicates, however, some of the scanners do not possess a uniform focal zone.

Four scanners in *price class 3* were tested. The graphic representation of the results by price groups highlights the quality improvement compared with lower-price instruments (**Fig. 1.20 a, b**). Looking at **Table 1.7**, however, we find considerable variation in the image field evaluation. One scanner has good contrast within the focal zone, but contrast becomes poor just 1 cm outside the focal zone (**Fig. 1.23 a, b**). A similar problem is seen with lateral resolution (**Table 1.7**, **Fig. 1.24 a, b**). Four of the

five targets are portrayed as separate objects in the focal region. The minimum spacing for achieving this separation is 1 mm. But 0.5 cm outside the focal zone, only objects spaced at 2 mm are separated; and 1–2 cm outside the focal zone, all the targets blend together. This means that the lateral resolution in that region is less than 4 mm. Even cysts are visualized only within the maximum focal region (**Fig. 1.25 a, b**), and multiple focusing provides acceptable image quality only within a narrow depth range (**Fig. 1.26 a, b**). This emphasizes the importance of accurate instrument settings.

Price class 4 shows a further quality improvement in terms of resolution and image field. The high image quality outside the focal zone is striking (**Table 1.7**). **Fig. 1.27 a–d** shows the high-

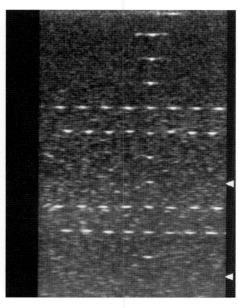

c, d

Fig. 1.22 c, d
c Acceptable lateral resolution. Four of the five horizontal wires are defined within the focal zone at a depth of 2 cm. Three of the five wires are still visible 2 cm deeper.
d The wire targets for image field evaluation are uniformly portrayed and show only slight linear smearing.

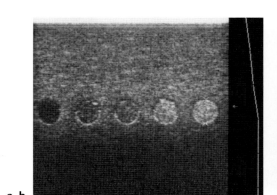
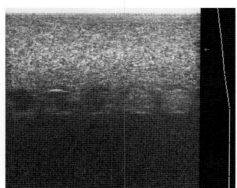

a, b

Fig. 1.23 a, b Image contrast of a class 3 scanner with a 7.5-MHz linear transducer and a balanced image field.
a Good contrast is obtained within the focal zone.
b When the focus is placed 1 cm above the targets, the contrast outside the focal zone is unsatisfactory.

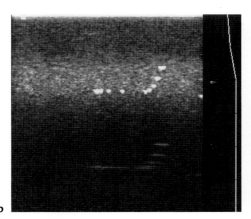
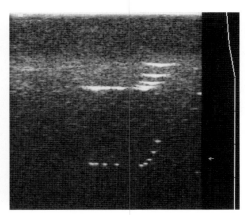

a, b

Fig. 1.24 a, b Lateral resolution of the scanner in Fig. 1.23.
a Four of the five wires are delineated within the focal zone.
b When the focus is deepened to 4 cm, four of the five wires at that depth are well defined, but the more superficial targets at 2 cm are blended together.

contrast resolution and uniform image field throughout the working range of one of the high-priced scanners. A balanced image field and acceptable lateral resolution beyond the focal zone are essential in breast examinations for the detection of nonpalpable lesions.

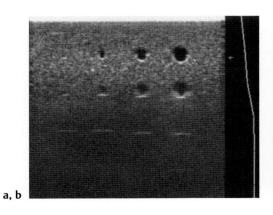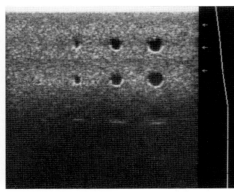

Fig. 1.25 a, b Cyst delineation with the scanner in Figs. 1.23, 1.24: comparison of single and multiple focusing.

a With a single focus placed at a depth of 1 cm, all four cysts (1–4 mm in diameter) are visualized at depths of 1 and 2 cm. The cysts at 3 cm are not defined.

b With multiple focusing in the near zone (0.5–2 cm), all four cysts are visualized at depths of 1 and 2 cm, but none of the deeper targets is defined.

a, b

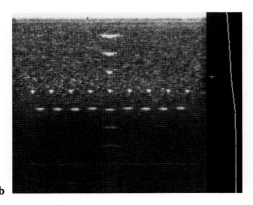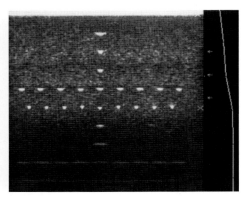

Fig. 1.26 a, b Image field test of the scanner in Figs. 1.23–1.25 with single and multiple focusing.

a Single focus at a depth of 1.5 cm.

b Multiple focusing at 1–2.5 cm. Neither focusing method provides a uniform image field.

a, b

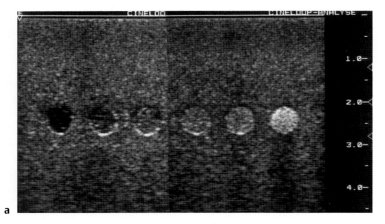

Fig. 1.27 a–d Example of a good scanner in price class 4.

a Image contrast.

b Cysts are resolved down to 1 mm within the focal zone (2 cm).

c Four wires are defined within the focal zone (2 cm) and at a depth of 4 cm.

d Image field with a single focus at a depth of 2 cm.

a

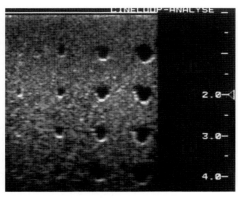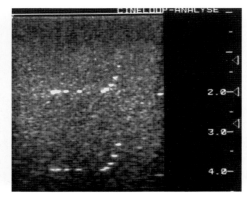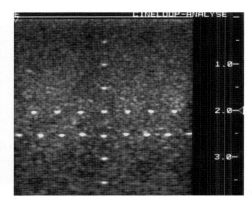

b

c, d

Clinical Relevance

In addition to standard scanners, there are high-resolution instruments that offer more sophisticated image processing and higher operating frequencies. According to the guidelines of the American College of Radiology and the American Institute of Ultrasound in Medicine (AIUM), frequencies of 7.5–10 MHz should be used for breast imaging, and preference should be given to higher-resolution transducers. At frequencies in the range of 7–10 MHz, however, the length of the transducer is generally less than 5 cm, and so these instruments do not conform to the guidelines of the German Association of Statutory Health Insurance Physicians for breast examinations. There are transducers higher than 5 MHz that provide an image field width of 5 cm or more and thus conform to German guidelines, but these instruments offer limited resolution due to their relatively unsophisticated signal processing systems.

Our goal in the study described here was to determine whether the performance of an ultrasound scanner could be meaningfully evaluated by a series of simple phantom tests that any physician can do. It is also hoped that the study will stimulate discussion on quality improvements in ultrasound imaging equipment.

As **Table 1.7** indicates, the cost of an ultrasound imaging system is closely related to image quality. If applications are limited strictly to the cystic/solid differentiation of large, palpable breast masses, the quality of the equipment is not a major concern. But given the inherent limitations of X-ray mammography in dense breasts and breasts with fibrocystic changes, there is a need for high-quality ultrasound technology that is capable of detecting small lesions. Resolution is extremely important in this type of investigation. Axial resolution is affected by transducer frequency and pulse length, and is generally acceptable at frequencies above 5 MHz. A bigger problem is lateral resolution, which depends on focusing and signal processing. Phantom tests demonstrate significant differences between different scanners (**Fig. 1.20 a, b**). Budget scanners (class 1) are not recommended for breast imaging because of the potential for missing a malignant tumor. Higher-priced scanners display satisfactory to good performance according to all criteria. The differences are greatest in the moderate-to-high price ranges. All the scanners provide good resolution in the focal zone, but major differences are seen outside the focal zone, again posing the risk that tumors will go undetected. This emphasizes the importance of testing the image field. Another factor to be considered in the selection of transducers is that sound absorption increases with transducer frequency. One of the two 10-MHz transducers tested was unacceptable because of insufficient penetration depth.

High-quality equipment and an understanding of how to optimize it are critical for accurate diagnoses Test phantoms permit objective evaluations, and clinical experience with the scanners confirms the validity of the results of phantom testing. Quality control and quality assurance are as necessary in breast ultrasound as they are in mammography, where they are required by United States federal law.

A recognition of the inherent limitations of mammography in depicting masses in dense fibroglandular tissue has sparked renewed interest in adjunctive modalities that might supplement mammography for breast cancer screening. Most important currently are MRI and ultrasound, and both are subjects of intense, active research.

Water-Path Scanning

Various devices for ultrasonic breast imaging were developed during the 1970s and 1980s. The single-focus real-time scanners and handheld mechanical transducers used at that time were unable to provide good lateral resolution. The design principle of water-path scanners is based on mechanical single-crystal transducers. These probes have a large diameter with a correspondingly large focusing radius. Thus, the sound beam narrows gradually over a long distance and provides good focusing over a longer range. This simple principle made it possible to achieve uniform image quality within the region of interest. An essential component was the water path interposed between the transducer face and the breast, accomplished either by using a water bag or by immersing the breast in water.

Water-Bag Technique

In this technique the patient is examined supine. A small water tank sealed at the bottom with plastic film is placed onto the breast. A single-crystal transducer is introduced into the tank from above and is motor-driven along a linear path (**Fig. 2.1a, b**), producing static longitudinal or transverse images. Image generation was relatively slow, however, and a complete survey of the breast was time consuming. The real-time examinations relied upon currently for lesion characterization and ultrasound-guided needle procedures were almost impossible. It was also difficult to obtain good contact at the periphery of the bag, particularly at the lateral aspect of the breast and the axilla. Scanning large breasts was also challenging. Thus, although this technique provided excellent anatomic detail, these systems are no longer available for clinical use in the United States.

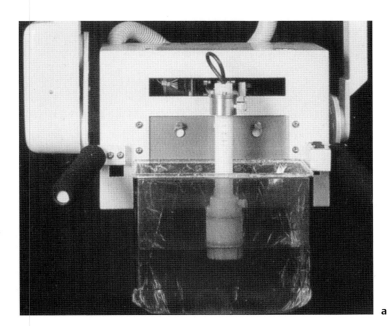

a

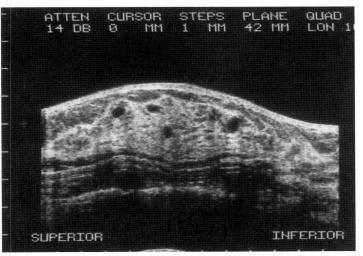

b

Fig. 2.1a, b Mechanical transducer used with a water bag for breast scanning in the supine patient.
a The motor-driven transducer is moved in a linear pattern and provides sectional images of the entire breast.
b Example of breast cysts.

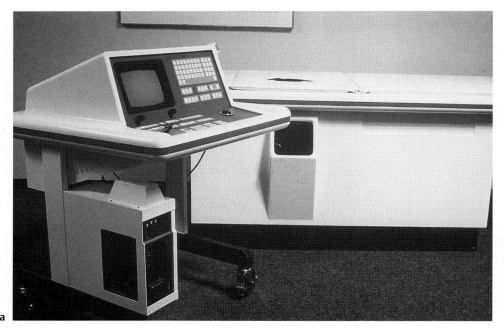
a

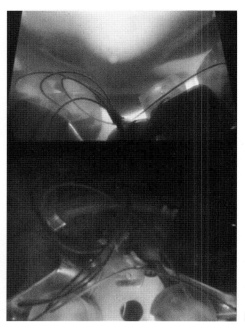
b

Fig. 2.2 a, b   Water-path immersion scanner.
a System 1 (Ausonics, Australia). The breast hangs through an opening into the water tank. Four motor-driven transducers inside the tank are moved in a pattern that systematically surveys the entire breast.
b View of the mechanical sector transducers inside the tank. The four transducer images are superimposed to produce a compound scan, or an image reconstructed by superimposing multiple scans from different directions. Alternatively, simple scans can be obtained by activating only one transducer. Although this and other older automated scanners are no longer available, there has been a revival of interest in automated scanners suitable for supplemental breast cancer screening of women with mammographically dense fibroglandular tissue and high risk of breast cancer.

Immersion Technique

Immersion scanning was once widely practiced, and as early as the 1970 s it was used for clinical studies at many centers throughout the world. The patient lay prone on a table over a large water tank (**Fig. 2.2 a, b**). The breast entered the tank through an aperture similar to that found in prone tables used today for stereotactic biopsies, and hung freely in the water. Motor-driven transducers on the floor of the tank generated sector scans in sagittal or transverse planes. The transducers could be moved horizontally by remote control to scan the breast systematically, section by section, to obtain complete breast coverage.

Some scanners had only one sector transducer which provided simple scans similar to those in real-time imaging but depicting a representative section of the whole breast (**Fig. 2.3 a, b**). These scanners were relatively easy to operate. Usually, some degree of breast compression was applied to improve sound penetration and eliminate refraction artifacts (**Fig. 2.4 a–d**). Compression alters sound propagation and can be used to distinguish artifactual attenuation from acoustic shadowing associated with carcinoma and other breast lesions, such as stromal fibrosis.

Higher-end systems were equipped with multiple transducers that could scan the breast from different directions. The images were then superimposed to produce a composite (compound) scan. A simple scan can only demonstrate structures that are insonated at a favorable angles, but a compound scan allows many more surfaces to be presented perpendicular to the transducer. As a result, compounding provides a sharper and more detailed depiction of breast anatomy (**Fig. 2.5 a, b**).

Acoustic enhancement and shadowing are posterior features included in ultrasound characterization of masses. The multiple

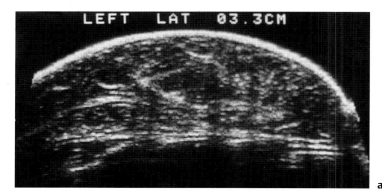
a

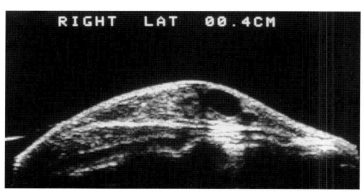
b

Fig. 2.3 a, b   Breast anatomy demonstrated by immersion scanning with one transducer (simple scan technique). The breast hangs freely into the water bath, providing an expanded view of anatomic structures. Compression alters but can improve the appearance of the image. Optimum compression was used in these examples.
a Fatty breast.
b Breast cysts.

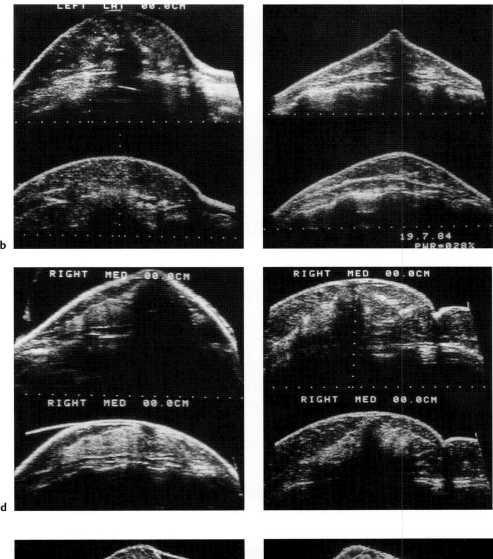

a, b

c, d

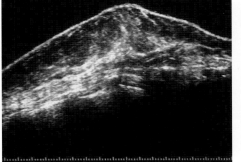
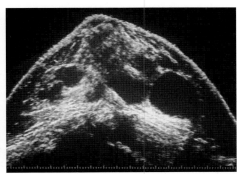

a, b

Fig. 2.4 a–d Comparison of noncompression and compression immersion scans. As the examples show, slight compression is usually necessary to improve image quality.
a Fatty breast. This breast is ≤ 25 % dense (BI-RADS category 1 density for mammography). The noncompression image (top) shows a central acoustic shadow. When light compression is applied (bottom), the acoustic shadow disappears and the central portion of the breast can be evaluated.
b Breast with scattered fibroglandular densities, 26–50 % dense (BI-RADS category 2 density for mammography). Without compression (top), a dense subareolar acoustic shadow is seen despite the paucity of breast parenchyma. Compression eliminates this artifact and reveals the continuity of breast architecture below the nipple.
c Adolescent breast is extremely dense—category 4 BI-RADS density (76–100 %). The noncompression image (top) shows a broad subareolar acoustic shadow. Compression eliminates the shadow obscuring the central breast, permitting evaluation.
d Breast carcinoma measuring 2.5 × 3 cm. The acoustic shadow caused by desmoplasia persists when compression is applied. The persistence helps confirm a hypoechoic, shadowing mass with irregular, ill-defined margins. Compression would have eliminated refraction artifacts at glandular interfaces, and there is little change in the appearance of the mass following compression.

Fig. 2.5 a, b Compound scan: need for scanning in at least two orthogonal planes.
a Normal appearance of an involuted breast, sagittal scan.
b Multiple cysts in the plane of the nipple, transverse scan.

angles of insonation in compound scanning caused reduced conspicuity of both enhancement and shadowing in the water immersion technique just as these features are less perceptible in real-time spatial compounding. In immersion breast examinations, it was common to obtain both simple and compound scans. The compound scan provided better anatomic definition and marginal detail of individual focal lesions, while a simple scan revealed the associated posterior features. (**Fig. 2.6 a–d**). Additional information was obtained in simple scans by selectively activating transducers at different positions and scanning the breast from various angles (**Fig. 2.7 a, b**).

In immersion scanning the breast was usually not compressed, but as in simple scanning there are instances where compression enhanced sound penetration and improved the compound image. This was accomplished by stretching a sheet of film across the tank to flatten the breast. Compression was necessary to confirm a suspected tumor, as **Figs. 2.8 a, b** and **2.9 a, b** illustrate.

> Water-bath immersion is outmoded because of cost, large numbers of images to review, and poorer spatial resolution compared with current real-time scanners, but the classic water-bath scan still has value as a teaching tool.

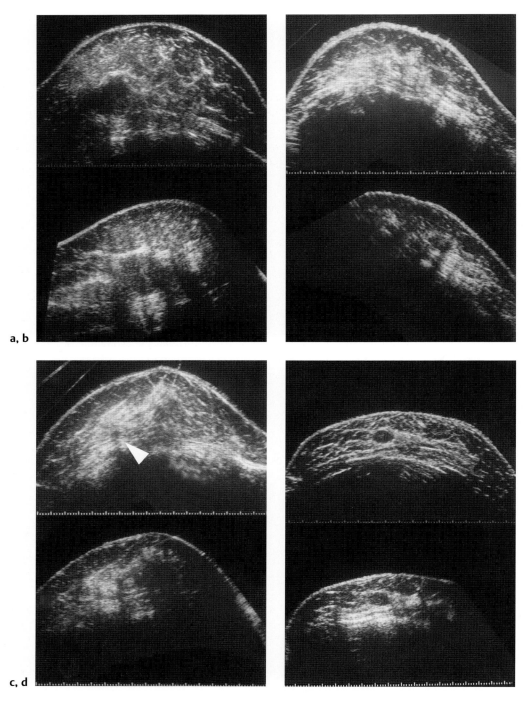

a, b

c, d

Fig. 2.6 a–d Comparison of compound and simple scans.

a Invasive breast carcinoma, 3 × 4 cm. Applicable to small field of view, high-resolution handheld ultrasound as well as to survey scanners, the compound scan (top) shows the irregular shape and angular, microlobulated margins of the tumor and the structures of the breast parenchyma better than the simple scan (bottom). If the mass were interpreted as circumscribed, on a simple scan using the conventional vertical beam, the diagnosis would have been missed. It is easier, however, to appreciate the posterior features, both the enhancing and attenuating effects of the tumor on sound transmission (**b**).

b Invasive ductal carcinoma, 2 × 1.5 cm. The compound scan (top) more clearly demonstrates the parenchymal anatomy of the dense breast and the combination of smooth and irregular tumor margins. Fewer anatomic structures are visible in the simple scan (bottom), but the acoustic phenomena are better appreciated. Among the diagnostic criteria for interpretation, posterior features hold less weight than shape and margins.

c Invasive breast carcinoma 7 mm in diameter (arrowhead). The compound scan (top) demonstrates the parenchymal structure of the breast and the irregular tumor. The simple scan reveals a tumor shadow but also shows shadowing in the adjacent breast parenchyma. The tumor is poorly delineated.

d This compound scan shows a solid, smooth, homogeneous mass whose margins can be clearly evaluated. The good sound transmission through the tumor and adjacent parenchyma are apparent in the simple scan. Thus, each scan complements the other in evaluating the mass. Using high resolution handheld transducers with spatial compounding, the posterior feature characteristics are less conspicuous but remain identifiable, sometimes with a conical appearance the apex of the cone at the posterior aspect of the scan.

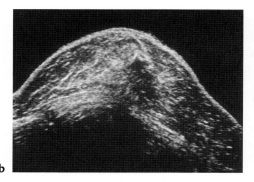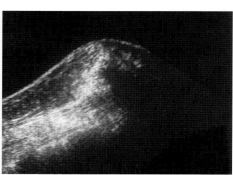

a, b

Fig. 2.7 a–d Effect of scanning direction on the acoustic shadow cast by an invasive breast carcinoma.

a Compound scan shows a 2.5 × 3.5 cm mass with irregular margins distorting the breast architecture.

b Scanning from the left side with transducer 1 (left) shows fewer structural details. A heavy acoustic shadow projects to the right from the mass.

Fig. 2.7 **c, d** ▷

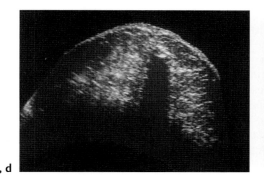
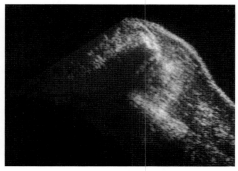

c, d

Fig. 2.7 c, d
c Scanning from the right front with transducer 3 demonstrates an acoustic shadow directed posteriorly and to the left.
d Scanning from the right side with transducer 4 demonstrates a shadow directed to the left. It is apparent from all images that the shadow emanates from the mass and is not caused by breast parenchyma.

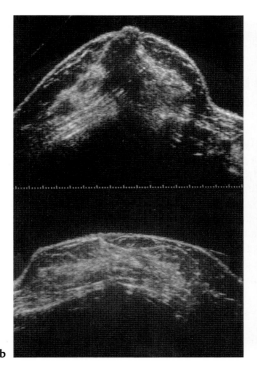
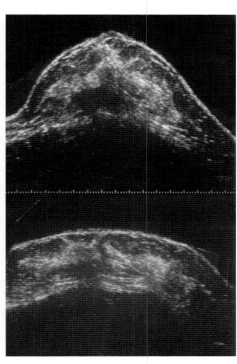

a, b

Fig. 2.8 a, b Compound scans: comparison of both breasts with and without compression in a patient with left breast carcinoma.
a Scan of the right breast without compression shows marked central sound absorption (top). Compression eliminates the hypoechoic region to depict the subareolar breast architecture (bottom).
b Left breast scan with minimal compression also shows prominent central attenuation. It is unclear whether the shadow is cast by a tumor or is an artifact caused by breast parenchyma. The compression scan (bottom) reveals a deeply situated, hypoechoic focal lesion with irregular margins, consistent with a large invasive carcinoma. It is also important that the focal zones should be set at the area of interest.

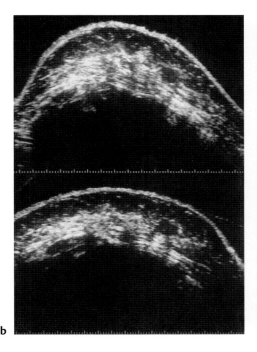
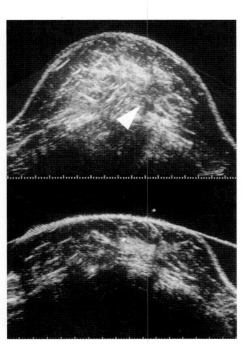

a, b

Fig. 2.9 a, b Noncompression and compression compound scans of breast carcinoma.
a Without compression a hypoechoic mass 2 × 1.5 cm can be seen (top). Compression of the breast does not alter the shape of the mass (bottom) identifiable now as a tumor. An artifact or fatty infiltration would have changed in response to tissue compression.
b Noncompression compound scan (top) shows a mass with irregular margins 2.5 × 1 cm in size (arrowhead). Internal echoes make the mass difficult to detect, but there is obvious local architectural distortion. Compression deforms the breast parenchyma, making the anatomic structures difficult to interpret (bottom). The mass, whose echogenicity is similar to that of the parenchymal tissue, is virtually undetectable.

❗ Comment:
This case illustrates the importance of using compression, but not excessively. Selective pressure is needed to improve sound penetration and determine compressibility.

Real-Time Examination

Patient Positioning

In real-time sonographic examination, only a small segment of the breast is visualized. In general, using a recommended high-frequency broad bandwidth linear transducer the field of view is approximately 5 cm² with a slice thickness of less than 1 mm. The small field of view is one reason that many examiners have not extended their sonographic studies beyond the focused ultrasound investigation of palpable or mammographically suspected masses ("lumpography"). Unlike water-path scanning where pressure exerted on tissue is constant, in real-time scanning the sonographer or sonologist applies variable pressure to the breast parenchyma with the ultrasound probe, and this pressure can alter the appearance of the tissue (**Fig. 2.10 a–c**). Thus, in real-time scanning, the examination technique should be adapted for each patient in order to optimize visualization of a specific lesion or area of interest. *Focused* or *targeted* scanning is here considered as the basic level of breast ultrasound. Its goal is to confirm a mass or other abnormality and to characterize it. Detection of nonpalpable lesions, or screening, is excluded from this type of scanning. Nevertheless, ultrasound depiction of a mass requires skill and an understanding of how to obtain a diagnostic ultrasound image.

> For the medial breast, the patient should be positioned supine with the hands clasped behind the neck (**Fig. 2.11 a–d**). This immobilizes the breast and makes the findings more reproducible. The flattening of the breast also improves sound penetration.

The supine position causes the breast to flatten on the chest wall, and elevating the arms places tension on the pectoralis muscles, further helping to flatten and immobilize the breast. This facilitates a complete, systematic examination and enhances the reproducibility of findings. The same position is used in breast surgery,

making it easier to identify and excise lesions that have been localized by breast ultrasound.

The flattening of the breast reduces the thickness of the tissue to be traversed by the acoustic beam, allowing for higher frequencies to be used and resulting in better spatial resolution in the area to be scanned. Also, the reduced tissue thickness and flattening of breast structures improve sound penetration, reducing the likelihood of troublesome acoustic shadows due to refraction effects.

For lesions in the lateral breast, or for large-breasted women, positioning the patient in a supine-oblique position with a pillow or firm wedge beneath her back and shoulder on the side to be scanned is also effective in minimizing the tissue thickness. The breast is additionally stabilized as the patient's arm is raised, bent at the elbow, and hand placed behind her neck. In this supine-oblique position, the breast falls contralaterally, thinning out the lateral breast tissue.

If a palpable mass cannot be located in the supine or supine-oblique position, ask the patient in what position she can most easily feel the mass. Ultrasound can be done with the subject in any position—standing, seated, or reclining—and moving the patient to a sitting position may enable the examiner to locate the lesion, stabilize it between two fingers, and place the probe directly over it. When a patient not in the supine or supine-oblique position is scanned, the patient's position should be labeled on the electronic image or film for reproducibility or follow-up. Although ultrasound characterization of a palpable mass, particularly in the upper breast, may be facilitated in an upright patient, it is difficult to conduct a systematic breast survey in the sitting position, because the breast is freely mobile and has a larger volume, and the lower breast is inaccessible.

Although the supine position may work well for small and average-size breasts, which tend to flatten uniformly and can usually be successfully examined, in larger breasts some of the parenchyma tends to shift laterally, creating a nonuniform tissue distribution. This makes it more difficult to conduct a systematic examination. In these cases, as in the examination targeted to

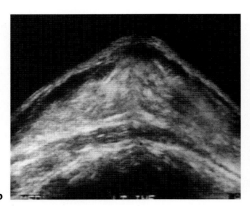 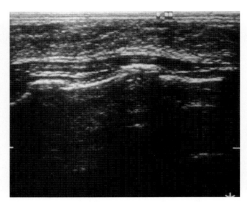 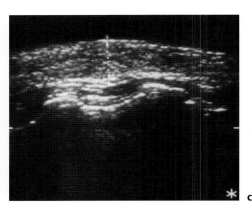

a, b   c

Fig. 2.10 a–c Comparison of water-bath immersion scan with real-time contact scan. The images illustrate a normal breast in a young woman.

a Compound scan. The breast tissues are fully expanded in the noncompression immersion scan. The thin layer of dark subcutaneous fat, the wispy, light gray glandular tissue, and the chest wall are clearly demonstrated.

b Examination of the same breast using a 5-MHz linear-array transducer 8 cm long. Current handheld transducers have much higher frequencies, with center frequencies ranging from 7 MHz to 10 MHz (or more). The supine position and the light transducer pressure give the breast a very

different appearance than in **a**. It should be noted, however, that only a small segment of the breast is visible.

c Same region as in **b**, scanned with a silicone standoff pad between the transducer and the breast.

❗ Comment:
The standoff pad provides better definition of the skin and parenchymal tissue. This improves the appearance of the image with this low-frequency probe. Currently, even with higher transducer frequencies (> 7.5 MHz), standoff pads improve visualization of the two-layered skin and the immediate subcutaneous layer.

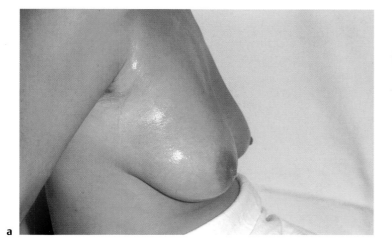
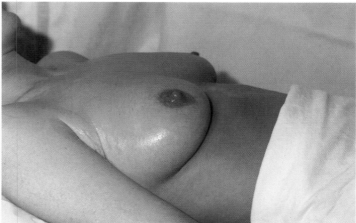

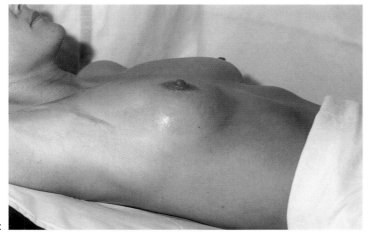
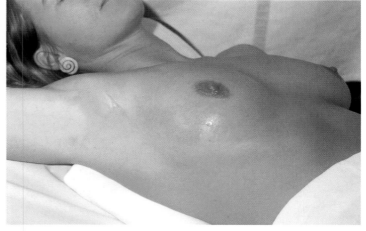

Fig. 2.11 a–d Positions for real-time breast scanning.
a Sitting position.
b Supine position.
c Supine with the arms elevated.
d Supine with a cushion elevating the side to be examined.

❗ Comment:
In the supine position, the breast flattens out on the chest wall. This improves sound penetration. Elevating the arms further flattens the breast and immobilizes it by tension from the pectoralis major muscle. Supine scanning is appropriate for small and normal-size breasts that can flatten uniformly; otherwise the side to be examined can be elevated on a triangular wedge or cushion.

lateral lesions described above, the supine-oblique position, and at times, nearly lateral position, will displace the breast tissue medially and obtain a more uniform tissue distribution. The patient's back and shoulder can be supported by a firm cushion or rolled towels (**Fig. 2.11 d, Table 2.1**).

Holding the Transducer

The transducer should be held at the base, and the examiner's forearm should rest lightly on the patient's torso. The transducer should be moved with the wrist, not with the entire arm

Table 2.1 Positioning the patient for breast ultrasound

▸ Supine position
▸ Arms elevated
▸ Hands clasped behind the neck
▸ In a patient with large breasts, the side to be examined is elevated on a cushion or triangular wedge

(**Fig. 2.12 a–c**). This improves the examiner's spatial sense and makes it easier to move the probe systematically over the convex surfaces of the breast with good tactile feedback while watching the monitor. Tactile sensation is better at the wrist than along the arm. This is important, because the transducer should be applied to the tissue with just enough pressure to maintain uniform contact as it glides along the skin surface. Slightly increased pressure is applied only if greater sound penetration is required, but at no time should the pressure of the probe be so excessive as to cause pain. Wrist-guided transducer movements also make it easier for the examiner to perceive subcutaneous masses and areas of increased breast firmness. Arm-guided movements can impair the spatial and tactile senses (**Fig. 2.13a–c, Table 2.2**). For this reason it is better to sit at the same level as the patient rather than standing above her or sitting too low so that the examination can be conducted in a relaxed posture. In setting up an ultrasound examination, it is important to consider ergonomic aspects to promote comfort during extended periods of scanning.

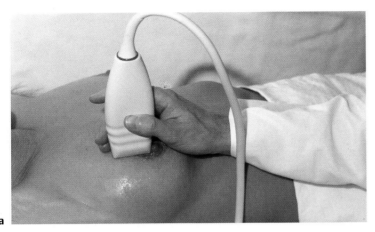

a

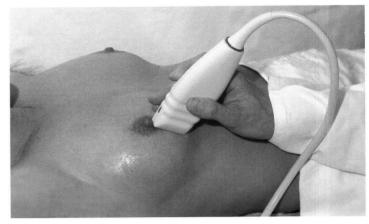

b

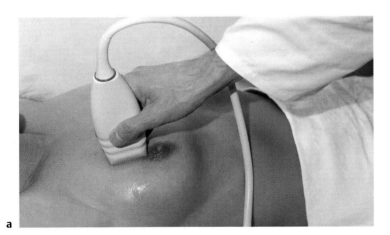

c

Fig. 2.12 a–c Correct way to hold the transducer: the probe is held at the base and guided with the wrist.
a Cranial right breast.
b Caudal.
c Lateral.

⚠ Comment:
The transducer should be grasped near the base and slid over the breast with gentle movements of the wrist. The arm rests lightly on the patient's body. This technique provides a good tactile and spatial sense. The transducer should be held perpendicular to the breast surface, especially at the periphery.

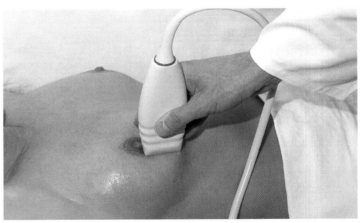

a

b

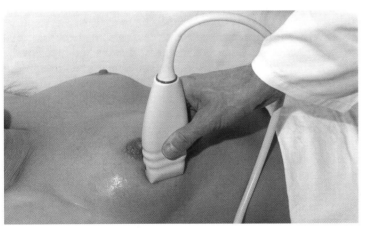

c

Fig. 2.13 a–c Wrong way to hold the transducer: the hand is placed too high, and the examiner is maneuvering the transducer from above with the wrist straight.
a Cranial right breast.
b Caudal.
c Lateral.

⚠ Comment:
A stiff, straight wrist does not provide the tactile feedback necessary for a dynamic examination and for accurately controlling transducer pressure. Also, guiding the probe with the arm does not provide the spatial sense that is obtained with wrist-guided movements, and it is more difficult to maintain a perpendicular probe angle when scanning over the lateral quadrants (as in **c**).

Table 2.2 Holding the transducer

- The transducer is held at the base
- The transducer is in maximal contact with the fingers and palm
- Transducer movements are controlled with the wrist
- The forearm rests lightly on the patient
- Just enough pressure is applied to maintain full contact
- The examiner sits at the level of the patient

Transducer Selection

The recommendation for breast ultrasonography is a broad bandwidth linear transducer whose center frequencies are above 7 or 8 MHz and whose frequency ranges may be as high as 17 MHz in the near field and as low as 5 MHz deeper in the image field to allow greater penetration of posterior breast tissue and pectoral muscle.

Older instruments, such as sector transducers and transducers of low frequency, e. g., 5 MHz, are not recommended. Rarely, a low-frequency transducer is useful for examining large, palpable masses deeply situated in large breasts (**Fig. 2.14 a, b**).

For efficient survey scanning, a high-frequency broad bandwidth probe with a relatively large footprint such as 38 mm, 50 mm or more is a good choice.

For superficial or dermal lesions, a small footprint (e. g., 18 mm), intraoperative or "hockey stick" high-frequency transducers can give good results. An offset is still required for superficial or intradermal lesions.

Coupling the Transducer

If the focal zone is set at a depth of 2–4 cm in older transducers, a standoff pad must be used to investigate superficial structures in or on the skin or in the subcutaneous fat lying just beneath the skin. The offset can be achieved with a gel pad or mound of coupling gel applied to the skin over the area to be scanned. Gel

pads are available in several thicknesses and with varying acoustic properties. Some of the pads require that overall gain be turned up (Kitecko, 3 M, Minneapolis, MN), whereas for others (Aquaflex, Parker Laboratories, Prescott, AZ) the gain must be decreased. The thickness of the standoff pad must be matched to the focal zone of the transducer; the thickness of the pad and depth of the lesion to be brought into focus should be added, and the focal zone or zones should be set at this depth. In general, a pad 1 cm thick is well suited to image the superficial breast. A mound of coupling gel is perhaps the most convenient type of offset. There is no point in using a standoff pad 2–3 cm thick on a transducer focused to a depth of 1 cm. This would move the optimum focal range outside the region of interest, and the beam would diverge within the tissue.

Gel pads, which are coupled to the skin with semiliquid gel and with gel between the transducer face and top of the pad, have a tendency to slide, and the operator often wishes to have more than two hands: one to hold the transducer, a second to hold the pad in place, and a third to annotate each image. Water-filled gloves or plastic pads have also been used as offsets, but they can cause problems due to air inclusions, and microbubbles in nondegassed water can hamper sound transmission. Some probes are manufactured with detachable clip-on offsets creating a scanning unit that is easy to handle and maneuver. It is important to adjust the TGC to compensate for the new position of the transducer face (**Fig. 2.14 b**).

> Standoff pads can improve the imaging of superficial lesions by placing the area or lesion of interest within the focal zone. These offsets may be unnecessary when short focal-length transducers are used, but thin standoff pads may nevertheless improve the image.

Older instruments and lower-frequency, lower-resolution transducers no longer provide the characterization of palpable masses, cysts, and mammographic densities that are relied upon for management decisions (**Figs. 2.15 a, b, 2.16 a, b**). Use of 5-MHz transducers is not recommended, and is currently below standard in

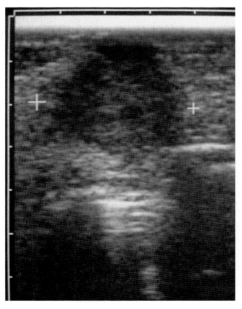 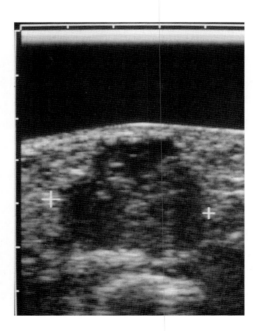

a, b

Fig. 2.14 a, b Invasive breast carcinoma 3.5 cm in diameter. The images were produced with a 5-MHz linear-array transducer with and without a standoff pad.
a Without standoff pad.
b With standoff pad.

❗ Comment:
Note how the standoff pad improves image quality. The tumor is located near the breast surface. The depth of the focal zone, at 3–4 cm, makes optimal use of the 2.5-cm standoff pad.

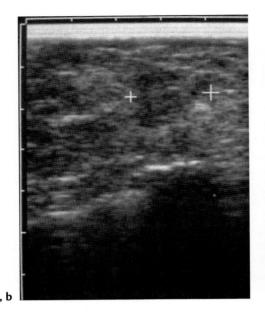
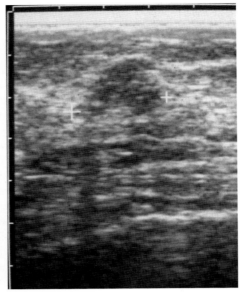

a, b

Fig. 2.15 a, b A 19-mm carcinoma imaged with a 5-MHz linear transducer.

! Comment:
The tumor is poorly demarcated from the breast parenchyma because of the low resolution of the scan.

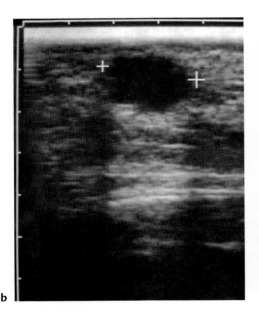
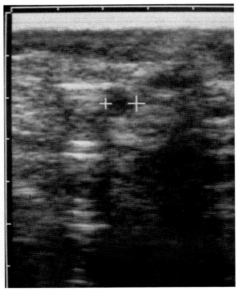

a, b

Fig. 2.16 a, b Cysts imaged with a 5-MHz linear transducer.
a A 10×2-mm cyst is plainly visible, but its margins are difficult to evaluate because of the poor resolution.
b Cysts smaller than 1 cm are difficult to detect or characterize with a 5-MHz transducer.

! Comment:
With the poor wall definition and poor demarcation from surrounding tissues, benign–malignant differentiation is difficult to accomplish with a low-frequency transducer.

the United States where transducers of higher frequencies improve image quality, allow more confident diagnoses of cysts less than 1 cm in diameter, and permit detection of small malignant masses, multifocal lesions, and intraductal processes (**Figs. 2.17a–d–2.20a–d**). These capabilities enable broadening of the indications for breast ultrasound.

Scanning Technique

In order to realize the full potential of today's high-resolution breast ultrasound systems, an appropriate examination technique is required (**Table 2.3**).

Because the breast contains few anatomic landmarks, it is necessary to employ a systematic pattern of transducer movements. The scans should overlap to achieve complete coverage and ensure that small lesions are detected.

Table 2.3 Standard scan planes for breast ultrasound

▸ Sagittal scan
▸ Transverse scan
▸ Radial and antiradial scan
▸ Parasternal sagittal scan (internal thoracic artery)
▸ Parasternal transverse scan (intercostal)
▸ Transverse axillary scan (axillary vein)
▸ Sagittal axillary scan (thoracodorsal artery and vein)

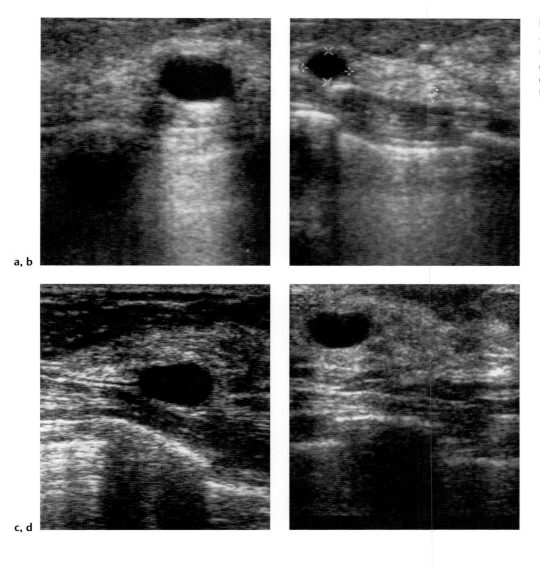

a, b

c, d

Fig. 2.17 a–d Cysts approximately 1 cm in diameter imaged with high-resolution instruments.
a, b High-resolution 5-MHz linear transducer.
c 7.5-MHz linear transducer, **d** 10-MHz linear transducer.

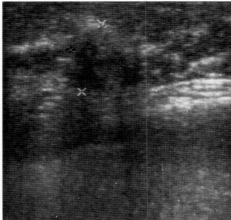

a, b

Fig. 2.18 a, b Invasive ductal carcinoma 1.7 cm in diameter, imaged with two different 5-MHz transducers.
a 5-MHz transducer of average quality.
b High-resolution 5-MHz transducer. Improved image processing provides better delineation of the tumor.

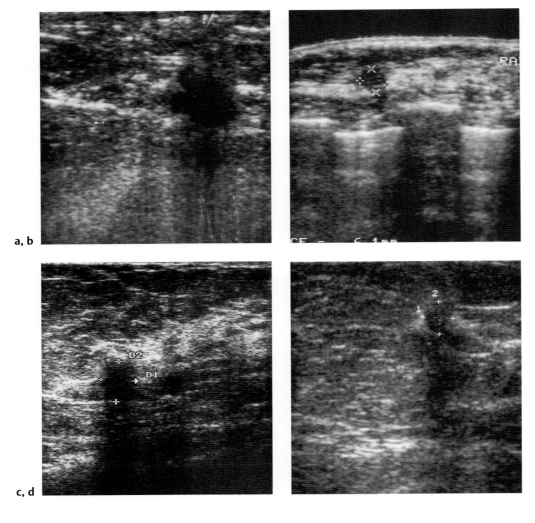

a, b

c, d

Fig. 2.19 a–d Carcinomas imaged with various high-resolution transducers.
a Tumor 15 mm in diameter, 5-MHz transducer.
b Tumor 7 mm in diameter, 5-MHz transducer with offset at skin.
c Tumor 9 mm in diameter, high-resolution 7.5-MHz transducer.
d Tumor 5 mm in diameter, high-resolution 10-MHz transducer.

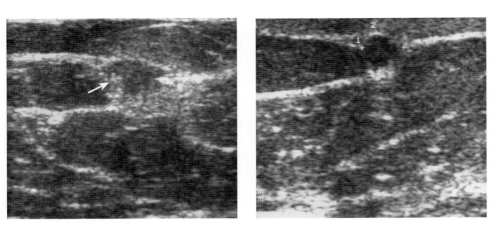

a, b

Fig. 2.20 a–d Multifocal carcinoma imaged with a high-resolution 10-MHz transducer.
a, b Two foci, 10 and 5 mm in diameter. Microcalcifications are seen in and adjacent to the mass in **a** (arrow).

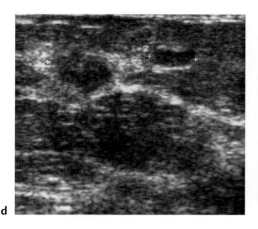
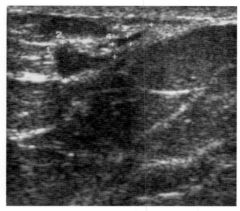

Fig. 2.20 c, d
c Two foci 12 and 8 mm in diameter.
d Dilatation of a subareolar duct caused by an intraductal carcinoma with incipient invasion. Maximum diameter 6 mm, total extent 10 mm.

c, d

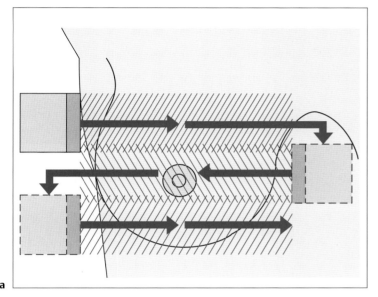
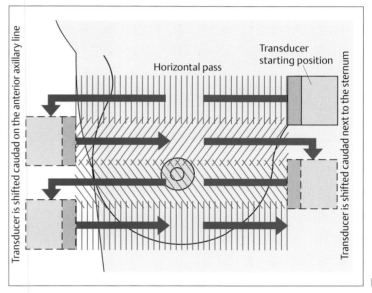

a

b

Fig. 2.21 a, b Scanning pattern for a systematic sagittal ultrasound survey of the breast. **a** Three-pass pattern (for transducers with an image field width of 5–6 cm). **b** Four-pass pattern (for smaller transducers with an image field width of approximately 4 cm).

Sagittal Scans

A complete survey of the breast is most easily accomplished with sagittal scans (**Fig. 2.21 a, b**). The number of passes depends on the size of the breast and the image field width of the transducer. After the gain, TGC, and focal settings have been adjusted, the transducer is placed on the axillary tail of the breast. From there it is moved anteromedially toward to the anterior axillary line and then in a lateral-to-medial direction to the parasternal region as sagittal scans are acquired. The rib cross sections provide landmarks that help the examiner move the transducer by slightly less than its own width in a caudad direction and then scan back laterally over the center of the breast to the anterior axillary line. At that point the transducer is again shifted caudad and moved back toward the sternum (**Fig. 2.22 a–i**). Three horizontal passes are sufficient with a large transducer, but smaller probes may require four or five excursions to cover the entire breast in overlapping sections.

> A complete, systematic survey of the breast is best accomplished with sagittal scans in overlapping planes. This ensures complete coverage of the mammary structures.

The transducer should always be held perpendicular to the skin surface. Angling the transducer away from the perpendicular leads to poor sound penetration. It is also important to be aware of the amount of transducer pressure being applied to the breast tissue. Applying too much pressure will deform and distort the anatomic structures of the breast, making them difficult to evaluate. Excessive pressure will also raise a small mound of breast tissue ahead of the transducer and may displace lesions out of the scan plane, causing them to be missed.

> The transducer should be applied to the breast with appropriate pressure. If greater sound penetration is needed, the pressure should be increased. The rule is to use as much pressure as necessary but no more than is required.

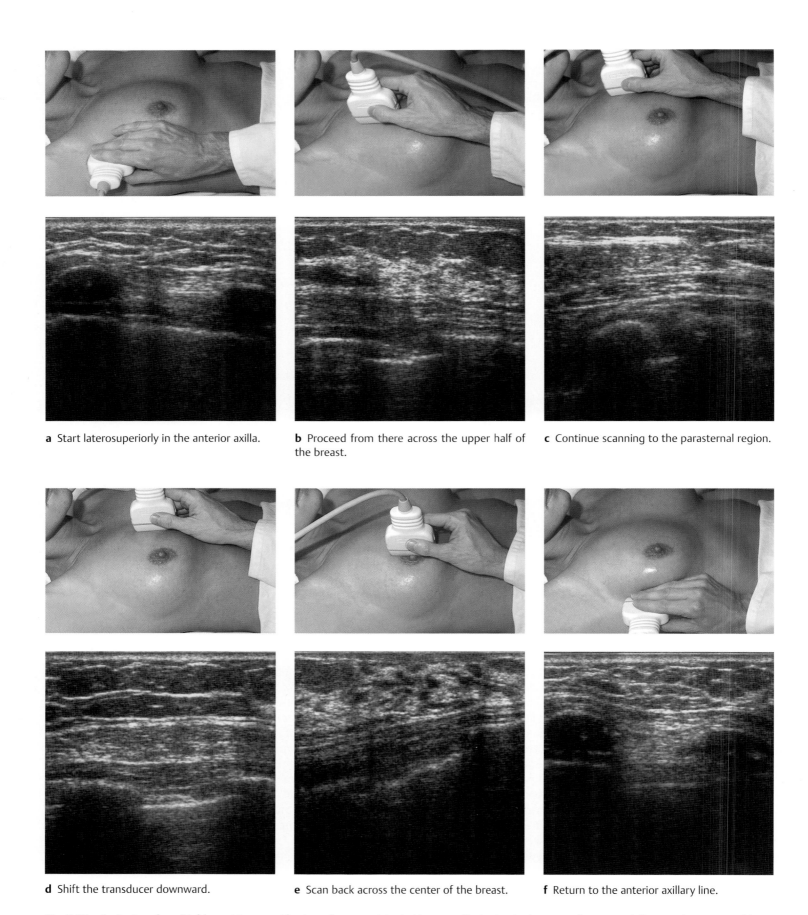

a Start laterosuperiorly in the anterior axilla.

b Proceed from there across the upper half of the breast.

c Continue scanning to the parasternal region.

d Shift the transducer downward.

e Scan back across the center of the breast.

f Return to the anterior axillary line.

Fig. 2.22 a–i Series of sagittal breast images. The transducer must be held perpendicular to the breast surface, especially over the outer and inner quadrants. Since the examiner watches the monitor during the examination, the breast structures and ribs provide important landmarks for making overlapping passes with the probe.

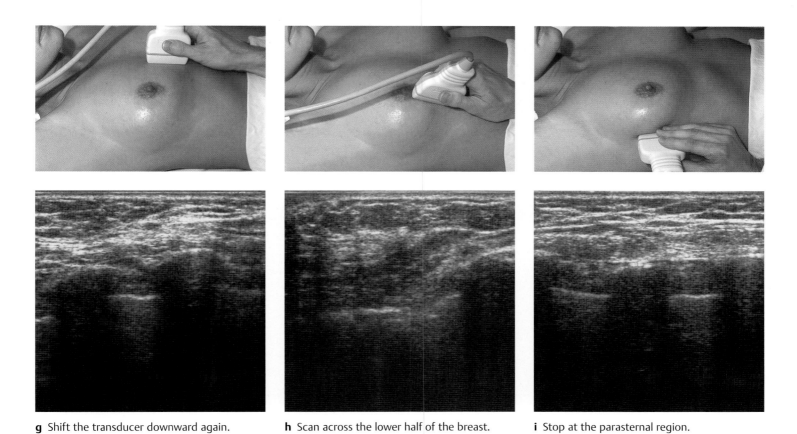

g Shift the transducer downward again.   **h** Scan across the lower half of the breast.   **i** Stop at the parasternal region.

Transverse Scans

Sagittal scans can be supplemented by imaging the breast in transverse (horizontal) planes, although experienced sonologists, confident that they have scanned every area of the breast in their sagittal surveys, may omit these transverse scans. Transverse scans are initiated by rotating the transducer 90° and scanning from medially to laterally in a meandering up-and-down pattern, shifting the probe by its own width for each successive pass (**Fig. 2.23**). In large breasts whose outer portions are difficult to evaluate with sagittal scans, the horizontal transducer placement may help to compress this region more uniformly and obtain a more systematic survey.

 Transverse scans are a useful adjunct for ensuring the seamless coverage of all breast structures.

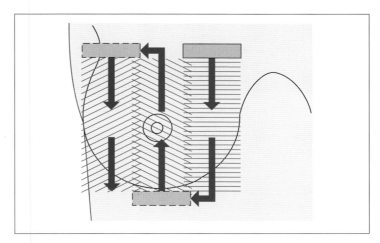

Fig. 2.23   Pattern for transverse (horizontal) scanning of the breast.

Radial Scans

Because the lactiferous ducts converge radially toward the central nipple–areolar complex from the periphery and terminate in the nipple, radial scans are useful for evaluating the ductal structures of the breast (**Fig. 2.24**). Some examiners prefer radial scans as their standard survey technique because they follow the natural anatomic course of the mammary ducts and lobules. The main drawback of radial scanning is that a radial, circular transducer pattern cannot cover all of the breast parenchyma. Multiple circular transducer passes would have to be made around the nipple areola and over the periphery to cover the entire breast, and centrally there is considerable overlap and duplication. It is difficult and time consuming to do radial scans systematically as the chief scanning method. It is much easier to locate focal lesions on sagittal or transverse scans and then do selective radial scans over the lesion to check for intraductal changes or tumor extension along the ducts (**Figs. 2.25–2.27**). The corresponding orthogonal antiradial scans can also show areas of duct ectasia or proliferative duct expansion, seen as well in transverse or oblique sectional images (**Fig. 2.28 a, b**).

 Radial scans are useful for investigating ductal abnormalities.

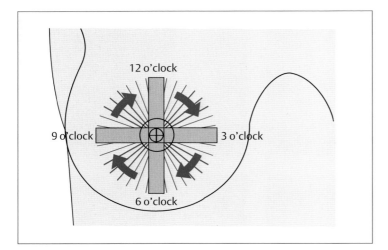

Fig. 2.24 Pattern for radial scanning of the breast.

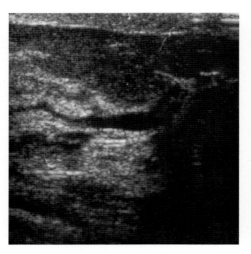

Fig. 2.25 Duct ectasia in a radial breast scan (nipple is on the right). A subareolar duct is dilated and tapers toward the periphery. Its anechoic contents are consistent with clear secretions.

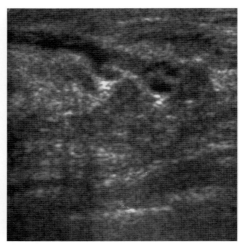

Fig. 2.26 Proliferative fibrocystic change. Radial scan (nipple on the left) shows irregular dilatation of peripheral ducts, which contain internal echoes.

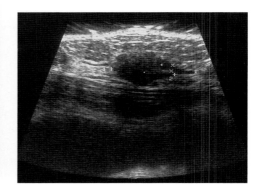

Fig. 2.27 Radial scan of invasive ductal carcinoma with an intraductal component. The tumor is 19 mm in diameter. Narrow, hypoechoic extensions 2 mm in diameter project from each side of the main tumor (calipers).

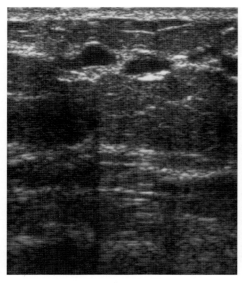

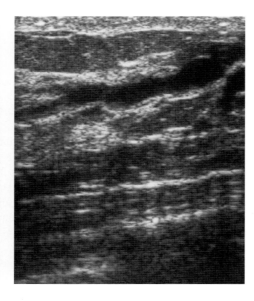

a, b

Fig. 2.28 a, b Comparison of sagittal and radial scans in duct ectasia.
a Parasagittal scan shows several dilated ducts in cross section. They resemble small cysts, but adjacent scans identified them as tubular structures.
b Radial scan shows the dilated ducts longitudinally.

Antiradial or Tangential Scans

Some examiners do tangential scans about the periphery of the breast, moving the transducer toward the center of the breast while keeping the scan angle perpendicular to the ducts (**Fig. 2.29**). The scans proceed clockwise around the breast in concentric circles. This technique is very time-consuming, because the scan planes diverge from one another toward the periphery and increasingly overlap toward the center of the breast. Even if the transducer passes are spaced closely together, there is a risk of missing small, peripheral focal lesions in the gaps between the scan planes. As a result, tangential scanning can be recommended as an adjunctive technique but should not be used alone. Antiradial scanning alone is not suitable for a rapid, systematic survey of the breast.

Targeted Ultrasound Assessment of Palpable Masses

When a palpable mass is present, a targeted ultrasound analysis of the mass should be done in addition to the general breast survey. This is important in making a final interpretation, which includes the determination of whether ultrasound can provide an explanation for a palpable mass, thickening, or mammographic finding. Often these masses are areas of fibrosis, which can be readily identified with ultrasound but are indeterminate by palpation. The examiner uses one hand to palpate and immobilize the mass between two fingers, then uses the other hand to place the transducer between the palpating fingers and move it slowly back and forth over the mass. At this time varying amounts of pressure can be applied to evaluate the compressibility of the mass.

Dynamic Examination

Evaluating Spatial Extent

Breast ultrasound is not a static, two-dimensional imaging technique but should be viewed as a dynamic modality that can cover the breast in all dimensions. The transducer can be angled and

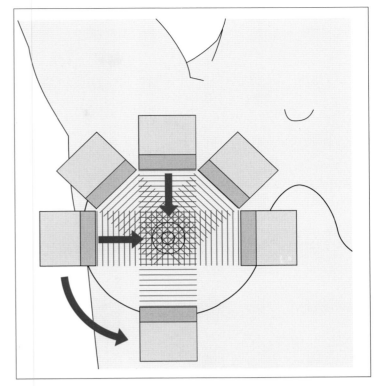

Fig. 2.29 Pattern for tangential scanning of the breast.

maneuvered to define the spatial extent of intramammary structures. This is particularly important in evaluating fatty tissue that has infiltrated the breast parenchyma. Often this tissue simulates a hypoechoic round or oval lesion that is confusing for the novice, because it is easily mistaken for a hypoechoic tumor. However, the moving, real-time image can provide a broadened anatomic setting for the fatty tissue that clearly distinguishes it from a circumscribed mass. Imaging the fat lobule in perpendicular planes during real-time scanning can show its elongation in one plane and possibly its connection with other fat lobules, convincingly excluding an abnormality and documenting its spatial extent. A real tumor, on the other hand, is discrete and is demarcated from normal surrounding tissues in more than one projection (**Figs. 2.30 a, b, 2.31 a, b**).

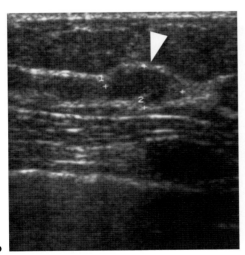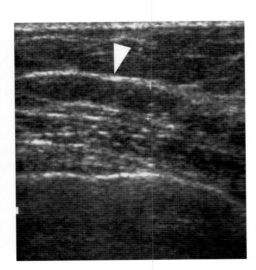

a, b

Fig. 2.30 a, b Pseudomass caused by fatty infiltration.
a Medial parasagittal scan shows a hypoechoic mass 13 × 7 mm in size.
b Transverse scan of the same lesion identifies it as a fat lobule, which can be traced toward the periphery.

❗ Comment:
Biplane scans can document the spatial extent of this normal anatomic structure.

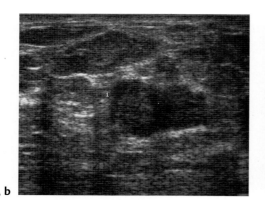 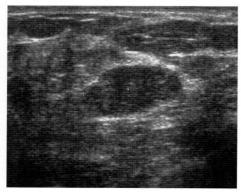

a, b

Fig. 2.31 a, b Proliferative fibroadenoma imaged in two planes.
a Parasagittal scan.
b Transverse scan. A comparison of both planes identifies the lesion as a circumscribed tumor.

⚠ Comment:
Because the tumor is isoechoic to fat, it could be misinterpreted as a fat lobule if just one image were evaluated.

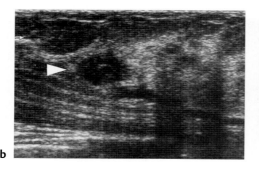 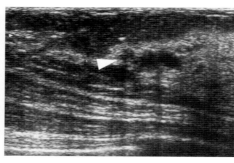

a, b

Fig. 2.32 a, b Compressibility of a focal mass.
a An area of fat appears as a hypoechoic pseudomass in the noncompression scan (arrowhead).
b The compression scan demonstrates the compressibility of the mass.

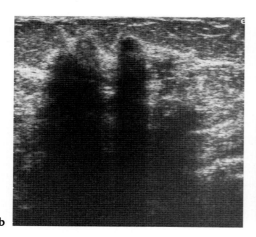 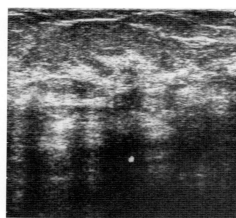

a, b

Fig. 2.33 a, b Improvement of sound penetration by compression.
a In the noncompression scan, fibrous tissue structures that cross the scan plane obliquely cause significant sound absorption, resulting in an equivocal image.
b Compression improves sound transmission and brings out anatomic details.

Compression

Varying degrees of transducer pressure can be applied to the breast surface to test the compressibility of intramammary structures. Fatty tissue, for example, is so soft that it is easily deformed by transducer pressure (**Fig. 2.32 a, b**). Another technique is to press down on the edge or narrow end of the transducer with the finger and observe the effect on underlying tissues. Glandular tissue and fat are easily deformed, whereas tumors have a firmer consistency and show little or no compressibility.

Compression can also establish whether areas of increased attenuation are caused by a sound-absorbing tumor or are artifacts caused by oblique beam incidence on normal connective tissue, parenchymal structures, or curved surfaces When the tissues are flattened by compression, these artifactual shadows fade as sound transmission is improved (**Figs. 2.33 a, b; 2.34 a, b**).

Elastography of tissues and tumors has been an active area of breast research for over a decade. Recently, several manufacturers have developed transducer adaptations suitable for clinical use in measuring tissue strain.

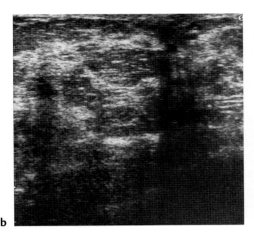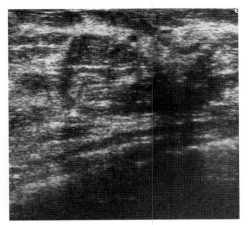

a, b

Summary

Opinions differ as to the best way to conduct a breast ultrasound examination. Whatever technique is used, it should be relatively easy to learn and should be carried out systematically. Reproducibility is a basic concern. The techniques that are necessary for an efficient, easy-to-learn breast examination are reviewed in **Table 2.4**. A systematic survey in the supine position (or supine-oblique for the lateral breast) with the arms elevated is preferred for routine examinations. This is an effective approach for evaluating the normal anatomic layers of the breast: skin, subcutaneous tissue, glandular tissue, ducts, retromammary fat, and chest wall. Because modern scanners permit the detection of small lesions, it is important to examine the entire breast, as is common in Europe and is becoming more prevalent in the United States. Transducer pressure is useful for testing local tissue compressibility and improving acoustic penetration.

Table 2.4   Recommended technique for breast ultrasound examination

▸ Supine position with the arms elevated to flatten and immobilize the breast
▸ Sagittal scans are performed in overlapping planes using a continuous, meandering pattern
▸ Sagittal survey may be supplemented by transverse and oblique scans
▸ Pressure is used to improve sound penetration and test the compressibility of breast masses
▸ Radial scans are obtained to investigate ductal changes

▶ The success of the breast examination depends on the dynamics of the scanning procedure: adjusting gain, TGC, and focal zones, varying the scan planes, evaluating the spatial extent of breast lesions, and testing their compressibility.

BI-RADS For Ultrasound

Development of the BI-RADS–US System

Along with the fourth edition for mammography and the first for breast MRI, the *Breast Imaging Reporting and Data System–Ultrasound* (BI-RADS–US) was published in 2003 by the American College of Radiology (ACR) after 5 years of development and validation. The project was supported in part by grants for protocol design for breast ultrasound research from the United States Public Health Service's Office on Women's Health and the National Cancer Institute. Topics that were designated for research included ultrasound for breast cancer screening, differentiation of benign/malignant solid masses, and the possible therapeutic applications of ultrasound, using ultrasound as a therapeutic agent (high-frequency ultrasound) as well as a guide for breast interventions.

An international Expert Working Group was assembled by the ACR that included the authors of this text. When the participants convened in Maine in 1998 they immediately recognized the need for a consistent and universally understood terminology to underlie projects using a modality as operator dependent as ultrasound, particularly when the projects involved the identification of criteria to apply in assessing an abnormality's likelihood of malignancy. Even at the time of the Maine meeting, ultrasound was entrusted only with cyst–solid differentiation. Encouraged by improvements in ultrasound systems and transducers, experienced breast ultrasonologists began to appreciate that if their technique were optimized and the language of interpretation standardized, ultrasound analysis of a mass might move beyond cyst vs. solid, and moreover, that a lexicon might aid in identifying feature patterns of benign solid masses as well as malignant lesions. Groups of characteristics analogous to those in mammography might emerge to allow follow-up for those masses with benign characteristics and biopsy for malignant-appearing or indeterminate lesions. The measure of success of a lexicon would be its potential to increase the specificity of solid mass assessments.

Shortly after the Maine meeting, a subcommittee of the ACR's BI-RADS Committee, then co-headed by Carl D'Orsi and Daniel B. Kopans, was formed to develop a BI-RADS for ultrasound. Ellen B. Mendelson chaired the subcommittee, which included Janet Baum, Wendie A. Berg, Christopher R. B. Merritt, and Eva Rubin. BI-RADS–US was modeled on the system used for mammography, in widespread clinical use in the United States. BI-RADS offered a method for quality assurance and outcome analysis, and its final assessment phrases had been incorporated into the Mammography Quality Standards Act of 1992. Anticipating breast imaging becoming increasingly multimodal in its approach, wherever the anatomic descriptors and feature categories of BI-RADS for mammography were applicable to ultrasound, we incorporated them into the ultrasound BI-RADS. The scheme was completed by adding feature categories and descriptors unique to ultrasound.

The proposed lexicon went through several versions, and the consensus document was presented and tested by breast imagers at several meetings, the first being the Society of Breast Imaging biennial meeting in San Diego, California in 2001. Kappa analysis of interobserver consistency confirmed good agreement among experienced and novice breast imagers for most descriptors within the various feature categories.

Basis of the BI-RADS–US System: Feature Analysis

Predicated on excellent, interpretable image quality, and acknowledging the importance of real-time ultrasound observations, BI-RADS assessments are based on analysis of combined features—using descriptors from several feature categories rather than any single one, with the most suspicious feature dominating the assessment and recommendation. The use of multiple features in the ultrasound analysis of breast lesions allows greater diagnostic confidence which, in turn, can increase specificity. For example, starting with one feature category, shape, an oval mass might be cystic or solid, benign or malignant. An oval mass oriented parallel to the skin ('wider-than-tall') does not limit possibilities much—the mass could still be benign or malignant, cystic or solid. Add a descriptor from the margin category, and the specificity jumps up. If the margin is circumscribed, the likelihood of malignancy diminishes, and descriptors from additional categories, such as echogenicity and posterior features, can be added to refine diagnostic possibilities further. If the mass were anechoic and posterior acoustic enhancement present, the diagnosis of a simple cyst could be made. If the margin were not circumscribed. (e. g., had spicules and microlobulations), and posterior acoustic shadowing were added, the mass would be incompatible with a simple cyst, and the analysis would lead the interpreter toward cancer or one of its mimics, with biopsy as the management recommendation. Primary feature categories for diagnosis include shape, margins, and unique to ultrasound, orientation with respect to the skin.

Additional feature categories that may help improve specificity include echogenicity, border zone, and posterior features as well as the BI-RADS category of "Effect on Surrounding Tissue." The effect, or lack of effect, of the mass on the tissue surrounding it, can provide supporting evidence, and it is important to assess the breast anatomy around a mass for an echogenic halo, disruption of fat planes, and duct derangements. When there is no mass and the lesion is itself architectural distortion, a beaded, ectatic duct, and skin thickening or edema, the anatomy and clinical history may provide clues to the lesion's etiology. In its feature analysis approach, BI-RADS–US employs similar methodology to that used for CT analysis of lung nodules, MRI for masses of the liver, and several imaging techniques for lesions of bone. As long as the definitions of terms are understood by the system's users, this standardized method of feature analysis for any abnormality makes possible structured reporting, a concise communication in which the significant points are clearly indicated and the assessment is yoked to a management recommendation. It also facilitates data tracking for self-audit of successes and failures, and a summary of outcomes, important at a time when healthcare dollars are challenged and the mantra is "pay for performance."

It is important to emphasize that descriptors within each feature category are selected after evaluation of at least two perpendicular views confirming reality of a lesion. When the performer is the interpreter, the analytic method is applied to a real-time assessment of the mass. Currently in development are computer-assisted diagnosis systems for breast ultrasound based on segmentation and feature extraction, initially using one view but now working with two perpendicular views. Lesion detection systems used with mammography are more difficult to apply to ultrasound because the US window is quite small; to date, the algorithms for ultrasound are applicable only to masses already detected.

Portions of BI-RADS–US are reproduced below with permission of the ACR. Definitions of the terms used and examples of each of the descriptors are provided. In assessing a lesion for diagnosis, in addition to analyzing the ultrasound images, correlation with mammography and MRI, if these examinations were done, physical findings, clinical history, the patient's age and other risk factors are important to consider. In feature analysis for breast ultrasound, the most important feature categories are shape, margin, and orientation taken together, and *the feature most associated with malignancy will dominate in the overall assessment.* An exam-

ple would be an oval mass, parallel to the skin, with circumscribed margin except where an acute angle is seen at one edge of the lesion. If the interpreter has not performed the scan, real-time observation would be indicated. If the angular margin is confirmed, it influences the assessment and management: greater likelihood of malignancy with biopsy indicated rather than follow-up.

Classification Categories in the BI-RADS–US System

Background Echotexture

As in mammography, great variability in tissue composition is the norm. The background texture of the breast may affect sensitivity to lesion detection, although further study is warranted.

Homogeneous Background Echotexture

– *Fat* lobules comprising the bulk of breast tissue. No discrete hypoechoic areas are present in the area scanned (**Fig. 3.1**).
– *Fibroglandular* tissue comprising the bulk of breast tissue (**Fig. 3.2**).

Heterogeneous Background

Heterogeneity can be focal or diffuse. Breast echotexture is characterized by multiple small areas of increased and decreased echogenicity. Shadowing may occur at interfaces of fat lobules and parenchyma. This pattern occurs in younger breasts and those with heterogeneously dense parenchyma seen mammographically. How and if this affects the sensitivity of sonography merits study, but technical maneuvers may help in interpretive issues of true lesion vs. pseudopathology (**Fig. 3.3**).

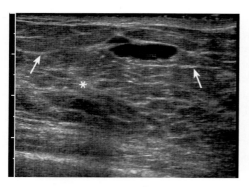

Fig. 3.1 Homogeneous echotexture: fat. Predominantly fatty breast tissue with well-defined fat lobules, hyperechoic Cooper ligaments and other connective tissue elements (arrows). Only a thin layer of more echogenic fibroglandular tissue is present (*). Anechogenicity of the simple cyst within the hypoechoic fat easily perceived with a high dynamic range and appropriate gain and contrast settings. With permission from ACR BI-RADS, 4th ed., 2003.

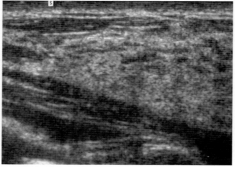

Fig. 3.2 Homogeneous echotexture: fibroglandular. Beneath a thin layer of subcutaneous fat lobules lies a uniformly echogenic layer of fibroglandular tissue. With permission from ACR BI-RADS, 4th ed., 2003.

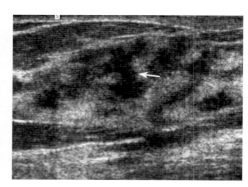

Fig. 3.3 Heterogeneous background tissue. The admixture of echogenic fibroglandular elements and hypoechoic ducts may prevent recognition of a small mass or may cause a group of ducts or a small fat lobule to be misinterpreted as an abnormality. Small hypoechoic area (arrow) was recognized as normal anatomic structure at real time imaging. With permission from ACR BI-RADS, 4th ed., 2003.

Masses

A mass occupies space and should be seen in two different projections. Masses can be distinguished from normal anatomic structures, such as ribs or fat lobules, using two or more projections and real-time scanning (**Fig. 3.4 a,b**; **Fig. 3.5 a,b**).

Shape

▸ *Oval*—a mass that is elliptical or egg-shaped (may include two or three undulations, i. e., "gently lobulated" or "macrolobulated") (**Fig. 3.6a–c**; **Fig. 3.7 a, b**).

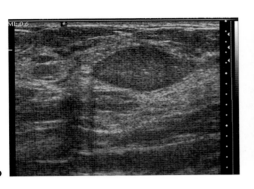 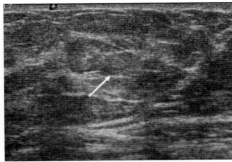

a, b

Fig. 3.4 a, b Fat lobule. Depending on the plane of section, a fat lobule may resemble a benign solid mass, such as a fibroadenoma (**a**). The fat lobule will elongate in the perpendicular view (arrow), excluding a mass (**b**). With permission from ACR BI-RADS, 4th ed., 2003.

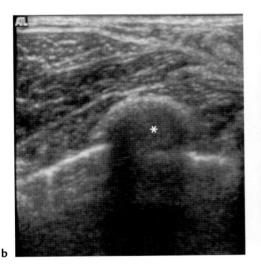 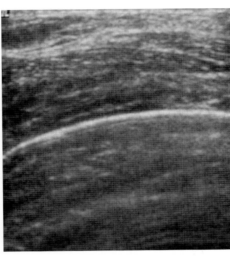

a, b

Fig. 3.5 a, b Ribs.
a Section through the short axis of a rib (*) depicts an oval, circumscribed, horizontally-oriented, shadowing mass that resembles a fibroadenoma.
b Anatomy provides the clue: the rib lies behind the pectoral muscle, not a site for primary breast cancer. The perpendicular projection shows the elongated, curved rib. With permission from ACR BI-RADS, 4th ed., 2003.

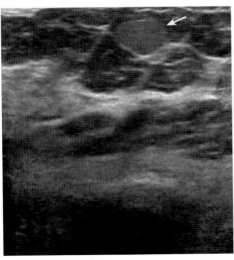 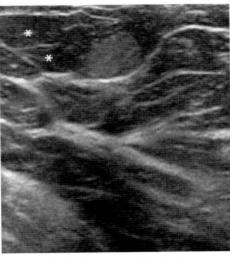 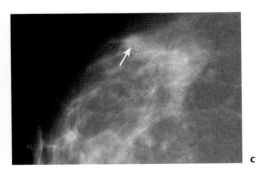

a, b
c

Fig. 3.6 a–c Oval, hyperechoic fibroadenoma. **a** Circumscribed oval mass, parallel to skin, noticeable only because of increased echogenicity (arrows). Its features all appear benign. **b** Perpendicular view shows mass surrounded by fat lobules (asterisks) except posteriorly, where it abuts a Cooper ligament. **c** Mammogram shows small mass correlating with US (arrow); the soft tissue density differentiates it from a lipoma, which would have fat density on the radiograph. Figures **a** and **b** with permission from ACR BI-RADS, 4th ed., 2003.

- *Round*—a mass that is spherical, ball-shaped, circular, or globular. A round mass has an anteroposterior diameter equal to its transverse diameter (**Fig. 3.8 a,b**).
- *Irregular*—a mass neither round nor oval in shape (**Fig. 3.9**).

Orientation

This feature of masses is unique to ultrasound imaging. Orientation is defined with reference to the skin line. A parallel or "wider-than-tall" orientation is a property of some benign masses, notably fibroadenomas; however, many carcinomas also have this orientation. Shape and marginal characteristics should help dictate the level of suspicion of malignancy.

- *Parallel*—the long axis of a lesion parallels the skin line ("wider-than-tall" or horizontal orientation) (**Figs. 3.10, 3.11 a,b**).
- *Not parallel*—the anteroposterior or vertical dimension is greater than the transverse or horizontal dimension. These masses can also be obliquely oriented to the skin line. Round masses are not parallel in their orientation. Synonyms: "taller-than-wide" or vertical (**Fig. 3.12**).

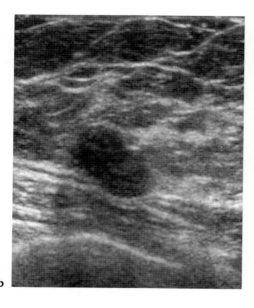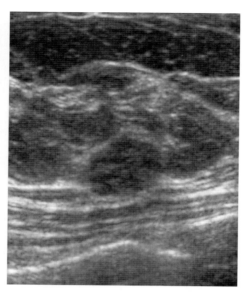

a, b

Fig. 3.7 a, b Oval shape—macrolobulated.
a Sagittal view of oval (macrolobulated) mass with circumscribed margins.
b Transverse view of this mass is round. Oval masses viewed orthogonally to their long axes will be seen as round. Core biopsy confirmed fibroadenoma. With permission from ACR BI-RADS, 4th ed., 2003.

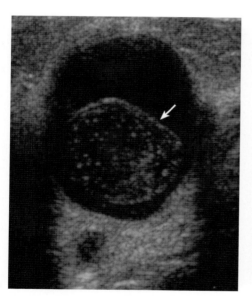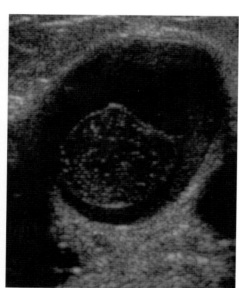

a, b

Fig. 3.8 a, b Round shape. Longitudinal (**a**) and transverse (**b**) views of a round complex cystic mass containing a small round, echogenic intracystic mass (arrow). The intracystic component is a thrombus that formed in a cyst that bled after aspiration. With permission from ACR BI-RADS, 4th ed., 2003.

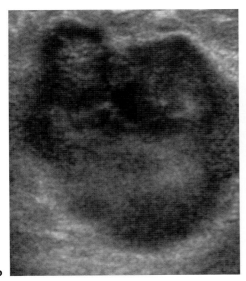 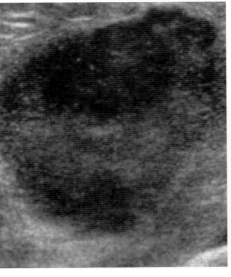

a, b

Fig. 3.9 a, b Irregular shape. Orthogonal views of a poorly differentiated infiltrating ductal carcinoma whose shape cannot be described by a geometric term. This irregular mass is hypoechoic compared with the surrounding fat lobules. Figure **a** with permission from ACR BI-RADS, 4th ed., 2003.

Fig. 3.10 Orientation—parallel. Simple cyst. Radial view of oval, parallel (wider-than-tall), circumscribed mass demonstrating diagnostic criteria of a benign cyst: anechoic, oval (or round) and circumscribed with posterior enhancement. With permission from ACR BI-RADS, 4th ed., 2003.

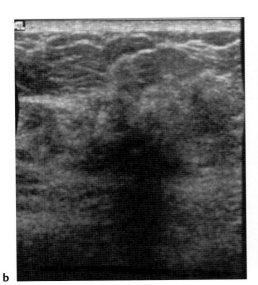 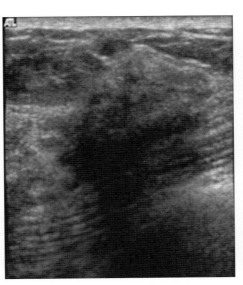

a, b

Fig. 3.11 a, b Orientation—parallel. Orthogonal views of a palpable mass with spiculation and posterior shadowing show that the mass in longitudinal projection is horizontal (wider-than-tall) or parallel in orientation. Histologic diagnosis is infiltrating lobular carcinoma. Longitudinal view (**a**), transverse view (**b**). With permission from ACR BI-RADS, 4th ed., 2003.

Fig. 3.12 Orientation—not parallel. Poorly differentiated invasive ductal carcinoma is diagnosis of vertically oriented oval mass whose long axis is not parallel to the skin line. Indistinct margins with short spicules anteriorly. At first glance the mass appears circumscribed, fibroadenomas will not have this orientation. Many poorly differentiated cancers demonstrate posterior enhancement rather than shadowing. With permission from ACR BI-RADS, 4th ed., 2003.

Margin

The margin is the edge or border of the lesion.

▸ *Circumscribed*—Margin well defined or sharp, with an abrupt transition between the lesion and surrounding tissue. Most circumscribed lesions have round or oval shapes (**Fig. 3.13 a,b**).

▸ *Not circumscribed*—If the margin is not circumscribed, a mass has one or more of the following features: indistinct, angular, microlobulated, or spiculated. "Irregular" is not used to group these marginal attributes because *irregular* describes the shape of a mass.

– *Indistinct*—No clear demarcation between a mass and its surrounding tissue. Boundary poorly defined (**Fig. 3.14 a, b**).

– *Angular*—some or all of the margin has sharp corners, often forming acute angles (**Fig. 3.15 a, b**).

– *Microlobulated*—short-cycle undulations impart a scalloped appearance to margin of mass (**Fig. 3.16 a, b; 3.17 a, b**).

– *Spiculated*—the margin is formed or characterized by sharp lines projecting from the mass (**Fig. 3.18 a, b**).

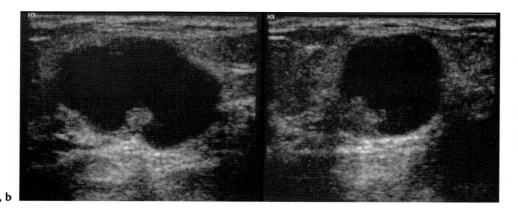

a, b

Fig. 3.13 a, b Margin—circumscribed. The margin of this intracystic papillary carcinoma is sharply defined at the interface of the cyst with the surrounding tissue. In **a**, the mass is pedunculated; in the orthogonal view (**b**), the lesion is sessile in the dependent position of the cyst. Sharp marginal definition of the small carcinoma within the cyst is explained by growth of this mass within fluid. With permission from ACR BI-RADS, 4th ed., 2003.

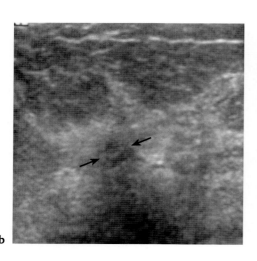
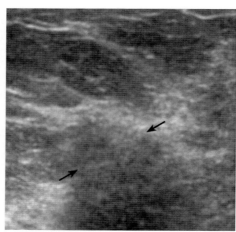

a, b

Fig. 3.14 a, b Margin—not circumscribed: *Indistinct*. This hypoechoic invasive ductal carcinoma (arrows) has an irregular shape and indistinct margins. It is infiltrating the surrounding breast parenchyma. Associated architectural distortion is manifested by destruction of tissue planes. With permission from ACR BI-RADS, 4th ed., 2003.

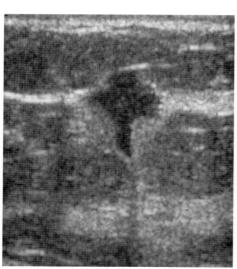
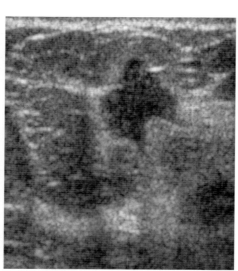

a, b

Fig. 3.15 a, b Margin—not circumscribed: *Angular*. Infiltrating ductal carcinoma. This angular mass, markedly hypoechoic compared with the surrounding fat lobules and parenchyma, has an irregular shape. Shape and marginal features of this mass suggest its malignant etiology. **a** transverse view; **b** longitudinal view. With permission from ACR BI-RADS, 4th ed., 2003.

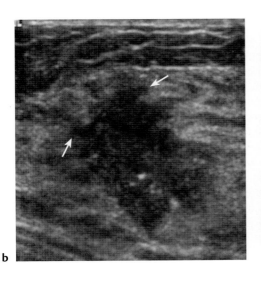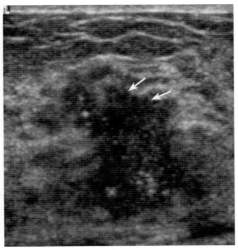

a, b

Fig. 3.16 a, b Margin—not circumscribed: *Microlobulated*. Markedly hypoechoic, irregularly shaped mass has numerous short cycle undulations (arrows) at its border with surrounding tissue. Microlobulation is frequently associated with malignancy. As in this case, where parts of the margin are angular and indistinct, a combination of marginal features is often present. Histology: infiltrating ductal carcinoma.
a transverse view; **b** longitudinal view. With permission from ACR BI-RADS, 4th ed., 2003.

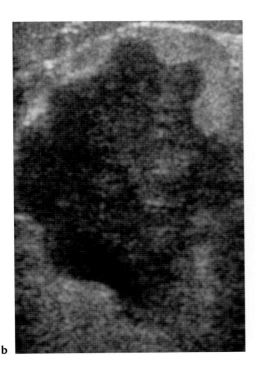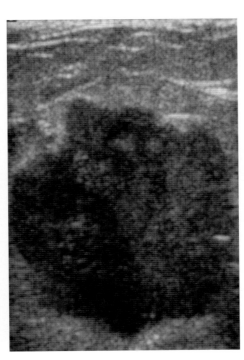

a, b

Fig. 3.17 a, b Margin—not circumscribed: *Microlobulated*. This large microlobulated mass in a male patient was DCIS. The marginal features and the irregular shape of this mass suggest its malignant etiology.
a, b orthogonal projections. With permission from ACR BI-RADS, 4th ed., 2003.

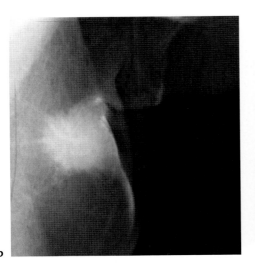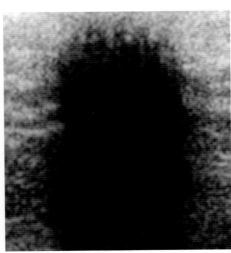

a, b

Fig. 3.18 a, b Margin—not circumscribed: *Spiculated*. Granular cell tumor.
a Dense mass present near the axilla on the tangential mammogram causes skin retraction and thickening.
b Hypoechoic, intensely shadowing mass with many anterior spicules on the corresponding ultrasound image. With permission from ACR BI-RADS, 4th ed., 2003.

Lesion Boundary

The lesion boundary describes the transition zone between the mass and the surrounding tissue.

▸ *Abrupt interface*—the sharp demarcation between the lesion and surrounding tissue can be imperceptible or a distinct, well-defined echogenic rim of any thickness (**Fig. 3.19 a,b**).

▸ *Echogenic halo*—there is no sharp demarcation between the mass and the surrounding tissue which is bridged by an echogenic transition zone. An echogenic halo is a feature associated with some carcinomas and abscesses (**Fig. 3.20**).

Echo Pattern

▸ *Anechoic*—without internal echoes (**Fig. 3.21 a, b**).
▸ *Hyperechoic*—having increased echogenicity relative to fat or equal to fibroglandular tissue (**Fig. 3.22 a,b**).
▸ *Complex*—a complex mass contains both anechoic (cystic) and echogenic (solid) components (**Fig. 3.23**).
▸ *Hypoechoic*—defined relative to fat; hypoechoic masses are characterized by low-level echoes throughout (for example, the appearances of complicated cysts and fibroadenomas) (**Fig. 3.24 a, b**).
▸ *Isoechoic*—having the same echogenicity as fat. Isoechoic masses may be relatively inconspicuous, particularly when they are situated within an area of fat lobules (**Fig. 3.25**).

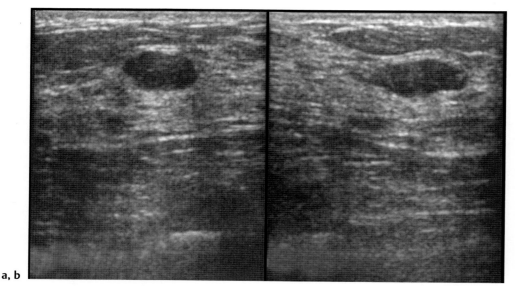

a, b

Fig. 3.19 a, b Lesion boundary—abrupt interface. Fibroadenoma. This benign, solid mass has an abrupt interface with the surrounding tissue; these boundary characteristics are identical to those of a simple cyst. **a** Radial and **b** antiradial views. With permission from ACR BI-RADS, 4th ed., 2003.

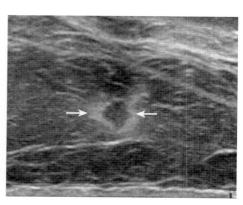

Fig. 3.20 Lesion boundary—echogenic halo. Foreign body granuloma. Indistinct echogenic halo (arrows) surrounds small, hypoechoic mass. Other features suggesting malignancy are irregular shape and angular margin of the central hypoechoic portion of this cancer mimic. With permission from ACR BI-RADS, 4th ed., 2003.

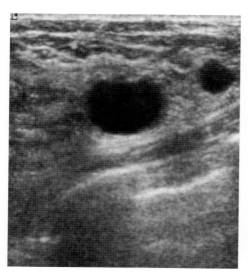
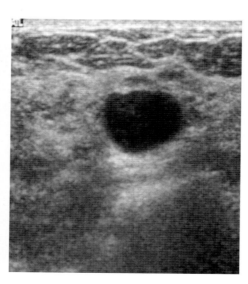

a, b

Fig. 3.21 a, b Echo pattern—anechoic. Cysts. A cyst should be anechoic, resembling a black hole. Other criteria for diagnosing simple cysts include circumscribed margins, round or oval shape and posterior acoustic enhancement. **a** Radial view; **b** antiradial view. With permission from ACR BI-RADS, 4th ed., 2003.

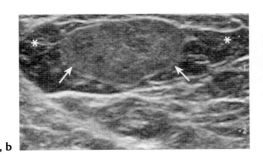
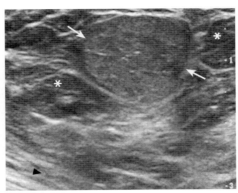

a, b

Fig. 3.22 a, b Echo pattern—hyperechoic. Lipoma. Small lipoma in longitudinal (a) and transverse (b) views (arrows) has the benign features of oval shape and circumscribed margins. The echogenicity of the mass exceeds that of the surrounding fat lobules (asterisks) and is isoechoic to fibroglandular parenchyma and hyperechoic to fat. The lipoma is adjacent to the pectoral muscle band in b (arrowhead). With permission from ACR BI-RADS, 4th ed., 2003.

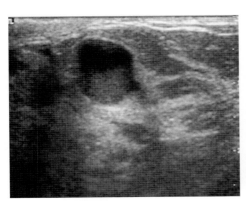
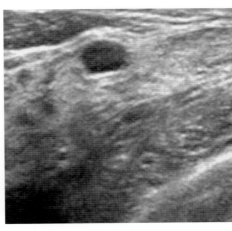
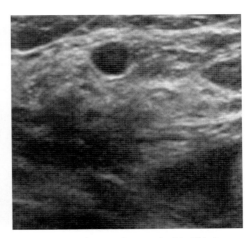

a, b

Fig. 3.23 Echo pattern—complex. Intracystic carcinoma. An echogenic focus is present in the dependent portion of the cyst. Diagnosis is intracystic papillary carcinoma, less common than an intracystic papilloma. These masses are not distinguishable with ultrasound, and a clot might have a similar appearance. With permission from ACR BI-RADS, 4th ed., 2003.

Fig. 3.24 a, b Echo pattern—hypoechoic. Complicated cyst. Orthogonal views (a, b). This hypoechoic mass situated in dense fibroglandular tissue appears solid and similar to a fibroadenoma because of its internal echoes, but greenish fluid was aspirated. In addition to low-level internal echoes, a complicated cyst may show a fluid–fluid level as seen in the small lesion at the top right corner of the image. Oval shape and circumscribed margins are consistent with a benign etiology. With permission from ACR BI-RADS, 4th ed., 2003.

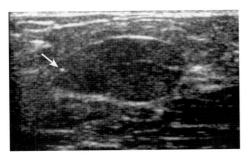

Fig. 3.25 Echo pattern—isoechoic. Fibroadenoma. The shape of this isoechoic fibroadenoma resembles that of a fat lobule. Were it not for the calcification (arrow), the fibroadenoma might have been overlooked. With permission from ACR BI-RADS, 4th ed., 2003.

Posterior Acoustic Features

Posterior acoustic features represent the attenuation characteristics of a mass with respect to its acoustic transmission.

▶ *No posterior acoustic features*—no shadowing or enhancement is present deep to the mass; the echogenicity of the area immediately behind the mass is not different from that of adjacent tissue at the same depth (**Fig. 3.26 a, b**).

▶ *Enhancement*—sound transmission is unimpeded in its passage through the mass. Enhancement appears as a column that is more echogenic (whiter) deep to the mass. One criterion for cyst diagnosis is enhancement (**Fig. 3.27 a, b**).

▶ *Shadowing*—posterior attenuation of the acoustic transmission. Sonographically, the area posterior to the mass appears darker. At the edges of curved masses, acoustic velocity changes and thin shadows are seen. This refraction or edge shadowing is of no significance and should be distinguished from central shadowing, which is a property of the mass. Shadowing is associated with fibrosis, with or without an underlying carcinoma. Postsurgical scars, fibrous mastopathy and cancers with a desmoplastic response will show posterior shadowing. Similar to a vertical (taller-than-wide) orientation, shadowing is a feature more helpful when present than when absent (**Fig. 3.28 a, b**). Many cancers will exhibit enhancement or no change in posterior features, just as many cancers are wider-than-tall. However, fibroadenomas are not vertically oriented (taller-than-wide).

▶ *Combined pattern*—Some lesions have more than one pattern of posterior attenuation. For example, a fibroadenoma containing a large calcification may demonstrate shadowing posterior to the calcified area but enhancement of the tissues deep to the uncalcified portion. A combined pattern of posterior features may also be seen in lesions that are evolving (**Fig. 3.29 a–d**). One such example is a postlumpectomy seroma, which enhances posteriorly. As the fluid is resorbed and scarring develops, the features of fibrosis become evident as spiculation of the margins and posterior acoustic shadowing.

a, b
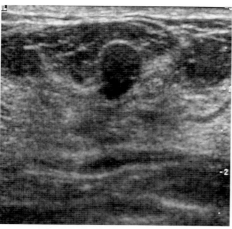 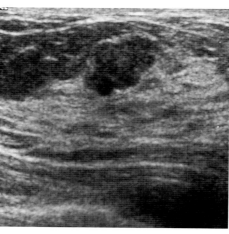

Fig. 3.26 a, b Posterior acoustic features—none. Compared with tissue at the same depth, orthogonal views show no difference in echogenicity deep to the mass. This mass has an irregular shape and microlobulated margins that are not circumscribed. Posterior features are less important than margin and shape. Histology: atypical ductal hyperplasia, fibroadenoma, and stromal fibrosis. With permission from ACR BI-RADS, 4th ed., 2003.

a, b
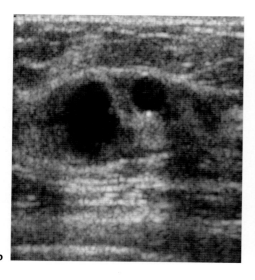 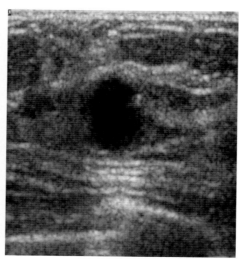

Fig. 3.27 a, b Posterior acoustic features—enhancement. Fibrocystic change. Complex cystic mass with cysts, calcification, and solid areas of fibrosis has circumscribed margins, oval shape, and parallel orientation on radial (**a**) and antiradial (**b**) views. The tissue immediately deep to the lesion enhances. With permission from ACR BI-RADS, 4th ed., 2003.

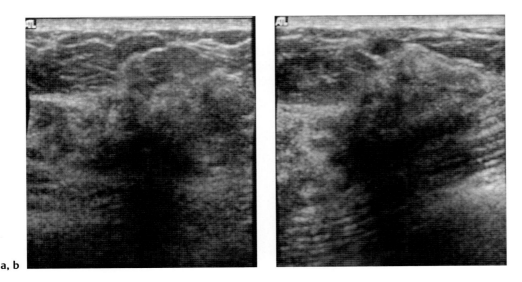

a, b

Fig. 3.28 a, b Posterior acoustic features—shadowing. Invasive lobular carcinoma. Spiculated, hypoechoic, irregularly shaped mass with parallel orientation causes acoustic attenuation (shadowing) deep to the mass. The shadowing obscures the posterior margin of the mass. **a** Radial and **b** antiradial views.

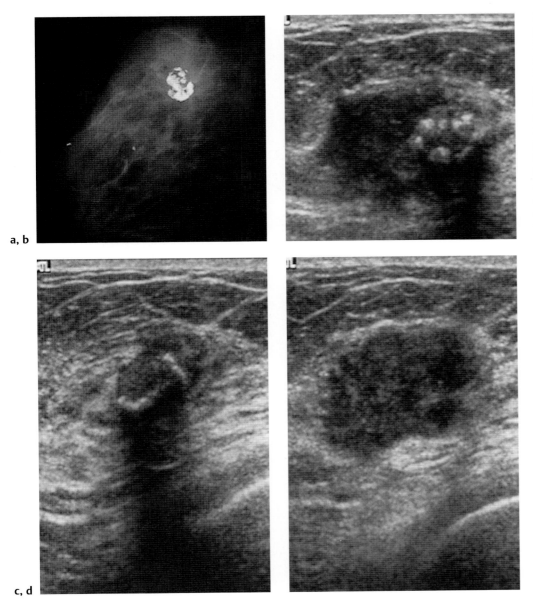

a, b

c, d

Fig. 3.29 a–d Posterior acoustic features—Combined pattern fibroadenoma and infiltrating ductal carcinoma: importance of integrating ultrasound, mammographic, and clinical information. Lateral mammographic view (**a**) showing typical "popcorn" calcifications of a fibroadenoma that could explain a palpable mass, but the elderly patient stated that the mass was new. In longitudinal view, shadowing is present posterior to the macrocalcifications of the calcifying fibroadenoma (**b**). Adjacent to the fibroadenoma is uncalcified tissue of irregular shape with microlobulated and spiculated margins. Mild enhancement is seen behind the carcinoma. In **c**, short axis view, only the shadowing fibroadenoma is seen, but **d** shows the malignant mass. Figures **a–c** with permission from ACR BI-RADS, 4th ed., 2003.

Surrounding Tissue

▸ *No effect* (**Fig. 3.30**).
▸ Effects of a mass on its surroundings are: compression of the tissue around the mass, obliteration of the tissue planes by an infiltrating lesion, straightening or thickening of Cooper ligaments and an echogenic halo. Edema may be present, caused by inflammatory carcinoma, radiation therapy, mastitis or a systemic process such as congestive heart failure.

– *Intraductal mass* (**Fig. 3.31 a, b**).
– *Ducts*—abnormal caliber and/or arborization (**Fig. 3.32 a, b**).
– *Cooper ligament changes*—straightening or thickening (**Fig. 3.33**).

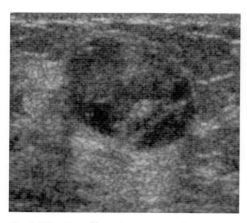

Fig. 3.30 No effect on surrounding tissue. This complex cystic, circumscribed, enhancing mass, a galactocele, has no effect on the tissue that surrounds it except for mild compression. A history of lactation is important clinical information and should be applied in formulating the differential considerations. If aspirated, the lesion will yield milky fluid.

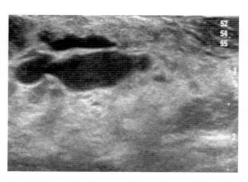

Fig. 3.31 a, b Surrounding tissue—identifiable effect: duct ectasia. Dilated portion of a duct near the nipple. Low-level internal echoes are present consistent with intraductal debris.
a Mediolateral oblique view of the right breast shows cystically dilated ducts posterior to the nipple correlating with the sonographic findings (**b**).

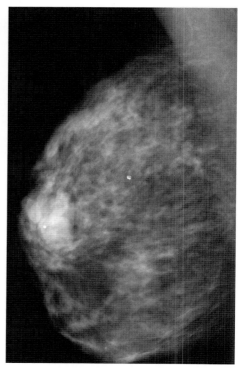

a, b

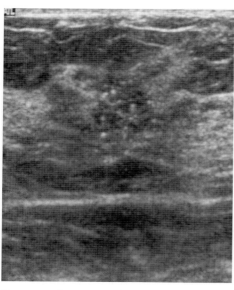

a, b

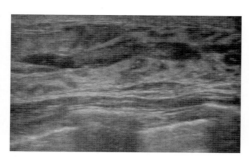

Fig. 3.32 a, b Surrounding tissue—identifiable effect: ducts. DCIS. Mildly dilated ducts containing grouped microcalcifications in linear array (**a**). The morphology of the microcalcifications is beyond the resolution of the L 12–5 MHz transducer and requires mammographic magnification. In another patient with DCIS, the duct is distended by the intraluminal epithelial proliferation (**b**). With permission from ACR BI-RADS, 4th ed., 2003.

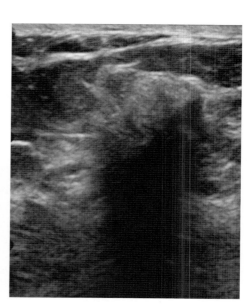

Fig. 3.33 Surrounding tissue—identifiable effect: Cooper ligament changes. Invasive lobular carcinoma straightens and truncates a Cooper ligament, seen as a horizontal hyperechoic line at the left lateral aspect of the mass.

- *Edema*—increased echogenicity of surrounding tissue and reticulation (angular network of hypoechoic lines) (**Fig. 3.34**).
- *Architectural distortion*—disruption of normal anatomic planes (**Fig. 3.35**).
- *Skin thickening*—focal or diffuse skin thickening. Thickness of normal skin is 2 mm or less except in the periareolar area and lower breasts (see **Fig. 3.34**).
- *Skin retraction/irregularity* (**Fig. 3.36**).

Calcifications

Calcifications are poorly characterized with ultrasound but can be recognized as echogenic foci, particularly when in a mass.

Macrocalcifications

Macrocalcifications are coarse calcifications that are 0.5 mm or more in size. As in other parts of the body, macrocalcifications will attenuate the acoustic beam and cause acoustic shadowing (**Fig. 3.37 a, b**).

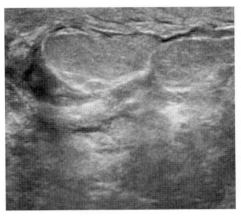

Fig. 3.34 Surrounding tissue—identifiable effect: edema and skin thickening in inflammatory carcinoma. Increased echogenicity of tissue deep to the skin and an angular reticulation of hypoechoic lines within and beneath the thickened skin are hallmarks of inflammatory carcinoma and other causes such as congestive heart failure, renal failure, and mastitis. In inflammatory carcinoma, tumor masses, masked by edema on mammograms, can often be depicted within the breast by ultrasound.

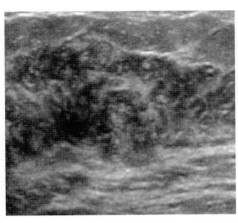

Fig. 3.35 Surrounding tissue—identifiable effect: architectural distortion. Mastitis can cause architectural derangement, here seen beneath the reddened skin as a hypoechoic ill-defined lesion in an area of pain reddened skin. Anatomic distinctions are blurred.

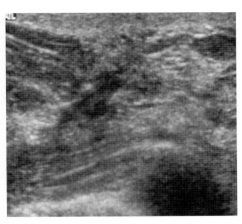

Fig. 3.36 Surrounding tissue—identifiable effect: skin retraction/irregularity, surgical scar. Localized skin irregularity and thickening are expected findings after lumpectomy and radiation therapy. The hypoechoic scar extends from the skin to the pectoral muscle. Directly over the scar, at the incision site, the skin is thickened and forms a V.

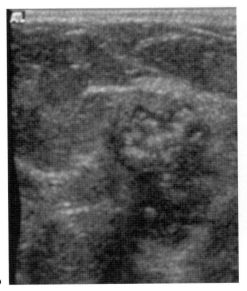

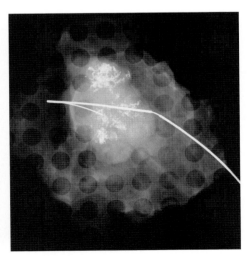

a, b

Fig. 3.37 a, b Calcifications—macrocalcifications. Ultrasound image **a** shows irregularly shaped malignant marginal characteristics in this mass with clumped calcifications, some of them shadowing posteriorly. **b** Plaque-like calcifications within mass excised after presurgical localization. Pathology: metaplastic carcinoma. With permission from ACR BI-RADS, 4th ed., 2003.

Microcalcifications

▸ *Microcalcifications out of a mass*—microcalcifications situated in fat or fibroglandular tissue are less conspicuous than those present in a mass. Small echogenic flecks grouped in tissue may sometimes be identified because they have patterns different from those of acoustic speckle or transversely sectioned Cooper ligaments, Because they occupy too small a portion of the acoustic beam, microcalcifications will not shadow. If calcifications are numerous enough for a pattern to be discerned, they may be perceived as scattered or grouped in the area of tissue being examined with ultrasound (**Fig. 3.38**).

▸ *Microcalcifications in a mass*—microcalcifications embedded in a mass are well depicted. The punctate, hyperechoic foci will be conspicuous in a hypoechoic mass (**Fig. 3.39**).

Special Cases

Special cases are those cases with a unique diagnosis or findings.

Clustered Microcysts

The lesion consists of a cluster of tiny anechoic foci, individually smaller than 2–3 mm, with thin (≤ 0.5 mm) intervening septations and no discrete solid component. If they are nonpalpable, clustered microcysts may be assessed as probably benign, with short-interval follow-up. Causes include fibrocystic changes and apocrine metaplasia (**Fig. 3.40**).

Complicated Cysts

The homogeneous low-level internal echoes that characterize the commonly encountered cyst may also have a layered appearance. Fluid–debris levels may shift slowly with changes in the patient's position. A complicated cyst may also contain brightly echogenic foci that scintillate as they shift. If aspirated, the cyst fluid may be a clear, yellow, or turbid green color. The term "complicated" describes the ultrasound appearance and does not indicate that pus or blood is responsible for the internal echoes. Complicated cysts do not contain solid mural nodules. A discrete solid component places the cystic lesion into the category of "complex mass," requiring aspiration or other intervention (**Fig. 3.41 a, b**).

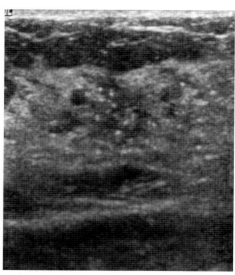

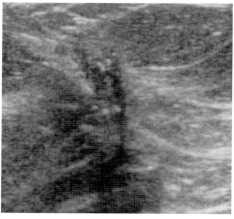

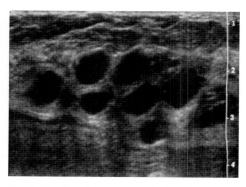

Fig. 3.38 Microcalcifications out of a mass. Numerous echogenic foci, microcalcifications, are seen beneath the subcutaneous fat in the fibroglandular layer. Pathology: DCIS. With permission from ACR BI-RADS, 4th ed., 2003.

Fig. 3.39 Microcalcifications in a mass. Echogenic foci within hypoechoic, irregularly shaped mass are microcalcifications. Pathology: recurrent invasive ductal and intraductal carcinoma.

Fig. 3.40 Special cases—clustered microcysts. Microcysts 2–3 mm in diameter are distended acini within the lobule. No solid component is present; a solid component requires further evaluation or biopsy.

Fig. 3.41 a, b Complicated cysts. **a** Circumscribed, benign-appearing mass containing low-level echoes within it and posterior enhancement, consistent with a complicated cyst, difficult to tell from a solid mass such as a fibroadenoma. When palpable, tender, new, or enlarging, aspiration should be considered. In another patient, the mass contains a fluid–fluid level which can shift during real-time scanning (**b**). If an intracystic solid mass is suspected, the lesion can be partially aspirated initially followed by biopsy of the solid component and placement of a marker clip.

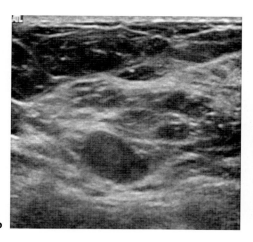

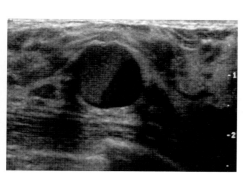

a, b

Mass in or on the Skin

These masses are usually clinically apparent and include sebaceous or epidermal inclusion cysts, keloids, moles, neurofibromas, and accessory nipples. It is important to recognize the interface between skin and parenchyma and to establish that the mass is at least partially within the thin echogenic bands of skin (**Fig. 3.42**).

Foreign Bodies

These include marker clips, coils, wires, catheter sleeves, silicone, and metal or glass related to trauma. History is usually helpful in establishing the presence and nature of foreign matter within the patient. Silicone within the parenchyma has a characteristic snowstorm appearance with echogenic noise, which propagates deep to the mass and obscures deep structures. Extravasated silicone or silicone gel bleed can travel through lymphatics and lodge in lymph nodes. An example of a foreign body is shown in **Fig. 3.43 a, b**.

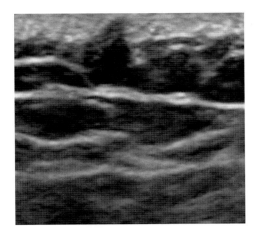

Fig. 3.42 Special cases—mass in or on skin. The largest portion of this epidermal inclusion or sebaceous cyst lies within the skin layer and has a tract leading to a pore on the skin. For confident diagnosis, it is important to demonstrate the relationship of the mass to the skin, showing the tract, best accomplished using a thin offset pad or thick layer of coupling gel.

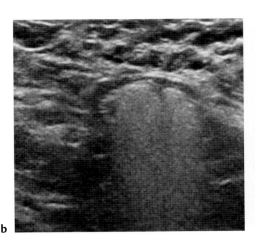

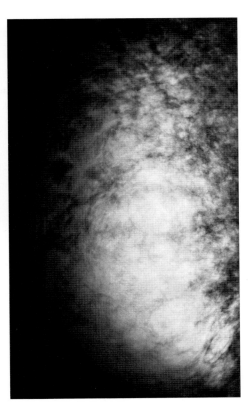

a, b

Fig. 3.43 a, b Special cases—foreign body. Sonogram shows characteristic silicone signature, the snowstorm pattern or echogenic noise, which obscures the lymph node (**a**). Only the very ends of the cortex are seen. This male patient undergoing gender change had injections of free silicone into his breasts for augmentation (**b**, mediolateral oblique mammogram). The lymphatics have taken up the silicone, which has collected in the lymph node.

Lymph Nodes—Intramammary

Lymph nodes are common findings in the breast, including the axillary tail. These circumscribed oval masses resemble miniature kidneys. When found in the breast, the usual location is the posterior upper two thirds, although medially located intramammary nodes are reported. The usual size of normal intramammary lymph nodes ranges from 3–4 mm up to approximately 1 cm.

When present within the breast or axilla, lymph nodes have a distinctive appearance with a hypoechoic cortex and echogenic fatty hilum. When the cortex is focally or diffusely thickened, or microcalcifications are present within the node, metastatic disease is a consideration along with infectious and inflammatory processes, lymphoma or leukemia, granulomatous disease, and connective tissue disorders such as rheumatoid arthritis and sarcoidosis (**Fig. 3.44**).

Lymph Nodes—Axillary

Axillary lymph nodes are often visible on mammograms. Normal nodes are smaller than 2 cm and contain hyperechoic fatty hilar areas. Larger nodes may be normal when a very thin cortical rim is seen around the hilar fat. Enlarged round lymph nodes or those with small or no fatty hilar area are abnormal, although there is no specific feature or finding to distinguish a nodal metastasis from a benign reactive node. Presence of fat in the nodal hilum does not exclude metastatic involvement; replacement of the node by tumor may be a gradual process best detected by interval change. In a patient with breast cancer, a cortical bulge or cortical area of increased echogenicity may suggest tumor involvement.

A normal lymph node can be up to 2 cm in longest dimension. Larger lymph nodes, 3 cm or longer, with very thin cortical rims and most of the node consisting of fat, are also normal. Large rounded nodes with a paucity of hilar fat or none at all, should be evaluated further and correlated clinically (**Fig. 3.45 a,b**).

Vascularity

Vascularity can be regarded as one more feature to apply in analyzing a mass. Comparison with a contralateral normal area or unaffected site in the same breast provides an important basis for comparison. No pattern is specific for any particular diagnosis. Vascularity is either present or not present.

▸ Vascularity immediately adjacent to the lesion.
▸ Diffusely increased vascularity in the tissue surrounding the lesion (**Fig. 3.46 a, b**).
▸ No vascularity. If a mass is avascular and other features are consistent with the diagnosis, a cyst is the most likely explanation. Some solid masses have little or no vascularity, possibly related to technical factors such as sensitive settings for color Doppler. Vigorous compression may occlude small vessels, and when scanning with color or power Doppler, little or no pressure should be applied.

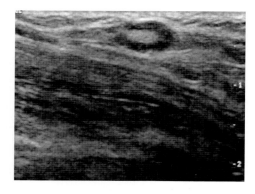

Fig. 3.44 Special cases—lymph nodes. Normal intramammary lymph node resembling a miniature kidney located in the upper outer quadrant demonstrates central hyperechogenicity and a thin hypoechoic cortical rim which should be less than 2–3 mm in thickness. As in a kidney, the nodal hilar fat is echogenic with the hypoechoic cortex similar in echogenicity to the subcutaneous fat lobules. These characteristics are also seen in axillary lymph nodes, which may be larger, up to 1.5 cm or even ≥3 cm if the cortex is very thin with most of the node replaced by fat. With permission from ACR BI-RADS, 4th ed., 2003.

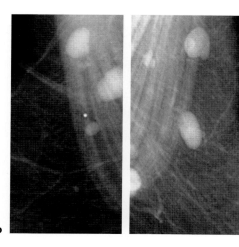

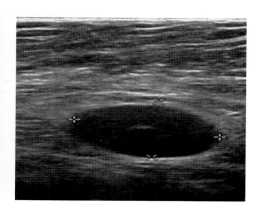

Fig. 3.45 a, b Sarcoidosis.
a Rounded, dense lymph nodes are present in both axillae.
b Decreased hilar fat and thickened cortex characterize this lymph node of normal size.

a, b

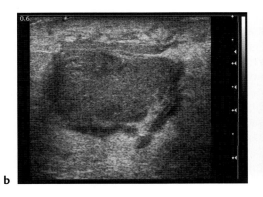
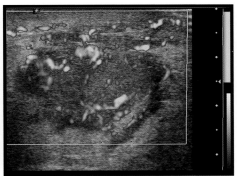

a, b

Fig. 3.46 a, b Vascularity. a Inflammatory carcinoma. Invasive ductal carcinoma, an irregular mass with angular and microlobulated margins. The increased echogenicity and network of intersecting, hypoechoic lymphatics or interstitial fluid are ultrasound findings suggesting inflammatory carcinoma. Power Doppler image (b) shows tangle of numerous vessels. With permission from ACR BI-RADS, 4th ed., 2003.

Assessment Categories in the BI-RADS–US System

Lesion analysis using BI-RADS should enable a diagnosis to be suggested and a management recommendation to be made. If ultrasound is performed along with mammography, the final assessment can combine findings of the two modalities giving an assessment based on the highest level of suspicion for malignancy. The final assessment phrases taken from the BI-RADS and required by the Mammography Quality Standards Act are (1) Negative; (2) Benign finding; (3) Probably benign; (4) Suspicious for malignancy; (5) Highly suggestive of malignancy. The management recommendations that ordinarily accompany these phrases are for categories (1) and (2) routine or annual follow-up for age; for the probably benign category (3), short-interval follow-up (current convention is for 6 months); and for suspicious for malignancy, category (4), tissue sampling; and for highly suggestive of malignancy (5), "appropriate action," ordinarily biopsy. Becoming standard in the United States, albeit slowly for some geographic areas and sites, is percutaneous, imaging-guided large-needle biopsy rather than open surgical biopsy for diagnosis.

BI-RADS–US is a living document, open to change and periodic revision. For example, elastography is of current interest. Until recently, it has not been made widely available for clinical use, and its diagnostic usefulness in ultrasound or MRI is an area of research. As additional studies are completed and reported, elastography may be established as another feature category.

Quality Assurance

Quality assurance programs have become an integral part of mammographic studies, and have contributed to the maintenance of high standards for diagnostic and screening mammograms.

In the United States, the American College of Radiology's Mammography Accreditation Program, a voluntary program, was begun in the late 1980 s and the ACR is accepted by the Food and Drug Administration (FDA) as an accrediting body. Most states still use this program, but some states have developed their own accreditation programs, and facilities are inspected annually by FDA agents. The need for similar programs for breast ultrasound is recognized but has been slow in acceptance. When the Mammography Quality Standards Act of 1992 is renewed, it may or may not

include breast ultrasound and MRI. In recent years, both the ACR and the American Institute of Ultrasound in Medicine (AIUM) have developed accreditation programs to improve the practice of breast ultrasound, and there is increasing participation in these voluntary programs which ensures that facilities meet and comply with minimum standards.

American College of Radiology Accreditation

The ACR has a practice guideline for performing breast ultrasound, and the organization has developed a voluntary accreditation program for ultrasound imaging and ultrasound-guided breast biopsy procedures which offers physicians the opportunity for peer review and evaluation of their qualifications, equipment, quality control and quality assurance programs, and image quality. Included is a component which details the requirements for the maintenance of competence in the performance of the breast ultrasound interventional procedures through continuing clinical activity and continuing medical education. For detailed information on the ACR breast ultrasound accreditation programs, contact the ACR office at 1891 Preston White Drive, Reston, Virginia, USA (*www.acr.org*).

American Institute of Ultrasound in Medicine Accreditation

The AIUM has collaborated with the ACR and has introduced a joint voluntary breast accreditation program to ensure that specific standards are met by medical staff and personnel who perform and interpret breast ultrasound examinations. The aim of the program is to ensure that practices conform to nationally accepted standards with regard to personnel education, training, and experience; physical facilities; document storage and record keeping; policies and procedures safeguarding patients; ultrasound personnel and equipment instrumentation and quality assurance; and case study and supporting document requirements. Training guidelines are set out for physicians, and these cover diagnostic ultrasound, interventional breast ultrasound, and continuing medical education requirements. For detailed information on the AIUM breast accreditation practice program, contact the AIUM office at 14750 Sweitzer Lane, Suite 100, Laurel, Maryland, USA (*www.aium.org*).

European Group for Breast Cancer Screening

Although ultrasound has been shown to be an important adjunct to mammography in the clinical assessment of both palpable and nonpalpable breast abnormalities, there is little scientific evidence which endorses the use of this imaging modality for the examination of asymptomatic women. The European Group for Breast Cancer Screening has therefore not included ultrasound for primary screening of asymptomatic women.

Nevertheless, several recent studies have demonstrated a relatively high detection rate of malignant breast lesions unsuspected in women who have been screened by mammography and clinical examination. Ultrasound screening of high-risk women with mammographically dense fibroglandular tissue has detected 3–6 additional cancers per 1000 women screened. Data are awaited from the ACRIN (American College of Radiology Imaging Network/NCI) multicenter study using ultrasound screening in addition to mammography. Patient participants are offered MRI as well at the time of the last follow-up mammography and ultrasound examinations. Results of the initial prevalence screen are not yet reported. The study should shed some light on the relative sensitivities of clinical examination, mammography, ultrasound and MRI. This study may support more extensive use of ultrasound adjunctively with mammography in breast cancer screening for women with dense breasts as a cost-effective alternative to contrast-enhanced breast MRI.

International Breast Ultrasound School

The International Breast Ultrasound School (IBUS) has published guidelines which form the basis of recommendations devised to improve the quality of breast ultrasound examinations. These guidelines cover equipment requirements, examination technique, interpretation, and accuracy and confidence. They are reproduced in the Appendix with permission of the International Breast Ultrasound School.

IBUS was formed in December 1991, and its office is located in Switzerland at the Kantonsspital Baden. It is a multidisciplinary organization with representation from the different medical disciplines dedicated to the detection, diagnosis, and management of breast disease. The aims of IBUS are: (1) to improve the standards of breast ultrasound for assessing the breast and its pathology; (2) to provide high-quality seminars and interactive workshops covering ultrasound, X-ray mammography, MRI, and other investigative techniques; (3) to evaluate the role of conventional and newer imaging techniques; and (4) to promote an international forum for the exchange of scientific and clinical breast imaging information.

In recent years, IBUS has provided teaching programs in many countries, based on formal lectures and interactive workshops at basic and advanced levels covering all aspects of breast imaging.

More detailed information on the IBUS guidelines and teaching faculty can be found in the Appendix and by visiting the website at www.ibus.org.

Summary and Conclusions

Development of a structured lexicon for breast ultrasound has been inspired by the reporting and data system for mammography, whose standardized descriptors within feature categories used in analyzing the primary findings of cancer on mammograms—masses and calcifications—helped create clear, unambiguous communications to referring physicians of the likelihood of malignancy and recommendations for patient management based on the imaging assessments. The feature categories and lexicon of descriptors within them also enable analyses of practice patterns and outcome measurements to be made, directing attention to areas needing improvement as well as providing a method to advance the art and science of lesion characterization with ultrasound.

4 Sonographic Anatomy of the Breast and Axilla

Gross Anatomy

Breast

Anatomically the breast is a modified sweat gland lying within the deep and superficial layers of superficial pectoral fascia. Viewing a schematic sagittal section of the breast turned 90° to correlate with ultrasonographic positioning, we observe the following anatomic structures (from anterior to posterior), which can also be visualized with ultrasound (**Tables 4.1, 4.2**): skin, subcutaneous fat, Cooper ligaments, the superficial mammary fascia, the breast parenchyma (with ducts and lobules), interlobar fibrofatty tissue, the deep mammary fascia, retromammary fat, muscle fascia, the pectoralis major and minor muscles, the ribs and intercostal spaces, and finally the pleura and lung (**Fig. 4.1**).

The breast consists of a varying mixture of tissue components, and its composition depends on age, hormonal influences, structural changes (congenital, degenerative, or pathologic), and individual characteristics (**Tables 4.3, 4.4**). As a general rule, the breast tissue of young women consists mostly of parenchyma and contains little fat. With aging, the glandular tissue of the breast is replaced by connective tissue and fat. But there is great individual variation, so that the breasts of young multiparous women who have nursed their infants are predominantly fatty, and even in young girls a substantial portion may consist of fat, especially if the breasts are large.

Conversely, the breasts of older women who receive postmenopausal hormone replacement may respond by increasing fibro-glandular density, and many older women may have mammographically dense breasts, the density reflecting the fibrous (rather than glandular) predominance of their breast tissue. This should be considered in breast examinations as it will influence the overall interpretation of clinical, sonographic, and mammographic findings.

> The structural composition of the breast varies with age, functional status, and individual differences in tissue distribution and quantitative make-up.

Table 4.1 Gross anatomy of the female breast (sequence of tissue layers from anterior to posterior)

- Skin
- Subcutaneous fat
- Cooper ligaments
- Superficial mammary fascia
- Breast parenchyma with
  - Lobules
  - Lactiferous ducts
  - Interlobar connective tissue
  - Fat
- Deep mammary fascia
- Retromammary fat
- Muscle fascia
- Pectoralis major muscle
- Pectoralis minor muscle
- Ribs and intercostal muscles
- Pleura

Table 4.2 Echogenicity of the various breast tissues

Anatomic structure	Echogenicity
Skin	Hyperechoic
Nipple	Hypoechoic
Parenchyma	Hyperechoic
Connective tissue	Hyperechoic
Subcutaneous fat	Hypoechoic
Fatty infiltration	Hypoechoic
Retromammary fat	Hypoechoic
Cooper ligaments	Hyperechoic
Lactiferous ducts	Anechoic*

* Intraductal secretions appear as echo-free fluid, but proliferative changes and inspissated secretions may produce low-level internal echoes.

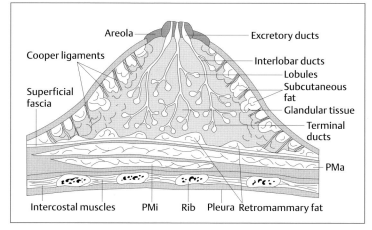

Fig. 4.1 Gross anatomy of the breast. PMa = pectoralis major muscle, PMi = pectoralis minor muscle.

Table 4.3 Principal components of the female breast

▸ Fat
▸ Parenchyma
   – Alveoli
   – Lactiferous ducts
   – Intralobar connective tissue (hormonally responsive)
▸ Interlobar connective tissue

Table 4.4 Parenchymal patterns in breast ultrasound

▸ Homogeneous hyperechoic pattern
   – Young women
   – Good readability
▸ Heterogeneous hyperechoic pattern
   – Scant fatty infiltration
   – Middle-aged women
   – Good or moderate readability
▸ Partially involuted or involuted pattern
   – Predominantly hypoechoic with connective-tissue septa
   – Older women
   – Moderate readability
▸ Fibrotic pattern (heterogeneously hypoechoic)
   – Young and middle-aged women
   – Poor readability

Parasternal Region

The internal thoracic artery descends on either side of the sternum (**Fig. 4.2**), identifiable in the intercostal spaces on sagittal and transverse ultrasound scans, providing a landmark for evaluating the parasternal chain of lymph nodes. This is important with inner-quadrant breast tumors, as they may metastasize to these nodes. As the nodes are deep to the muscle fascia, they cannot be evaluated clinically and usually are not removed at surgery, setting the stage for progression or an apparent early parasternal recurrence. If the nodes are detected sonographically, they can be selectively removed at operation. The sagittal ultrasound examination of the breasts described above will generally cover the

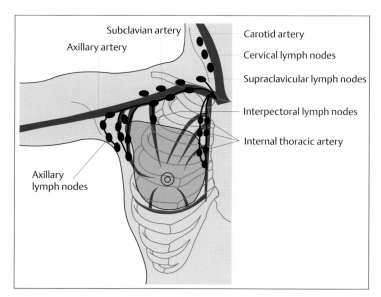

Fig. 4.2 Lymphatic drainage and blood vessels of the breast and axilla.

parasternal regions if scanning is done from axilla to sternum (see **Fig. 2.21**). If contrast-enhanced breast MRI is done preoperatively or before neoadjuvant chemotherapy, axial sections should be scrutinized for enlarged lymph nodes in the internal mammary chains.

Axilla

The anatomic boundaries of the axilla are visible externally with the arm raised. The axilla is defined superiorly by the lower border of the pectoralis major, which passes laterally to the humerus from the chest wall and tapers toward its site of insertion. Below it is the pectoralis minor. With the arm raised to the horizontal, the axillary artery runs below and parallel to the pectoralis minor, and inferior to that vessel is the larger-caliber axillary vein. The thoracodorsal neurovascular bundle descends in a parasagittal plane at right angles to the axillary vessels. Most lymph nodes in this region are embedded in the axillary lymphatic tissue and fat (**Fig. 4.2**). The thickness of this area and its proportion of axillary fat can vary markedly. The thicker the tissue, the more difficult it is to palpate axillary lymph nodes and the poorer the ultrasound visualization of deeper structures, limiting our ability to evaluate the axillary region fully. Positional changes such as moving from supine-oblique to a standing or sitting position, arm elevated, may help to alter tissue relationships enough for sonographic observation of deeper axillary lymph nodes, but sometimes mammography may be more successful at depicting these lymph nodes.

Sonographic Morphology

Breast

Breast structures display various echo characteristics (**Table 4.2**). The sonographic anatomy of the breast is illustrated with immersion scans (**Figs. 4.3–4.5**), which are excellent for depicting general anatomic features. As noted in Chapter 2, compression of the breast can significantly alter its sonographic appearance (**Fig. 4.5**). In describing the degree of echogenicity, the reference tissue for breast ultrasound is fat, characterized by low-amplitude echoes. Fat is *hypoechoic* and on ultrasound images is dark gray. Skin and connective tissue fibers such as Cooper ligaments give rise to high-amplitude echoes. When the scanner is properly adjusted, these *echogenic* or *hyperechoic* structures should appear bright on the monitor. Fluid within cysts or ducts is generally anechoic and appears black, although inspissated fluid contains internal echoes. Breast parenchyma is moderately echoic (compared with fat) and is displayed in varying shades of light gray.

Breast anatomy can also be evaluated in real-time images despite a small field of view (**Table 4.4**). An extended sectional view can be obtained by splicing several longitudinal scans that progress from the upper to the lower portion of the breast (**Figs. 4.6, 4.7**). Similarly, the scope can be broadened in systems that offer wide or panoramic fields of view. Individual images may be sufficient for evaluating glandular structure, depending on the width of the visual field and the experience of the examiner (**Figs. 4.8, 4.9**).

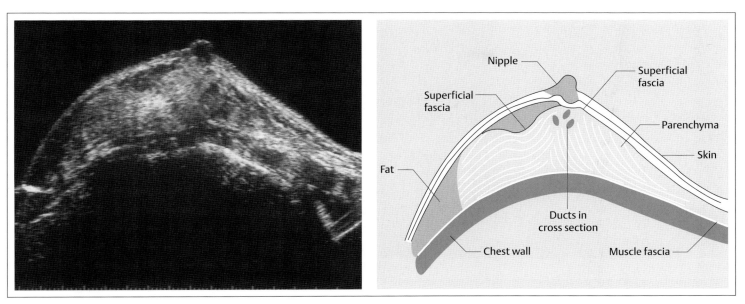

Fig. 4.3 Immersion scan of a dense adolescent breast. Transverse scan through the center of the breast. The breast is composed of parenchyma of varying echogenicity and small amounts of subcutaneous fat. Mammary ducts are visible in cross section in the subareolar region.

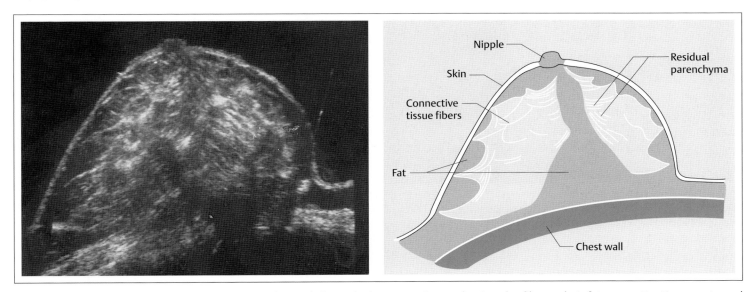

Fig. 4.4 Immersion scan of an involuted breast. Midsagittal plane. The breast consists predominantly of hypoechoic fat, connective tissue septa, and small hyperechoic islands of residual parenchyma.

Relatively low echo amplitudes are characteristic of normal and adolescent breast tissue (**Fig. 4.10**). The low echogenicity is partly due to hormonal influences producing a spongy, hydrated structural pattern. A similar pattern is observed in menopausal women on hormone replacement therapy and in edematous parenchyma in the early stage of inflammatory disease (Chapter 9). As the breast ages and fibrocystic changes become more pronounced, the parenchyma becomes more echogenic due to an increased proportion of connective tissue, and the breast appears brighter (**Fig. 4.11**, see also Chapters 6 and 7). Meanwhile, deeper portions of the breast often appear hypoechoic because of increased sound absorption. Compression of the breast improves sound transmission, increasing echogenicity and delineation of deeper tissues.

The ducts should be visible in the subareolar region, at least with a high-resolution transducer operating above 7.5 MHz. Converging behind the nipple, ducts appear as tubular, anechoic structures,

linear, branching, round and oval, depending on the angle of insonation. In more peripheral areas of the breast, their segmental distribution pattern is best defined on radial scans (Chapters 2 and 6).

The parenchymal zone of the breast is bounded posteriorly by the fascia of the pectoralis major muscle. This fascia appears as an echogenic line bordering the chest wall (**Figs. 4.3, 4.5**). Muscle fibers are visible between the anterior and posterior fascial planes. The underlying ribs appear on sagittal scans as rounded, hypoechoic structures that appear partially anechoic at their cartilaginous sternal attachments. Because they are ossified, the more distal rib segments resemble circumscribed, hypoechoic masses that cast acoustic shadows (**Fig. 4.12 a, b**). It is important to maintain proper orientation so that these normal anatomic structures, when seen alone in an image, are not mistaken for intramammary tumors. It is helpful to recognize the surrounding anatomy: ribs

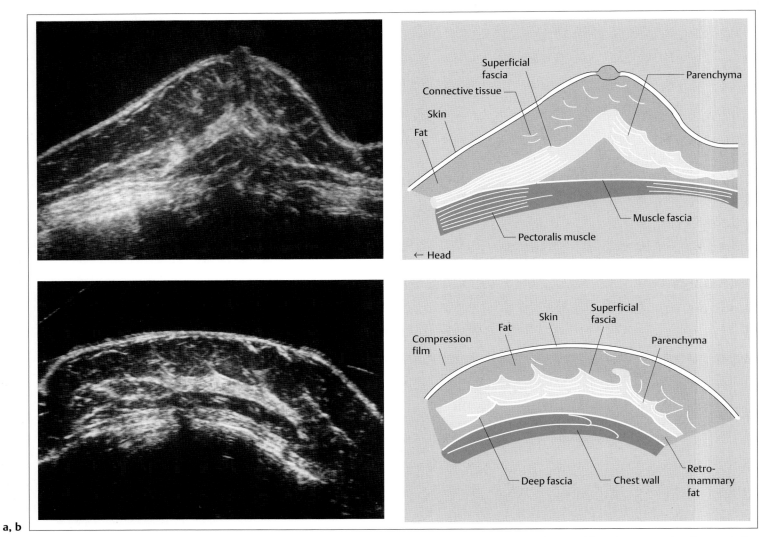

Fig. 4.5 a, b   Immersion scan of a partially involuted breast. **a** Midsagittal plane, without compression (top) and **b** with compression (bottom). The images show thick layers of subcutaneous and retromammary fat with echogenic glandular tissue between them.

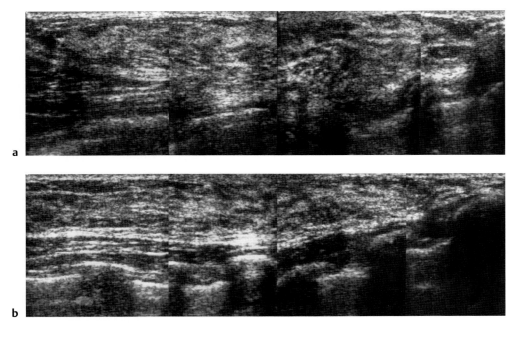

Fig. 4.6 a, b   Real-time scans in a dense adolescent breast.
a Right breast.
b Left breast. Multiple midsagittal scans along the craniocaudal axis are spliced to give an extended view of breast anatomy. The nipple–areola complex is at the center.

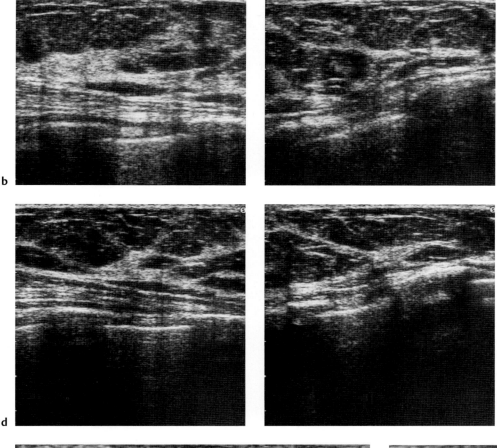

Fig. 4.7 a–d Real-time midsagittal scans in an involuted breast.
a Right breast, cranial extension.
b Right breast, caudal extension.
c Left breast, cranial extension.
d Left breast, caudal extension. The cranial breast extension is shown at the left, the nipple and areola at the center, and the caudal extension at right.

a, b

c, d

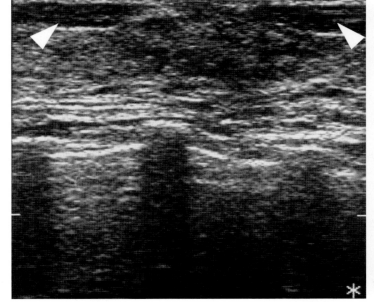

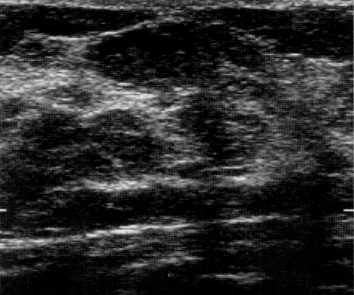

Fig. 4.8 Real-time scan at the center of a dense breast, showing scant subcutaneous fat (arrowheads).

Fig. 4.9 Sagittal scan at the center of a partially involuted breast shows hypoechoic fat permeated by connective-tissue septa and small, scattered islands of parenchyma.

posterior to muscle, not a site for primary breast carcinomas (or fibroadenomas) to occur. In addition, real-time scanning enables one to document the repetitive pattern of ribs.

> Breast diagnosis with ultrasound requires a knowledge of normal sonographic anatomy and its variations, recognition of architectural distortion, and the ability to distinguish circumscribed anatomic features from focal abnormalities.

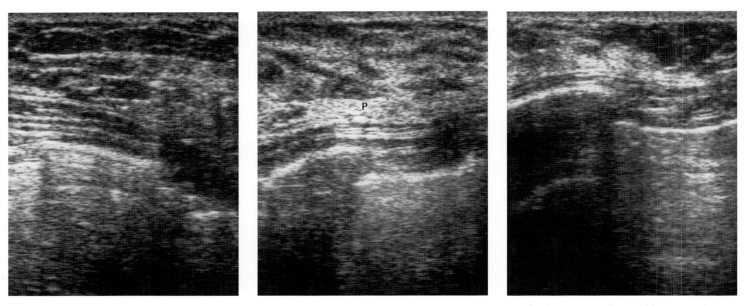

Fig. 4.10 Midsagittal scans of a dense adolescent breast. The cranial and caudal scans show areas of subcutaneous fat, and between them is parenchymal tissue (P).

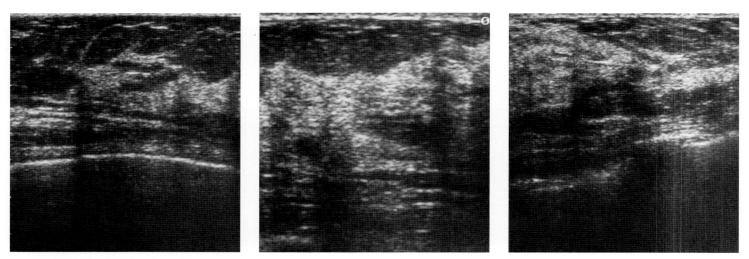

Fig. 4.11 Midsagittal scans of a partially involuted breast with fibrotic changes. The glandular breast tissue is coarser and more echogenic than in **Fig. 4.10** above. The abundant connective tissue increases sound absorption, causing deeper portions of the breast to appear hypoechoic and shadow. Compression increases sound transmission and tissue echogenicity, helping to separate artifact from abnormality.

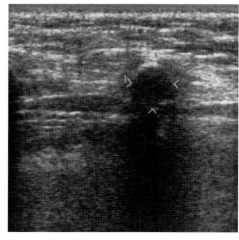 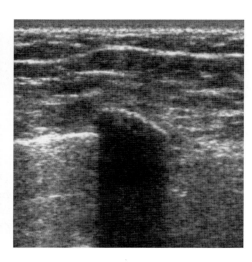

Fig. 4.12 a, b Sagittal scans in the medial portion of the breast show a rib in cross section.
a Parasternal scan shows the nearly anechoic cartilaginous portion of the rib.
b More lateral scan shows the ossified portion of the rib. Only the anterior surface appears bright. Just below it is the acoustic shadow cast by the dense bone.

a, b

Parasternal Region

The parasternal lymph nodes distributed along the internal thoracic artery are small and usually are not visualized with ultrasound, but the artery can be seen deep to the fascia and ribs just anterior to the pleura (**Fig. 4.13**). Metastatic lymph nodes appear as hypoechoic masses of varying size that resemble a rib imaged in cross section (**Fig. 4.14**). By moving the transducer and comparing sagittal and transverse parasternal scans, the examiner can definitively distinguish ribs from lymph node metastases (**Table 4.5**).

Axilla

A transducer placed obliquely along the lower rim of the pectoralis major muscle can be moved in the caudad direction to evaluate the principal lymphatic drainage of the axilla (level I nodes, **Figs. 4.15–4.20**). The thoracodorsal neurovascular bundle is imaged in cross section; usually only the larger-caliber vein can be seen within the hypoechoic axillary fat. A more complete survey is obtained by positioning the transducer over this vessel in a sagittal orientation. Most lymph nodes in the axilla are isoechoic to axillary fat and contain an echogenic hilum. Palpable axillary lymph nodes are frequently normal or a result of nonspecific reactive enlargement; they are easily correlated with sonographic findings. Although the cortex of a reactive lymph node may be uniformly thickened beyond the 3 mm normal, metastatic nodes may manifest echogenic or hypoechoic focal cortical bulges (**Fig. 4.21 a, b**). Sequential studies may show decrease in or disappearance of the

Table 4.5 Echogenicity of parasternal structures

Anatomic structure	Echogenicity
Ribs	Hypoechoic
Intercostal muscles	Hypoechoic
Internal thoracic vessels	Anechoic
Pleura	Hyperechoic
Lung	Diffuse shadow
Lymph node metastases	Hypoechoic

echogenic hili of these nodes. Presence of hilar fat is not dependable as a sign that the lymph node has no metastatic involvement. Localizing these nodes in relation to the axillary vessels is important in the surveillance of axillary lymphadenopathy.

Higher-level lymph nodes are also easy to locate with ultrasound (**Fig. 4.22 a, b**). If the transducer is moved medially and horizontally from the pectoralis major muscle, the narrower pectoralis minor muscle can be seen directly below it. The transducer can then be angled cephalad to demonstrate the axillary vein. The level II nodes that drain the axilla can be traced farther medially between the pectoralis minor muscle and axillary vein. The muscle tapers appreciably in its course toward the midclavicular line. Medial to the pectoralis minor is the level III region. Because of significantly increased risk of lymphedema, this region usually is not included in surgical resections unless there is clinical or sonographic evidence of lymphadenopathy at that level (**Table 4.6**).

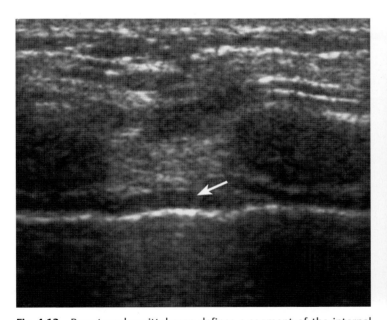

Fig. 4.13 Parasternal sagittal scan defines a segment of the internal thoracic artery between the ribs and pleura.

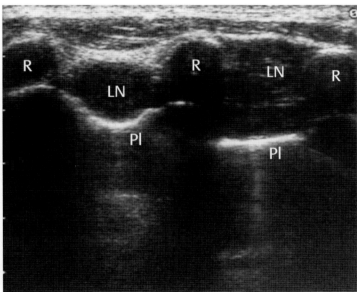

Fig. 4.14 Parasternal sagittal scan of lymph node metastases in the region of the internal thoracic artery. Three ribs are visible in cross section, and between each adjacent rib pair is one metastatic lymph node in the intercostal space. Both lymph nodes form impressions in the underlying pleura. R = Rib; LN = Lymph node; Pl = Pleura.

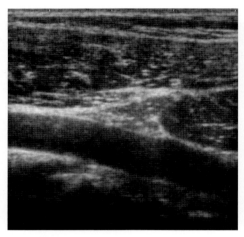

Fig. 4.**15**

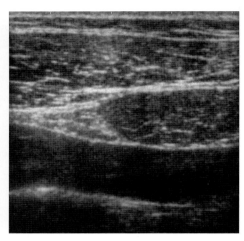

Fig. 4.**16**

Fig. 4.15 Transverse scan of the right axilla at the level of the axillary artery.

Fig. 4.16 Transverse scan of the right axilla at the level of the axillary vein.

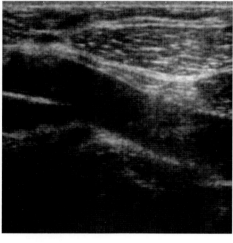

Fig. 4.**17**

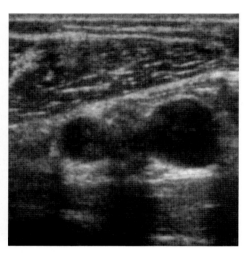

Fig. 4.**18**

Fig. 4.17 Transverse scan of the lateral axilla *(right)* at the level where the axillary vein receives the brachial veins.

Fig. 4.18 Sagittal scan through the axilla. The axillary artery and vein are imaged in cross section.

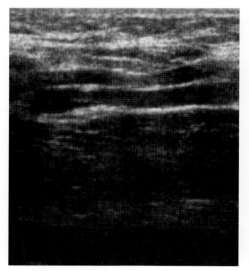

Fig. 4.**19**

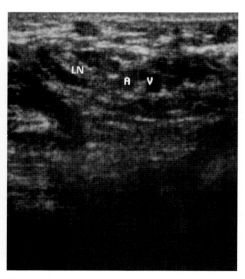

Fig. 4.**20**

Fig. 4.19 Sagittal scan below the axillary vein. The thoracodorsal artery and vein are imaged in longitudinal section.

Fig. 4.20 Transverse scan of the right axilla in the region of the thoracodorsal artery and vein. The scan demonstrates both vessels (A, V), and lateral to them is a reactive lymph node (LN).

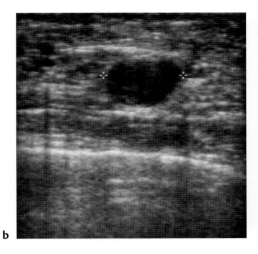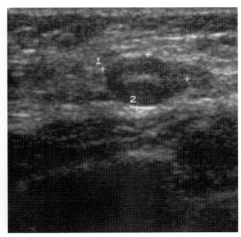

Fig. 4.21 a, b Typical lymph node findings in the axilla.
a Hypoechoic metastatic lymph node. The fatty hilum is not seen.
b Reactive lymph node with minimal concentric cortical thickening is not suspicious for malignancy.

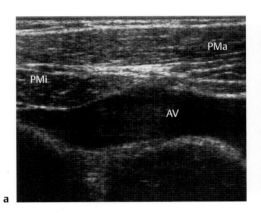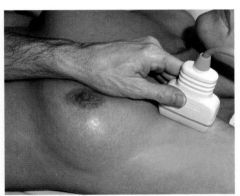

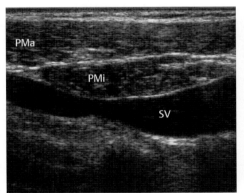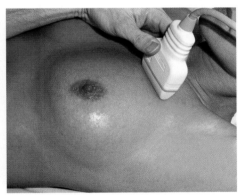

Fig. 4.22 a, b Lymph nodal drainage pathways (levels I–III) in the left axilla, transverse scan.
a Axillary vein (AV) in longitudinal section. Above the vein is the lateral extension of the pectoralis minor muscle (PMi) and the pectoralis major muscle (PMa). The region lateral to PMi is defined as level I (three surgically defined levels of axillary anatomy). Between axillary vein and PMi is level II.
b The transducer is moved farther proximally along the subclavian vein (SV). Above the vein are the pectoralis major muscle and the medial extension of the pectoralis minor (PMi) providing visualization of levels II and III.

Table 4.6 Echogenicity of axillary structures

Anatomic structure	Echogenicity
Pectoralis major muscle	Hypoechoic
Pectoralis minor muscle	Hypoechoic
Axillary artery and vein	Anechoic
Thoracodorsal artery and vein	Anechoic
Fat	Hypoechoic
Connective tissue	Hyperechoic
Humeral head	Bright entry echo with acoustic shadow

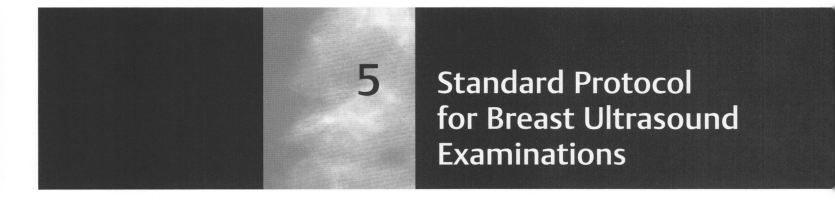

5 Standard Protocol for Breast Ultrasound Examinations

Patient History

A thorough history should be taken prior to clinical examination, sonography, or any other imaging studies. Many practices ask patients to complete a questionnaire as a means of obtaining pertinent personal, clinical, and family history. The first question to be answered is the reason for the visit: mass, focal pain, thickening, nipple discharge. The history should include allergies, medical and surgical history, history of breast or other carcinomas, medications (hormone replacement or oral contraceptive use, risk reducers or breast cancer treatment such as tamoxifen or chemotherapy), and reproductive history. The majority of women who undergo mammography regularly are asymptomatic and complying with screening recommendations, but ultrasound examinations are most often done for problem-solving. Ultrasound screening remains a research focus in the United States, although there is recognition from individual studies that survey ultrasound can increase the yield of carcinomas above and beyond those identifiable clinically or by mammography.

It is of great importance at the outset to determine a patient's risk of breast cancer. Factors associated with the highest risk include personal history of breast cancer, prior radiation therapy to the mediastinum for lymphoma or to the thorax for tuberculosis, genetic aberrations (BRCA1 and 2 genes), family history of breast carcinoma in a premenopausal first-degree relative (mother, sister, or daughter), and histological findings of lobular carcinoma in situ, atypical lobular hyperplasia, or atypical ductal hyperplasia on previous biopsies. Other factors that increase breast cancer risk, although of lower relative risk than the preceding, include personal history of ovarian or endometrial carcinoma (and prostatic carcinoma in male relatives), nulliparity or first pregnancy after the age of 30 years, and family history of breast cancer in a first-degree relative, not premenopausal.

Prior surgical history can be helpful in correlating sonographic with mammographic or clinical findings. Expected sonographic changes following lumpectomy for carcinoma followed by radiation therapy are discussed in Chapter 11. Reduction mammoplasty is a common procedure that may result in areas of scarring or fat necrosis, and sonographic findings associated with intra- or extracapsular ruptures of breast implants placed for reconstruction or augmentation are known.

The patient should also be questioned about previous surgery on other organs, given the potential for metastases to the breast and lymph nodes from tumors at other locations. Previous gynecologic disorders are also important, as they may direct attention to hormonal changes that affect the breast (**Table 5.1**).

Table 5.1 Information included in the clinical history

▸ Menarche, menopause
▸ Menstrual history
▸ Obstetric history
▸ Medications, including hormones
▸ Family risk factors
▸ Prior operations and histology
▸ Prior gynecologic disorders
▸ Reason for seeking medical attention

Table 5.2 Description of findings on inspection

Findings	Localization
Breast size	Symmetry
Skin redness, edema	Right, left, bilateral
Skin dimpling or protrusion	Diffuse, circumscribed
Skin thickening	Quadrant, clock-face position
Nipple: Paget, eczema, retraction	Central, peripheral Distance from the nipple (in cm)

Table 5.3 Description of palpable findings

Findings	Localization
No palpable abnormalities	Symmetry
Mild nodularity	Right, left, bilateral
Moderate nodularity	Diffuse, circumscribed
Coarse nodularity	Quadrant, clock-face position
Indurations	Central, peripheral
Masses: soft, firm, rubbery, smooth, lobulated, irregular, mobile, fixed	Distance from the nipple (cm)

Clinical Examination

The findings from physical inspection and palpation should also be documented (**Tables 5.2, 5.3**). Spontaneous pain and diffuse or focal tenderness should be noted. It should be determined whether the pain is constant, sporadic, or cyclic in its occurrence, and its severity should be noted. It is important to know when visible or palpable changes first appeared and how they have

Table 5.4 Interpretation of mammographic findings

Breast parenchyma	ACR density I (parenchyma <25%, involution), II (25–50%), III (50–75%), IV (parenchyma >75%, dense breast tissue)
Focal densities	Round, oval, smooth, sharp, ill-defined, spiculated
Macrocalcifications and micro-calcifications	Disseminated, focal clusters, clumped, rounded, pleomorphic
Benign–malignant differentiation	BI-RADS categories I–V

Table 5.5 Interpretation of ultrasound findings

Architecture	Homogeneous/heterogeneous
Background echotexture	Fat Fibroglandular Mixed pattern
Proportion of fat	According to ACR mammography classification (I–IV)
Ducts	Diameter (mm) Smooth, irregular Anechoic, low-level internal echoes

progressed over time. Surgical scars should be diagrammed, and the date of the procedure and its histologic findings should be noted. If the breasts have not been examined prior to sonography, physical examination to correlate with the ultrasound findings is opportunely done by the sonologist at the time of sonography.

Prior Mammograms

If sonography is directed to evaluation of a mammographic finding, mammograms and reports should be available for review. Whether or not the prior mammograms were normal, the breast density should be noted according to the mammography BI-RADS categorization (fat, scattered fibroglandular density, heterogeneously dense, extremely dense; see Chapter 3), the sensitivity of mammography decreasing as the breast density increases. Federal legislation in the United States requires that breast density be reported along with the mammographic findings. The sonograms should be placed in context of mammographic findings, the relative importance of the ultrasound examination increasing concomitantly with progressive breast density on mammograms.

In addition to diffuse changes, symmetry of the breasts can be an important diagnostic criterion. Nonspecific asymmetric densities may correlate with sonographically visible abnormalities or patterns of fibroglandular parenchyma. All circumscribed focal lesions as well as diffuse and clustered microcalcifications should be characterized using BI-RADS descriptors (**Table 5.4**).

Other Studies

The results of previous ultrasound and other examinations (e.g., Doppler scans, MRI, percutaneous aspiration or needle biopsy, radionuclide scans, CT scans, and PET and other special studies) should be accounted for and correlated with findings of the current ultrasound examination.

Ultrasound Findings

It is important to appreciate the normal breast anatomic pattern in a given patient (see **Table 4.1**) since architectural distortion can provide important evidence of abnormality (**Table 5.5**). In most cases the breast architecture can be assessed (**Fig. 5.1 a–d**). Islands of fat that simulate focal lesions in the breast parenchyma can be identified by applying compression or by rotating the transducer to define the extent of the fat lobule, which frequently elongates in the orthogonal view. These steps should be documented with images so that they can be reproduced later by a different examiner.

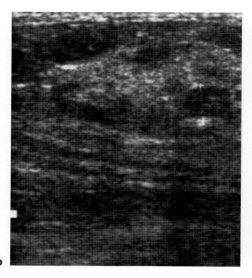
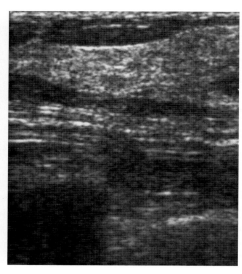

a, b

Fig. 5.1 a–d Sonograms of a normal breast with homogeneous glandular structure.
a Noncompression sagittal scan of the upper outer quadrant of the right breast shows a hypoechoic focal lesion (fatty infiltration).
b Compression causes flattening of the fatty tissue.

Fig. 5.1 c, d ▷

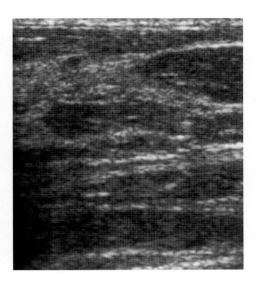

c, d

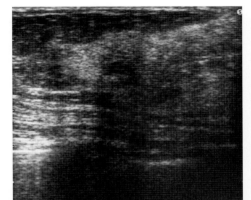

a, b

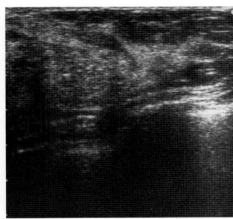

c, d

Fig. 5.1 c, d

c Fatty infiltration (calipers) in the upper outer quadrant of the right breast, noncompression sagittal scan.

d When the transducer is rotated, the transverse scan identifies the hypoechoic lesion as a tongue-shaped area of fatty infiltration.

Architecture	Homogeneous
Background echo-texture	Fibroglandular
Proportion of fibro-glandular tissue	ACR 3 (50–75%)

! Comment:

The glandular tissue in this young woman (age 33 years) is easily evaluated with ultrasound. Adjunctive techniques serve to confirm the diagnosis of fatty infiltration.

Fig. 5.2 Sound attenuation by fibrocystic breast changes.

a Sagittal scan in the upper right breast.

b Sagittal scan in the lower right breast.

c Sagittal scan in the upper outer quadrant of the right breast, without compression.

d Sagittal scan in the upper outer quadrant of the right breast, with compression.

Architecture	Heterogeneous
Background echo-texture	Fibroglandular
Proportion of fibro-glandular tissue	ACR 3 (50–75%)

! Comment:

The fibrosis increases sound attenuation, reducing the penetration depth and giving the parenchyma a heterogeneous appearance. Again, compression can be used to improve sound penetration and help differentiate fatty tissue from a hypoechoic tumor.

If an adequate evaluation cannot be made because of shadowing caused by fibrocystic changes, this should be documented as it reduces the reliability of the ultrasound findings (**Fig. 5.2 a–d**). The percentage distribution of glandular tissue and fat is important in comparing ultrasound findings with mammograms (**Fig. 5.3 a–d**). The fatty breast is transparent on mammograms, but a dense breast that contains little fat is difficult to evaluate, increasing the value of complementary sonography. As noted above, there are four categories of breast density described by the mammographic ACR BI-RADS system (**Table 5.4**). These categories can also be estimated by ultrasound.

The breast parenchyma can be classified on the basis of its echogenicity as homogeneous with a predominantly fatty or fibroglandular echotexture or heterogeneous, which is more difficult to interpret (**Figs. 5.1 a–d, 5.2 a–d**). Fibrosis attenuates the ultrasound beam and limits the penetration depth when a high-frequency transducer is used. The ducts should also be evaluated as part of the normal breast anatomy (**Figs. 5.3 a–d, 5.4 a, b**).

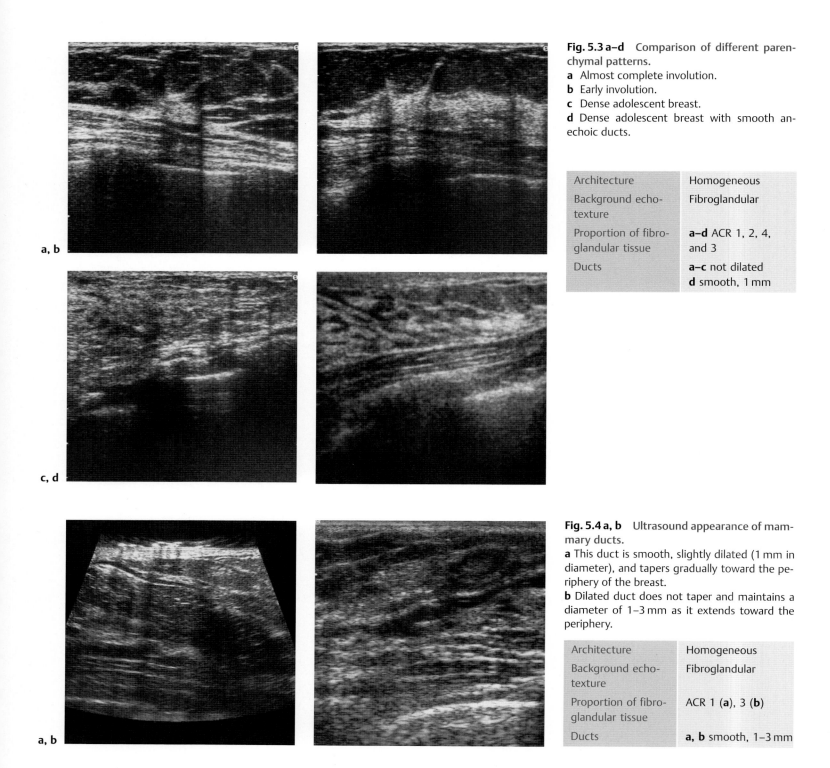

Fig. 5.3 a–d Comparison of different parenchymal patterns.
a Almost complete involution.
b Early involution.
c Dense adolescent breast.
d Dense adolescent breast with smooth anechoic ducts.

Architecture	Homogeneous
Background echo-texture	Fibroglandular
Proportion of fibroglandular tissue	**a–d** ACR 1, 2, 4, and 3
Ducts	**a–c** not dilated **d** smooth, 1 mm

Fig. 5.4 a, b Ultrasound appearance of mammary ducts.
a This duct is smooth, slightly dilated (1 mm in diameter), and tapers gradually toward the periphery of the breast.
b Dilated duct does not taper and maintains a diameter of 1–3 mm as it extends toward the periphery.

Architecture	Homogeneous
Background echo-texture	Fibroglandular
Proportion of fibroglandular tissue	ACR 1 (**a**), 3 (**b**)
Ducts	**a, b** smooth, 1–3 mm

Circumscribed breast lesions are most accurately described according to the ACR ultrasound BI-RADS classification system (**Table 5.6**): shape, orientation, margin, lesion boundary, echo pattern, posterior acoustic features, surrounding tissue, calcifications and vascularity (**Figs. 5.5–5.7**). In addition several special cases have been defined with typical ultrasonic appearance.

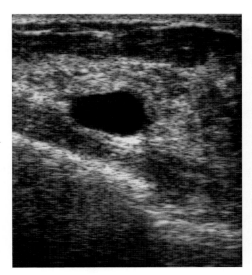

Fig. 5.5 Typical cyst.

Shape	Oval
Orientation	Parallel
Margin	Circumscribed
Echo pattern	Anechoic
Posterior acoustic features	Enhancement
Surrounding tissue	–
Calcifications	–
Vascularity	Not present

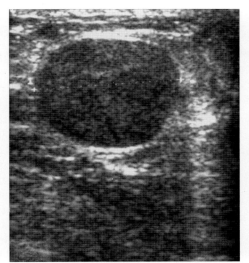

Fig. 5.6 Typical fibroadenoma.

Shape	Oval
Orientation	Parallel
Margin	Circumscribed
Echo pattern	Hypoechoic
Posterior acoustic features	Enhancement
Surrounding tissue	–
Calcifications	–
Vascularity	Not present

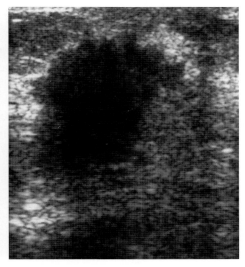

Fig. 5.7 Typical invasive carcinoma.

Shape	Irregular
Orientation	Not parallel
Margin	Not circumscribed
Echo pattern	Hypoechoic
Posterior acoustic features	Shadowing
Surrounding tissue	–
Calcifications	–
Vascularity	Not assessed

! Comment:
Simple cysts can be confidently diagnosed with ultrasound. Atypical cysts lead to problems of differential diagnosis (Chapter 7).

Table 5.6 Ultrasound evaluation of focal breast lesions

Shape	Round, oval, irregular
Orientation	Parallel, not parallel
Margin	Circumscribed, not circumscribed (indistinct, angular, microlobulated, spiculated)
Lesion boundary	Abrupt interface, echogenic halo
Echo pattern	Anechoic, hypoechoic, hyperechoic, complex, isoechoic
Posterior acoustic features	No posterior acoustic features, enhancement, shadowing, combined pattern
Surrounding tissue	Duct changes, Cooper ligament changes, edema, architectural distortion, skin thickening, skin retraction/irregularity
Calcifications	Macrocalcifications, microcalcifications out of mass, microcalcifications in mass
Vascularity	Not assessed, not present, present in lesion, present immediately adjacent to lesion, diffusely increased vascularity in surrounding tissue

Benign–Malignant Differentiation

After a lesion has been described, it should be assigned one of six assessment categories according to the degree of suspicion for a malignant tumor (**Table 5.7**). If other imaging studies have been done at the same facility, their results should be combined, and a single BI-RADS assessment provided. This assessment should re-flect the highest level of suspicion in any of the imaging studies. If more than one imaging study has been done, patient management should rely on the correlated findings and the most specific imaging depiction of a lesion. For example, with ultrasound, an area of fat necrosis may have characteristics indistinguishable from those of carcinoma, but the mammographic appearance of oil cysts with calcifications in their rims allows a benign assessment to be made.

Table 5.7 Levels of suspicion for sonographic breast lesions

0	Additional imaging needed
I	Normal breast that is confidently evaluated
II	Benign-appearing lesion (simple cysts, normal intramammary lymph nodes, breast implants, stable scars, and fibroadenomas unchanged on successive ultrasound studies)
III	Probably benign finding, short-interval follow-up suggested, including all solid masses (fibroadenomas, lipomas, fibromas, complicated cysts, and clustered microcysts). <2 % risk of malignancy
IV	Suspicious abnormality, biopsy should be considered. 3–94 % risk of malignancy
V	Highly suggestive of malignancy, appropriate action should be taken. >95 % risk of malignancy
VI	Known, biopsy- proven malignancy

Final Evaluation and Recommendation

For final evaluation, the ultrasound findings are interpreted along with the clinical and mammographic findings. In particular, ultrasound may support the need to further evaluate a palpable breast mass or indeterminate mammographic lesion or it may establish that nothing further may need to be done (**Table 5.8**). If the sonograms are to be interpreted by someone other than the sonologist who did them, i.e., someone who has not had the opportunity for real-time observation, the quality and reliability of the ultrasound scans should be assessed. Depending on the index of suspicion, the interpreting physician may recommend additional imaging studies such as MRI, short interval follow-up studies, aspiration/core biopsy, or excisional biopsy (**Tables 5.9–5.13**).

Table 5.8 Final evaluation

- ▸ Evaluation of the ultrasound findings in relation to:
  - – Palpable findings
  - – Clinical presentation
  - – Mammographic findings
  - – Reliability of ultrasound findings (on a case-by-case basis)

Table 5.11 Limitations of mammography

- ▸ Static examination technique
- ▸ Poor soft-tissue discrimination
- ▸ Superimposition of fibroglandular tissues
- ▸ Ionizing radiation
- ▸ Difficult to compress small and dense breasts

Table 5.9 Possible recommendations on completion of the ultrasound examination

- ▸ Ultrasound follow-up at … week(s), month(s), or year(s)
- ▸ Repeat mammograms at … week(s), month(s), or year(s)
- ▸ Clinical follow-up at … week(s), month(s), or year(s)
- ▸ MRI, Doppler, or other special examinations
- ▸ Percutaneous biopsy (aspiration or core biopsy)
- ▸ Excisional biopsy
- ▸ Tumor excision
  - – Directed by palpation or by sonographic/mammographic wire localization
  - – With specimen mammography or sonography
  - – With or without frozen-section control of margins

Table 5.12 Advantages of ultrasound

- ▸ Dynamic examination
  - – Compressibility
  - – Evaluating spatial extent
- ▸ Sound penetration in dense glandular tissue
  - – Contrast between parenchyma and lesions
  - – Young women
  - – Benign breast diseases
  - – Postmenopausal women on hormone replacement
- ▸ Sectional images
  - – Can detect tumors in dense glandular tissue
  - – Can exclude tumors in patients with equivocal mammograms
  - – Allow for precise measurement of tumor extent
  - – Can detect multifocal lesions
- ▸ Availability
  - – Widely available technology
  - – Mobile equipment
  - – Universal applications
  - – Cost-effective technique
- ▸ Differentiation of cystic and solid masses
- ▸ Good soft-tissue discrimination with broad gray-scale
- ▸ No radiation exposure, may be repeated as often as desired
- ▸ Accurate real-time guidance of interventional procedures
  - – Needle localization under real-time guidance
  - – Specimen ultrasonography
  - – Guidance of tissue sampling by:
    - • Fine-needle aspiration (cytology)
    - • Core biopsy (histology)
    - • Preoperative localization

Table 5.10 Advantages of mammography

- ▸ Standardized technique
- ▸ Systematic breast coverage in two planes
- ▸ Independent interpretation and examination
- ▸ Short examination time
- ▸ In fatty breasts:
  - – High diagnostic accuracy
  - – Better compression than in dense breasts
  - – Good contrast resolution
  - – Detection of microcalcifications
  - – Suitable for screening examinations

Table 5.13 Disadvantages of ultrasound

- ▸ Operator-dependent
  - – Experience, examination technique
- ▸ Equipment-dependent
  - – Quality, transducer, settings
- ▸ Reproducibility, follow-up more difficult (small window)
- ▸ Difficult to standardize
- ▸ Length of examination
- ▸ Large fatty breasts (poor contrast between lesion and fat)
- ▸ Microcalcifications
- ▸ Screening efficacy not established

Documentation

Image documentation is necessary in addition to the written report. There has been considerable discussion in the United States as to what, if anything, should be recorded when sonography is normal. Some breast imagers suggest that an image with the patient's name and a unique identifier is sufficient; others propose that one scan from the center of each breast be recorded, and others suggest hard copy consisting of one image from each quadrant as an indication of the scope of the study (this is required for the ACRIN study of ultrasound for breast cancer screening in women of high risk with dense breast tissue).

If a focal lesion is detected, it should be documented in two planes and measured in three, or at least two, dimensions. Because measurements may obscure the margins of a mass, a set of images without calipers should also be recorded. If a malignancy is found or suspected, any axillary abnormalities should be noted and their number and sizes reported. This also applies to the parasternal nodes.

 A formal written report is required. Options include computerized structured reporting, a preprinted report form, or a dictated report. Reports should be brief but complete. Component sections are clinical history and reason for the examination, findings, an assessment, and a management recommendation. Quality audits and outcome data should be derivable from the reports.

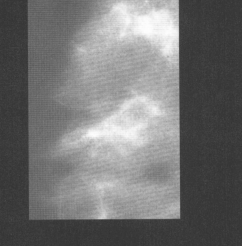

INTERMEDIATE COURSE

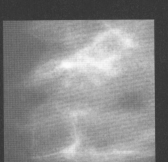

6 Fibrocystic Change   81

7 Cysts and Intracystic Tumors   99

8 Breast Implants   117

9 Abscesses   131

10 Benign Solid Tumors   141

11 Scars—The Treated Breast   157

12 Carcinoma   167

13 Lymph Nodes   191

Fibrocystic Change 6

Clinical Significance

Around the age of 35, degenerative structural changes begin to develop in the glandular tissue of the breast. Involution, with replacement of parenchyma by fat, is accompanied variably by fibrous tissue proliferation, micro- and macrocyst formation, and adenosis. Fibrocystic change is so common that, in the absence of troublesome symptoms, it should not be referred to as "fibrocystic disease" as it once was, to the consternation of women who were denied medical insurance coverage because of a "pre-existing condition." Although not always definitive, imaging plays an important role in helping to distinguish fibrocystic change from atypical or malignant lesions. Mammography and ultrasound are complementary.

The heterogeneous conglomeration of conditions known as *fibrocystic change* has several synonyms: fibrocystic disease, diffuse benign breast disease, mastopathy. It is commonly associated with a cyclic pattern of recurring and remitting pain and with diffuse or circumscribed areas of breast firmness (**Table 6.1**). Generally there is no need for treatment, and most patients with fibrocystic changes can tolerate the symptoms when given appropriate reassurance. Treatment is occasionally warranted if pain is severe. If so, the specific causes should be ascertained (**Tables 6.2, 6.3**).

Fibrosis may involve the entire breast or may be regional, with anatomic variations affecting, for example, the periductal tissues more than the interlobar tissues. As ducts narrow and become obliterated, an imbalance develops between secretion and reabsorption. Expanded by trapped secretions, some ducts may undergo cystic dilatation attributed to disturbances in menstrual regulation and to individual predisposing factors.

Areas of firmness in a dense fibrous breast or palpable circumscribed masses can be difficult to interpret on physical examination. Fibrocystic change is detected histologically in approximately 50 % of all women 40–50 years of age and in a smaller percentage of younger women. For biopsy specimens, the pathologist is charged with assigning not only a diagnosis of fibrocystic change but also with indicating the level of increased risk of breast cancer, if any. Frequently the fibrocystic change is a histologic mixture that might contain simple degenerative or fibrotic changes, epithelial proliferations in the ducts or lobules that can be graded as mild, florid, or atypical, the last a high risk marker most often managed with excision. These proliferative processes correspond respectively to benign breast disease grades I–III in the Prechtel classification (**Table 6.4**). The distinctions are important for the clinician as well, since grade I is not associated with an increased risk of breast cancer. In women with grade II change, the relative risk of

breast cancer is 2.5 times higher than in women of the same age without this risk factor. Grade III is associated with a 3–5-fold increase in the cancer risk. High relative risk is a significant factor that should be taken into account in managing the patient.

Table 6.1 Clinical symptoms of fibrocystic change

Manifestations	Features
Tension	Unilateral or bilateral
Feeling of heaviness	Circumscribed or diffuse
Pain	Cyclic or noncyclic
Firmness	Usually increases in the premenstrual period
Nodularity	Cyclic or persistent

Table 6.2 Causes of fibrocystic change

- ▸ Estrogen stimulation
  - – Increase in total levels
  - – Increase in free estrogens
- ▸ Progesterone deficiency
  - – Luteal insufficiency
  - – Anovulatory cycles
- ▸ Prolactin stimulation
  - – Pituitary
  - – Pharmacologic
- ▸ Thyroid hormone and iodine deficiency
  - – TSH ↑→ TRH ↑→ prolactin ↑
  - – Secondary luteal insufficiency

Table 6.3 Treatment options for fibrocystic change

Mild therapies	Hormonal therapies
▸ Withdrawal of methylxan- thines (coffee, tea)	▸ Estrogen reduction
▸ Low-fat diet	▸ Progestin (cyclic)
▸ Evening primrose oil	▸ Danazol
▸ Phytoestrogens	▸ Dopamine agonists
▸ Diuretics	▸ Tamoxifen
▸ Cold compresses	▸ GnRH analogs
▸ Local progesterone gel	▸ Thyroid hormones
▸ Acupuncture	

Diagnosis with Ultrasound

The criteria for the ultrasound diagnosis of fibrocystic change are shown in **Table 6.5**.

Common Findings

The fibrotic parenchyma appears hyperechoic, and its echotexture is coarser than that of normal glandular tissue (**Fig. 6.1 a, b**). The fibrosis increases the reflection and refraction of sound, leading to greater sound absorption. This can hamper the evaluation of large breasts because of poor image quality and acoustic shadowing at deeper levels, but compression and change in the patient's position can be used in these cases to improve sound penetration and for better delineation of deeper structures. Changes such as duct dilatation are often found in the subareolar area, and particular care is required in evaluating this region (**Fig. 6.2 a, b**). Here, sliding the areolar skin to one side will diminish artifact and allow clear insonation of the area behind the nipple. High-resolution scanning will often reveal microcysts 0.5–2.0 mm in size, many of which cannot be detected with the type of equipment that is no longer recommended for breast scanning (**Fig. 6.3 a, b**). Aggregations of microcysts or macrocysts can be associated with proliferative forms of fibrocystic changes, often but not always with apocrine metaplasia (**Fig. 6.4 a, b**). Frequently ductal dilatation is associated (**Figs. 6.5 a, b, 6.6 a, b**).

A good-quality scanner used with a 10-MHz or higher transducer frequency will often define the lactiferous ducts as tubular structures converging toward the nipple (see **Fig. 6.8**).

Table 6.4 Histopathologic classification of fibrocystic change

Histologic grade	Proliferation	Relative cancer risk
I	None	Not increased
II	Proliferation without atypia	Risk factor of 2–2.5
III	Proliferation with atypia	Risk factor of 3–5

Table 6.5 Criteria for the diagnosis of fibrocystic change

Shape, extent	Diffuse or oval lesions
Orientation	Parallel
Margin	Indistinct or circumscribed
Lesion boundary	Abrupt interface
Echo pattern	Hypoechoic or hyperechoic
Posterior acoustic features	Shadowing
Surrounding tissue	No changes, but fibrosis may limit readability
Calcifications	Microcalcifications may be present in mass
Vascularity	Diffusely increased vascularity in (surrounding) tissue
Ducts:	
Caliber	1–2 mm
Margins	Circumscribed
Echogenicity	Anechoic

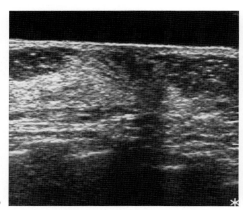 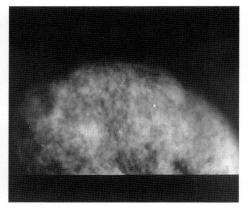

a, b

Fig. 6.1 a, b Sonographic and mammographic features of fibrotic change.
a Midsagittal ultrasound scan demonstrates the parenchymal cone, flanked by fat, which tapers anteriorly toward the nipple and thickens toward the periphery. A standoff pad was used to improve skin definition. Despite compression, the subareolar region appears hypoechoic and is obscured by acoustic shadows. Fibrous tissue proliferation coarsens the structure of the breast parenchyma and increases its echogenicity.
b The mammogram shows patchy areas of increased breast density (7.5-MHz transducer).

Shape, extent	Diffuse, no focal abnormality
Orientation	–
Margins	Indistinct
Lesion boundary	–
Echo pattern	Mixed hyperechoic and hypoechoic
Posterior acoustic features	Shadowing
Surrounding tissue	No changes
Calcifications	None
Vascularity	Not present

❗ Comment:
The radiographic density of the fibrocystic breast limits the sensitivity of mammography. Ultrasound clearly demonstrates the parenchyma, but the fibrotic changes lead to increased sound attenuation and the shadowing makes the image difficult to interpret.

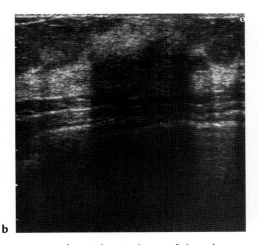
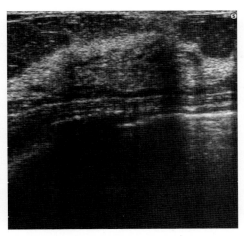

Shape, extent	Diffuse, non-mass
Orientation	–
Margins	Indistinct
Lesion boundary	–
Echo pattern	Mixed hyperechoic and hypoechoic
Posterior acoustic features	Shadowing
Surrounding tissue	No changes
Calcifications	None
Vascularity	Not present

a, b

Fig. 6.2 a, b Midsagittal scan of the subareolar region in a breast with fibrotic change, noncompression and compression views.
a Intense shadowing centrally in the noncompression scan prevents evaluation of the parenchymal structure.

b Compression improves sound transmission so that the ducts and deeper glandular tissues can be seen. It is not totally effective, however, in compensating for the increased sound absorption due to fibrosis (10-MHz transducer).

❗ Comment:
As is reported for mammography, an assessment of interpretability of the images should be noted. It is important to weigh the reliability of the ultrasound examination against that of mammography, and to give weight to the more accurate study or the one where the likelihood of malignancy is greater.

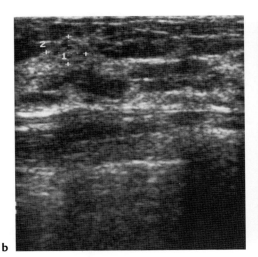
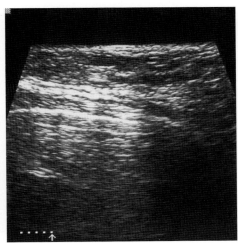

Shape	Oval
Orientation	Parallel
Margins	Circumscribed
Lesion boundary	Abrupt interface
Echo pattern	Anechoic to hypoechoic in hyperechoic background
Posterior acoustic features	None
Surrounding tissue	No changes
Calcifications	Not present
Vascularity	None
Special case	Clustered microcysts

a, b

Fig. 6.3 a, b Fibrocystic focus with microcysts 0.5 mm in diameter.
a High-resolution ultrasound scan (10-MHz transducer).

b Scan with a 5-MHz transducer.

❗ Comment:
Comparison of the images shows that the microcysts are detectable with high-resolution ultrasound or higher frequency but not with the 5-MHz transducer, which should no longer be used for breast sonography

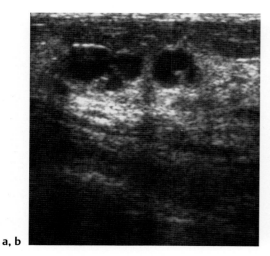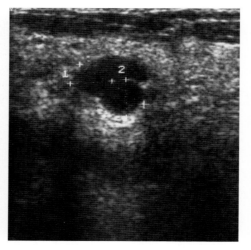

Shape	Oval
Orientation	Parallel
Margins	Circumscribed, lobulated
Lesion boundary	Abrupt interface
Echo pattern	Anechoic
Posterior acoustic features	Enhancement
Surrounding tissue	No changes
Calcifications	None
Vascularity	Not present
Special case	Clustered micro-cysts

a, b

Fig. 6.4 a, b Breast cysts aggregated in grape like pattern.
a Sagittal scan.
b Transverse scan (10-MHz transducer).

❗ Comment:
The scans show hyperechoic parenchymal fibrosis, within which is embedded a grapelike cluster of small cysts.
It is important to correlate the ultrasound findings with mammograms, as these foci are often associated with clustered microcalcifications. If there is no mammographic correlative finding, ultrasound-guided aspiration may be carried out to exclude proliferative disease.

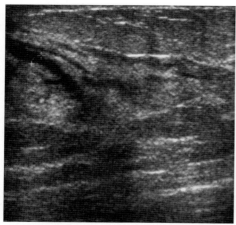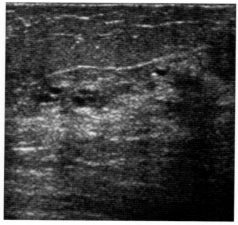

Shape (**b**)	Oval
Orientation	Parallel
Margins	Circumscribed
Lesion boundary	Abrupt interface
Echo pattern	Anechoic
Posterior acoustic features	Enhancement
Surrounding tissue	No changes
Calcifications	Microcalcifications within lesion (microcysts)
Vascularity	Not present
Special case	Clustered micro-cysts
Ducts (**a**):	
Caliber	2 mm
Margins	Circumscribed
Echo pattern	Anechoic

a, b

Fig. 6.5 a, b Fibrocystic change with microcysts and duct ectasia.
a Appearance of duct ectasia on a radial scan.
b Peripheral scan in the upper outer quadrant shows fibrotic changes in the parenchyma with an aggregation of several microcysts (10-MHz transducer).

❗ Comment:
The radial scan (**a**) shows smooth-walled ectatic ducts up to 2 mm in diameter with no abrupt caliber changes. **b** The right half of the image shows increased fibrosis with acoustic shadowing. Sound transmission in that region can be improved by increasing the TGC or by applying compression. The microcysts are clearly visible in the hyperechoic parenchyma and contain scattered punctate microcalcifications.

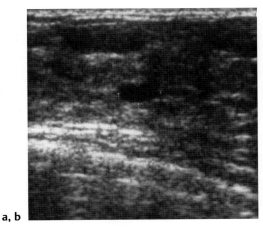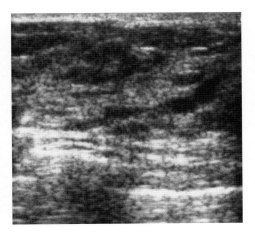

a, b

Shape (**a**)	Oval
Orientation	Parallel
Margins	Circumscribed
Lesion boundary	Abrupt interface
Echo pattern	Anechoic
Posterior acoustic features	None
Surrounding tissue	No changes
Calcifications	None
Vascularity	Not present
Ducts (**b**):	
Caliber	2–4 mm
Margins	Circumscribed
Echo pattern	Mixed anechoic and hypoechoic

Fig. 6.6 a, b Duct ectasia.
a The ectatic duct resembles a cyst when imaged in cross section.
b A radial scan defines the course of the ectatic duct as it approaches the nipple. Adjoining the expanded, anechoic duct segment are hyperechoic, irregularly dilated segments that suggest intraductal proliferation. Histology: fibrocystic change without atypia (7.5-MHz transducer).

❗ Comment:
The lesion mimics a cyst on the sagittal image. The radial scan identifies it as an ectatic duct. Additionally, the duct displays abrupt caliber changes and echogenic foci of intraductal proliferation.
An ectatic duct viewed in cross section may be mistaken for a cyst. Even in cross section, however, the transducer can be moved along the duct to define it as a tubular structure.

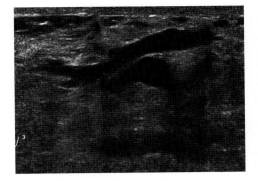

Fig. 6.7 Dilated, secretion-filled duct with smooth walls and slight caliber variations (12-MHz transducer).

Shape	No focal abnormality
Orientation	–
Margins	–
Lesion boundary	–
Echo pattern	–
Posterior acoustic features	–
Surrounding tissue	No changes
Calcifications	None
Vascularity	Not present
Ducts:	
Caliber	3–4 mm
Margins	Circumscribed
Echo pattern	Anechoic

❗ Comment:
Despite the slight caliber variations, this duct has smooth walls and contains no internal echoes. There is no evidence of proliferative change.

The ducts have smooth borders and taper toward the periphery where they may be less than 1 mm in diameter. There is wide variability in what is considered to be normal ductal caliber (**Fig. 6.7**). In women with ovarian cycles and those receiving hormone replacement therapy the ducts contain anechoic secretions. As the breast involutes at menopause, the ducts collapse and are less conspicuous although ectatic ducts more than 3–4 mm in diameter are not uncommon as a degenerative finding and are not suspicious for proliferative change if they have smooth walls and contain anechoic secretions (**Fig. 6.8**). These ducts may contain within them the thick, linear calcifications, commonly known as "secretory calcifications" and at times referred to as "plasma cell mastitis." These calcifications have no clinical significance and are to be distinguished from the groups of linear, branching microcalcifications linearly arrayed that may represent ductal carcinoma in situ (DCIS) and require biopsy.

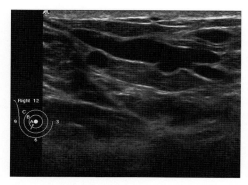

Fig. 6.8 Subareolar duct ectasia (12-MHz transducer).

Shape	No focal abnormality
Orientation	–
Margins	–
Lesion boundary	Abrupt interface
Echo pattern	–
Posterior acoustic features	–
Surrounding tissue	No changes
Calcifications	None
Vascularity	Not present
Ducts:	
Caliber	4–5 mm
Margins	Smooth
Echogenicity	Anechoic

! Comment:
Even pronounced duct ectasia is not considered suspicious if the duct has smooth walls and does not contain internal echoes.

Less Common Findings

The diagnostic criteria for less common forms of fibrocystic change are listed in **Table 6.6**.

Localized areas of fibrocystic change may present as hypoechoic focal lesions with indistinct margins and shadowing (**Fig. 6.9 a, b**). Shadowing can make it difficult to evaluate the breast architecture, and scanning at frequencies higher than 10 MHz can prevent the adequate visualization of deeper structures. This limitation is compensated for by the broad bandwidths and wide frequency ranges of most currently available probes used for breast imaging. Electronic focusing automatically reduces the frequencies of these transducers to enable them to penetrate deeper areas of breast tissue. In addition, greater transducer pressure usually has to be applied to the breast to achieve adequate, uniform sound penetration with care taken not to cause discomfort to the patient. Even with hypoechoic foci of fibrocystic change, the parenchyma-like internal structure of the lesion can usually be appreciated when adequate compression is applied. Compression is particularly helpful in investigating foci that are palpable as patchy areas of increased breast firmness or coarse nodularity and vaguely increased density on mammograms.

One special form of focal fibrocystic change is sclerosing adenosis which often shows some suspicious characteristics (**Fig. 6.10 a–d**). Some lesions of nodular sclerosing adenosis may have indistinct margins that mimic carcinoma, but many have circumscribed margins similar to those of a fibroadenoma (**Fig. 6.11**).

Diabetic mastopathy or fibrosis is another carcinoma-mimicking benign lesion associated with juvenile or long-standing insulin-dependent diabetes. Fibrosis can be very extensive, present as a firm mass or masses, and cause problems in differential diagnosis (**Fig. 6.12 a, b**). Even with a history suggesting diabetic fibrosis, bilateral ultrasound examinations can be helpful in detecting additional areas, but core needle biopsy must be carried out.

Table 6.6 Criteria for diagnosing atypical foci of fibrocystic change

Shape	Irregular
Orientation	Parallel
Margin	Not circumscribed (indistinct)
Lesion boundary	Abrupt interface
Echo pattern	Hypoechoic
Posterior acoustic features	Shadowing
Surrounding tissue	Architectural distortion, difficult to interpret
Calcifications	Microcalcifications may be present in mass
Vascularity	Present immediately adjacent to lesion or diffusely increased in surrounding tissue
Ducts:	
Caliber	>2 mm
Margin	Indistinct
Echogenicity	Hypoechoic with solid structures

Ducts in Fibrocystic Change

A proliferative lesion should be suspected if ultrasound shows variations in the caliber of peripheral duct segments, irregular wall contours, or intraluminal masses or debris.

Intraductal proliferation and secretory activity lead to enlarged ducts with increased internal echoes, irregular contours, and local variations in caliber (**Fig. 6.13 a, b**). In some cases internal echoes are confined to localized duct segments (**Fig. 6.14 a, b**). Ducts that expand rather than taper toward the periphery are particularly suspicious for proliferative changes (**Figs. 6.13 a, b, 6.14 a, b**). The internal echo pattern is suggestive of, but does not prove, solid intraductal vegetations or tumors, such as papillomas. Inspissated secretions produce intraductal echoes, even in the absence of proliferation. This emphasizes the importance of an accurate differential diagnostic investigation. Experienced examiners can accomplish this by means of ultrasound-guided aspiration. If correlative mammograms are not already available, they should be obtained beforehand so that the aspiration will not cause changes that would make it difficult to interpret subsequent mammograms.

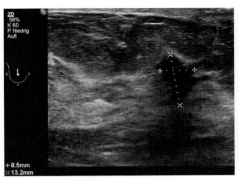
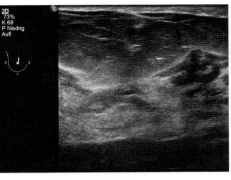

Shape, extent	Irregular, lesion disappears after compression (b)
Orientation	Not parallel
Margins	Indistinct
Lesion boundary	Abrupt interface
Echo pattern	Hypoechoic, increasing echogenicity in response to compression
Posterior acoustic features	Shadowing disappears after compression
Surrounding tissue	Without compression architectural distortion and duct changes. Under compression no abnormal changes visible
Calcifications	None
Vascularity	Not present

Fig. 6.9 a, b Effect of minimal and strong compression on the sonographic appearance of fibrocystic change.
a Light pressure on the breast with the transducer does not significantly increase sound transmission through the fibrotic parenchyma, creating the appearance of what appears to be an ill-defined, hypoechoic mass.
b Increasing the transducer pressure improves sound penetration through the fibrotic parenchyma (12-MHz transducer). No lesion is present.

⚠ Comment:
Strong sound attenuation creates the impression of a hypoechoic mass, which disappears when greater pressure is applied. The pseudomass is no longer seen, and the parenchymal structure can be evaluated.

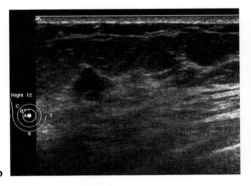
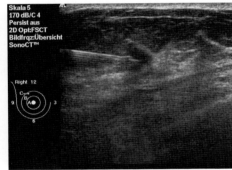
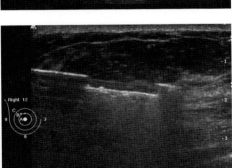

Fig. 6.10 a–d Tumor-forming sclerosing adenosis.
a Ultrasound scan.
b Fine-needle aspiration cytology.
c Lesion removal by vacuum-assisted biopsy.
d After complete removal (12-MHz transducer).

Shape, extent	Irregular
Orientation	Parallel
Margins	Angulated
Lesion boundary	Abrupt interface
Echo pattern	Hypoechoic
Posterior acoustic features	None
Surrounding tissue	Architectural distortion
Calcifications	None
Vascularity	Not present

⚠ Comment:
Fig. 6.10 a shows a suspicious lesion in the right breast, seen as an ill-defined density on mammography. FNAB (**Fig. 6.10 b**) revealed highly proliferative cells. Histology was recommended. As the patient wanted to avoid open excision biopsy, the lesion was removed by vacuum-assisted large-core biopsy (**Fig. 6.10 c–d**). Nodular sclerosing adenosis was found by histology.

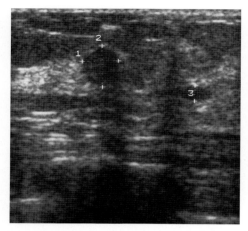

Shape	Oval
Orientation	Not parallel
Margins	Circumscribed
Lesion boundary	Abrupt interface
Echo pattern	Hypoechoic
Posterior acoustic features	Shadowing
Surrounding tissue	No changes
Calcifications	None
Vascularity	Not present

! Comment:
This type of lesion may be mistaken for a fibroadenoma.

Fig. 6.11 The lesion on the left is a solid fibrocystic nodule that resembles fibroadenoma. The lesion on the right is a small cyst (10-MHz transducer).

a, b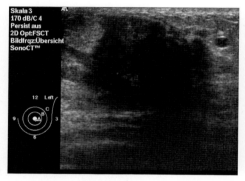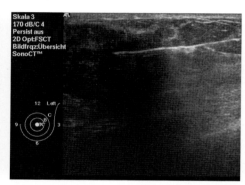

Fig. 6.12 a, b Diabetic mastopathy. In area of firm, palpable mass, a large hypoechoic lesion with ill-defined margins is seen in a patient with juvenile diabetes. Despite maximum transducer compression the mass remains visible. Because the finding was considered equivocal, ultrasound-guided core biopsy was done. Histology revealed tumor-forming benign breast disease (12-MHz transducer).

Shape	Irregular
Orientation	Parallel
Margins	Indistinct, angulations and spiculations
Lesion boundary	Abrupt interface
Echo pattern	Hypoechoic, no increase of echogenicity in response to compression
Posterior acoustic features	Shadowing
Surrounding tissue	Architectural distortion
Calcifications	None
Vascularity	Not present

! Comment:
This type of lesion may be mistaken for carcinoma and must be biopsied. It is unsafe to attribute such findings to diabetic mastopathy even when the clinical history supports the diagnosis. The mass grew considerably within 1 year. The lump was firm, immobile, and painful to palpation and was obscured by extremely dense fibroglandular tissue on mammography. Core biopsy specimens showed connective tissue with few glandular components. Concordance was questioned, and the excised lesion confirmed the core biopsy results, consistent with diabetic fibrosis.

Mammograms in patients with proliferative disease frequently show microcalcifications (defined as 0.1–0.5 mm in diameter) that are scattered throughout one or both breasts, regional or grouped (**Fig. 6.15 a**). Isolated or clustered calcifications are also commonly found in association with microcysts. When the microcysts are imaged with a high-resolution scanner, mural microcalcifications may be observed (**Fig. 6.15 b**). On mammograms, microcystic lesions may be completely obscured by dense fibroglandular tissue or may be visible as a focal asymmetry. Milk of calcium within microcysts can be identified on 90° lateral mammograms as curvilinear opacities or "teacup" calcifications in the dependent portion of these tiny dilated acini. On craniocaudal mammograms, they are seen as rounded opacities with smudged borders, the densest portion on mammograms correlating with the deepest part of the microcyst. Microcystic lesions are frequently, but not always, associated with apocrine metaplasia.

Around the area of microcysts, microcalcifications may sometimes be seen within the breast parenchyma (**Fig. 6.16**). If there is a

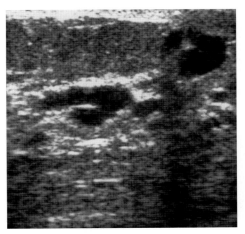 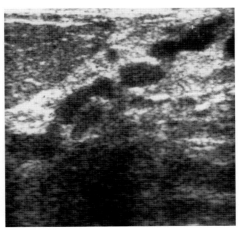

a, b

Fig. 6.13 a, b Atypical proliferative fibrocystic change. Two radial scans in the upper outer quadrant of the right breast show enlarged ducts with caliber fluctuations, internal echoes, and irregular borders. Clustered microcalcifications were also present, and therefore excisional biopsy was carried out (10-MHz transducer).

Shape, extent	No focal abnormality
Orientation	–
Margins	–
Lesion boundary	–
Echo pattern	–
Posterior acoustic features	–
Surrounding tissue	No changes
Ducts:	
Caliber	3–5 mm
Margins	Microlobulated
Echo pattern	Hypoechoic

! Comment:
Percutaneous needle biopsy may be inconclusive in cases with suspicious sonographic and mammographic findings, and the lesion, which may be upgraded on the surgical specimen, should be excised.

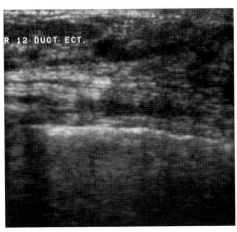 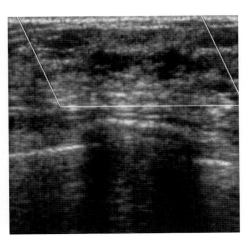

a, b

Fig. 6.14 a, b Proliferative fibrocystic change involving a duct segment. The sagittal scan (**a**) and corresponding transverse scan (**b**) show subareolar ductal pathology at the 12 o'clock position. (10-MHz transducer)

Shape, extent	No focal lesion
Orientation	–
Margins	–
Lesion boundary	–
Echo pattern	–
Posterior acoustic features	–
Surrounding tissue	No changes
Ducts:	
Caliber	2–4 mm
Margins	Irregular
Echogenicity	Hypoechoic

! Comment:
The scans show caliber irregularities of the duct, whose terminal portion is filled with secretions. Distally, a 4-mm segment of the duct contains internal echoes. The lesion was excised because of nipple discharge and intraductal filling defects observed at ductography.

group, their concentration in a given area helps distinguish these echogenic particles from acoustic speckle. Mammographic and sonographic findings should always be correlated, and the need for additional diagnostic procedures is determined by the assessment of combined mammographic, sonographic, and clinical findings.

Intraductal papillomas are epithelial proliferations within the walls of ducts (**Fig. 6.17 a, b**). Papillomas arising in large ducts may be pedunculated. Their fibrovascular stalks may undergo torsion as the masses grow. Papillomas may be isolated or multiple, and

may develop in one or more ducts centrally or in a peripheral location. Occasionally they are manifested by a bloody nipple discharge, and intraductal papillomas are the most common cause of a spontaneous nipple discharge.

The workup may include testing the discharge for occult blood and cytologic evaluation of a nipple smear, although the necessity for this test has been questioned because of its insensitivity. Ductography, either retrograde from nipple punctum or antegrade with ultrasound-guided injection into the duct responsible for the discharge, can help map the extent to guide surgical planning.

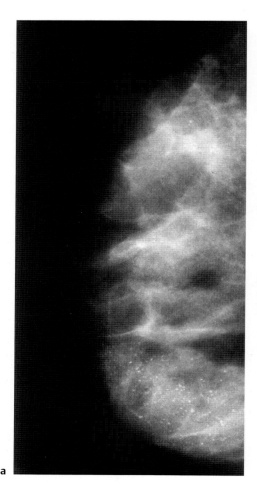

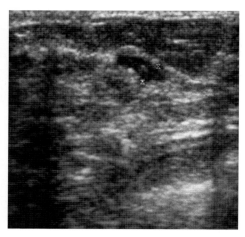

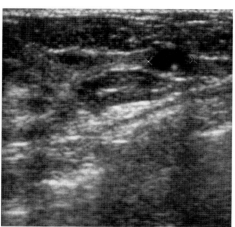

Fig. 6.15 a–c Microcalcifications in benign breast disease with atypical proliferations.
a Mammogram shows extensive rounded and pleomorphic microcalcifications in the lower portion of the breast.
b Ultrasound shows multiple circumscribed sites of ductal dilatation (top) and small cysts (**c**, bottom) with mural microcalcifications, which appear as bright punctate echoes (10-MHz transducer).

Shape, extent	Oval
Orientation	Parallel
Margins	Circumscribed
Lesion boundary	Abrupt interface
Echo pattern	Anechoic
Posterior acoustic features	No changes
Surrounding tissue	No changes
Calcifications	Micocalcifications within lesion (microcysts and ducts)
Vascularity	Not present
Ducts:	
Caliber	2–4 mm
Margins	Smooth
Echogenicity	Anechoic with mural microcalcifications

❗ Comment:
The morphology of the microcalcifications cannot be evaluated with ultrasound. It is important, therefore, to correlate the ultrasound images with mammograms.

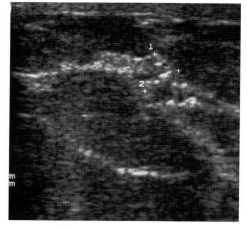

Shape	Irregular
Orientation	Parallel
Margins	Angular
Lesion boundary	Abrupt interface
Echo pattern	Complex
Posterior acoustic features	None
Surrounding tissue	No changes
Calcifications	Microcalcifications in mass
Vascularity	Not present

❗ Comment:
Microcalcifications are more difficult to detect in the echogenic parenchyma than in cysts or ducts. If a mammographic abnormality is found, ultrasound often demonstrates a correlate and permits sonographically guided core biopsy or vacuum-assisted needle biopsy. Ultrasound-guided preoperative localization can also be done with wire placement in or adjacent to the lesion confirmed by mammography. After the lesion has been excised, a specimen radiograph should be obtained to document removal of the microcalcifications and mass, if present.

Fig. 6.16 Clustered microcalcifications within the breast parenchyma in atypical proliferative benign disease. Mammograms showed clustered pleomorphic microcalcifications. Ultrasound shows numerous punctate, high-level echoes within the parenchymal tissue. Because the mammograms were equivocal, the lesion was excised (10-MHz transducer).

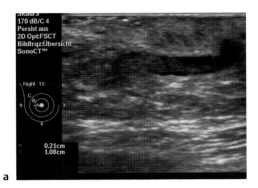

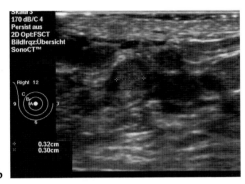

Shape (intraductal)	Oval
Orientation	Parallel
Margins	Circumscribed
Lesion boundary	Abrupt interface
Echo pattern	Hyperechoic
Posterior acoustic features	None
Surrounding tissue	No changes
Ducts:	
Caliber	2–3 mm
Margins	Circumscribed with abrupt caliber change
Echogenicity	Anechoic with a circumscribed area of higher echogenicity

Fig. 6.17 a, b Intraductal papilloma (15-MHz transducer).

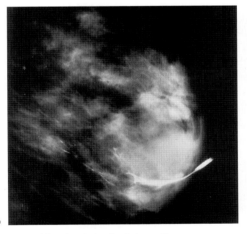

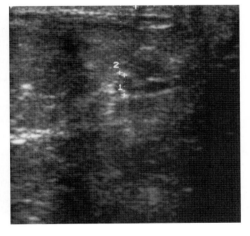

a, b

Fig. 6.18 a, b Intraductal papilloma.
a Ductography shows an obstructed duct in the lower inner quadrant of the left breast.
b Ultrasound reveals a circumscribed mass in the obstructed duct (10-MHz transducer).

Shape (intraductal lesion)	Rounded
Size	3 × 3 mm
Orientation	Parallel
Margins	Circumscribed
Lesion boundary	Abrupt interface
Echo pattern	Hyperechoic
Posterior acoustic features	None
Surrounding tissue	No changes
Calcifications	None
Vascularity	Not present
Ducts:	
Caliber	2–3 mm
Margins	Circumscribed with localized abrupt caliber change
Echogenicity	Anechoic with a circumscribed area of higher echogenicity within the duct

* Because of the small size of the lesion, its margins are difficult to evaluate.

■ Comment:
Ultrasound demonstrates a smooth, locally expanded duct containing a papilloma. Neither ductography nor ultrasound can provide a definitive diagnosis, and core needle bipsy, vacuum-assisted biopsy, or surgical excision is required. Ductography serves to confirm the finding and may depict additional intraductal lesions situated more peripherally.

This is usually accomplished by ductography (**Fig. 6.18 a**), but high-resolution ultrasound is often successful in localizing the intraductal masses, dilatation, or localized mural thickening (**Fig. 6.18 b**).

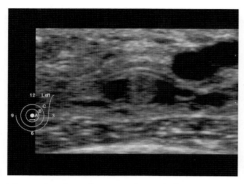 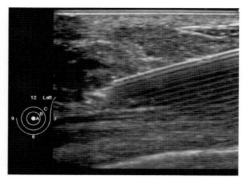

a, b

Shape	Oval
Size	3 mm diameter (**a**)
Orientation	Not parallel
Margins	Circumscribed,
Lesion boundary	Abrupt interface
Echo pattern	Hyperechoic
Posterior acoustic features	None
Surrounding tissue	No changes
Calcifications	None
Vascularity	Not present
Ducts:	
Caliber	2–3 mm
Margins	Circumscribed
Echogenicity	Anechoic with hyperechoic lesion within the duct

Fig. 6.19 a, b Ultrasound-guided preoperative localization of an intraductal papilloma. **a** Intraductal papilloma, **b** needle positioning for preoperative dye injection (15-MHz transducer).

❗ Comment:

This ultrasound-guided intervention was done for preoperative localization rather than cytologic sampling. Fine-needle aspiration is usually inconclusive in these cases, and vacuum-assisted or core needle biopsy is preferred for percutaneous image-guided sampling. Vacuum-assisted biopsy devices can also remove imaging evidence of the lesion's presence. Alternatively, the patient may go directly to surgical excision.

Sometimes intraductal abnormalities are detected incidentally with ultrasound, even in the absence of nipple discharge. Ultrasound can be used in these cases to direct fine-needle aspiration cytology, core biopsy, or even vacuum-assisted percutaneous removal of the affected duct. Most often, however, following the delineation of abnormal ducts, presurgical localization and excision are generally done regardless. (**Fig. 6.19 a, b**). Recently, for nipple discharge unexplained by mammographic or sonographic findings, contrast-enhanced breast MRI has been able to identify a cause and indicate an abnormal area. Percutaneous biopsy can be done with MRI guidance.

Diagnosis and Management, Pitfalls, and When to Biopsy

Increased sound attenuation frequently compromises the ultrasound evaluation of large breasts. Hypoechoic foci of fibrocystic change or stromal fibrosis may be mistaken for malignant tumors

Table 6.7 Differential diagnosis of breast carcinoma

Finding	Cause	Solution*
Hypoechoic lesion	Sound absorption	Compression to increase sound penetration
Posterior acoustic features	Shadowing	Compression, aspiration if required
Indistinct margin	Sound absorption	Compression, aspiration if required
Microcalcifications	Proliferation	Surgery or aspiration
Irregular ducts	Proliferation	Surgery or aspiration

* All cases require correlation with mammographic findings.

(**Table 6.7**). Compression will usually improve sound transmission and permit the evaluation of parenchymal structures (see **Fig. 6.9 a, b**). Changing the position of the patient slightly or altering the probe angle against the tissue may help to reduce artifact. Digital palpation under ultrasound control can demonstrate the compressibility of a focal hypoechoic lesion helping to support a benign diagnosis. Before recommending follow-up, a microcystic lesion should be evaluated with real-time ultrasound to exclude a solid component or a nodular area that persists under compression (**Fig. 6.20 a, b**). Core or vacuum-assisted biopsies of these lesions should be carried out percutaneously with ultrasound guidance.

Histologically, the underlying pathology may consist of simple fibrocystic change or a florid proliferation. If atypia is found, surgical excision is the current standard. The clinical and mammographic findings may prompt definitive evaluation by percutaneous or excisional biopsy. Duct irregularities combined with echogenic intraductal material may run the gamut from benign proliferation to papilloma, or to intraductal carcinoma. Ductal dilatation may be difficult to assess both sonographically and mammographically. If there is no definite mammographic finding to explain the findings, such as clustered or linearly distributed pleomorphic microcalcifications, the ultrasound images should be closely scrutinized to determine whether the lactiferous ducts have smooth contours and a normal arborization pattern, and whether or not they contain inspissated material. (**Fig. 6.21, Fig. 6.22**). When a patient presents with spontaneous clear or bloody nipple discharge, ductography may reveal the cause of the symptoms. Ultrasound-guided aspiration of the duct may also elucidate the etiology of the findings, and if ductal atypia or a papillary lesion is found, surgical biopsy may be indicated.

Nevertheless, although it is true that higher grades of proliferative disease lead to more pronounced ductal changes, even severe degrees of ductal dilatation may have a benign cause. On the other hand, intraductal carcinoma may spread along ducts in a thin layer only a few cells thick without causing obvious ductal changes. If findings are equivocal or discordant, expressed duct secretions may be examined cytologically; this is usually more successful

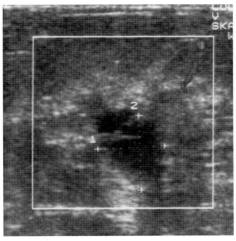 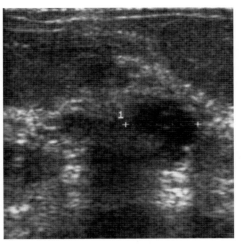

Shape	Oval
Orientation	Not parallel
Margins	Not circumscribed (partly)
Lesion boundary	Abrupt interface
Echo pattern	Hyperechoic
Posterior acoustic features	Combined pattern
Surrounding tissue	Architectural distortion
Calcifications	None
Vascularity	Not present

a, b

Fig. 6.20 a, b Equivocal fibrocystic lesion. Ultrasound shows a suspicious area with mixed solid and microcystic features, increased sound attenuation by the adjacent and overlying parenchyma, and distal enhancement. It is unclear whether the area consists of multiple small cysts or is a solid, hypoechoic tumor with microcysts. Histology indicated proliferative fibrocystic change with microcysts. **a** Sagittal scan, **b** transverse scan (10-MHz transducer).

❗ Comment:
Fibrocystic tissue permeated by clusters of microcysts often presents as a hypoechoic mass requiring further evaluation. If there is not a high index of suspicion for a tumor, fine-needle aspiration or core biopsy should be done to avoid needless surgery.

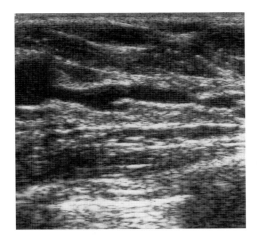

Shape	Oval
Orientation	Parallel
Margins	Circumscribed
Lesion boundary	Abrupt interface
Echo pattern	Hypoechoic
Posterior acoustic features	None
Surrounding tissue	No changes
Calcifications	None
Vascularity	Not present
Ducts:	
Caliber	2 mm
Margins	Smooth
Echogenicity	Hypoechoic

Fig. 6.21 Small cyst and a dilated duct with internal echoes caused by hemosiderin in the intraductal fluid. Both lesions were drained at aspiration. Cytology showed no proliferative changes (10-MHz transducer).

❗ Comment:
The hemosiderin-containing fluid mimics solid internal echoes. Intraductal or intracystic proliferation cannot be excluded on the basis of ultrasound morphology, but negative aspiration cytology reliably excludes proliferative disease.

for lesions close to the nipple than for those in the periphery of the breast, or on cellular material sampled by ultrasound-guided aspiration of the duct.

 Suspicious mammographic findings, such as clustered pleomorphic microcalcifications, require histologic evaluation even if the ultrasound findings are normal.

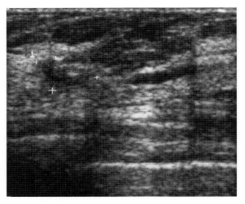

Shape	Irregular
Orientation	Parallel
Margins	Indistinct
Lesion boundary	Abrupt interface
Echo pattern	Hypoechoic
Posterior acoustic features	None
Surrounding tissue	Architectural distortion
Calcifications	None
Vascularity	Not assessed
Ducts:	
Caliber	2 mm proximally, up to 5 mm distally
Margins	Circumscribed proximally, irregular distally
Echogenicity	Anechoic proximally, hypoechoic distally

Fig. 6.22 Early invasive ductal carcinoma with an irregular duct. Screening mammograms in a 49-year-old woman showed clustered microcalcifications. Ultrasound shows a smooth, secretion-filled duct, 2 mm in diameter, just below the areola. A more distal portion of the duct (left side of image) shows ill-defined thickening with a hypoechoic, noncompressible focal lesion (10-MHz transducer).

! Comment:
A marked difference, caused by early invasive ductal carcinoma, is observed between the normal subareolar portion of the duct and the irregular dilatation of the more distal portion.

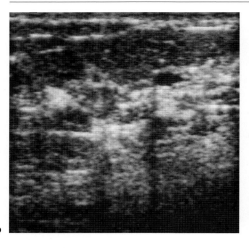
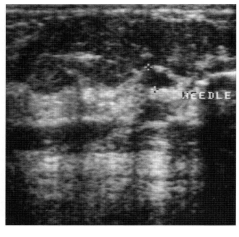

a, b

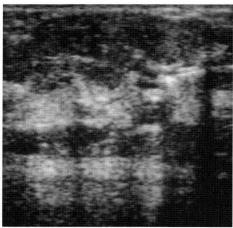
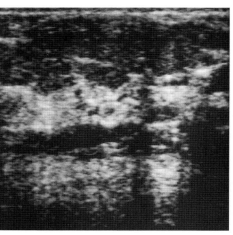

c, d

Fig. 6.23 a–d Suspected proliferative fibrocystic change in a 62-year-old woman (10-MHz transducer). The mammograms were unremarkable. Ultrasound showed a dilated duct above the nipple with mixed anechoic and hypoechoic features (**a, b**). Intraductal proliferation was suspected, and the duct was aspirated under ultrasound guidance. Image **b** shows the needle placed in front of the lesion, and **c** shows the needle inside the lesion during the aspiration. A small amount of fluid was aspirated (postaspiration view in **d**), and cytology revealed nuclear enlargement and dyskaryosis. Despite the suspicion of proliferative change, surgery was withheld because the mammograms were negative. Two years later, a 2-cm invasive carcinoma was found.

! Comment:
Ultrasound and cytology were equivocal. Despite the negative mammograms, follow-up at 3–6 months would have been advised. Cytology cannot positively distinguish between intraductal carcinoma and proliferative fibrocystic change. Because the latter implies an increased cancer risk, there should be little hesitation in recommending excisional biopsy.

Shape	Oval
Orientation	Parallel
Margins	Circumscribed
Lesion boundary	Abrupt interface
Echo pattern	Complex
Posterior acoustic features	None
Surrounding tissue	No changes
Calcifications	None
Vascularity	Not present
Ducts:	
Caliber	3–6 mm
Margins	Circumscribed
Echogenicity	Mixed anechoic and hypoechoic

Case 1

Breast ultrasound in a 62-year-old woman demonstrated irregularly dilated ducts at the 12 o'clock position in the right breast (**Fig. 6.23 a–d**). Prior mammograms were normal. Ultrasound-guided fine-needle aspiration cytology showed enlarged nuclei with suspicion of proliferative change. Because the mammograms were normal, surgery was withheld. The patient was scheduled for a 6-month follow-up, but it was 2 years before she returned, at which time a 2-cm invasive carcinoma was detected at the same location. It is unclear whether the tumor was already present 2 years before, when aspiration cytology was negative. It is possible that the carcinoma developed during the interval from a focus of proliferative change. Presumably the course would have been more favorable if percutaneous or surgical biopsy had been done 2 years earlier.

▶ If equivocal ultrasound findings correlate with negative mammograms, the ultrasound features should be scrutinized to determine whether it is sufficient to follow the suspicious area or whether it should be evaluated by fine-needle aspiration or core biopsy. If the features are suspicious for proliferation, core biopsy should be recommended even if clinical and mammographic findings are normal. MRI may be indicated if mammography or ultrasound are inconclusive.

Case 2

Screening mammograms in a 48-year-old premenopausal women with no clinical symptoms revealed clustered microcalcifications in the right breast with otherwise normal-appearing but heterogeneously dense breast tissue. Because of the microcalcifications, the patient was referred for surgery. Ultrasound scans of the right breast in the area of the calcifications showed only fibrocystic change with microcysts (**Fig. 6.24 a**). Ultrasound also showed a hypoechoic, irregularly shaped, angular incompressible mass in the lower inner quadrant of the left breast (**Fig. 6.24 b**). Histology revealed benign fibrocystic change in the right breast and invasive ductal carcinoma in the left breast.

▶ Mammograms showed no abnormalities in the left breast, yet invasive carcinoma was found. This illustrates the principle that although it must take into account the findings of other studies, ultrasound may have a role in screening. Ultrasound features such as irregular shape, noncircumscribed margins, and nonparallel orientation can stand on their own merit in assessment of the lesion as suspicious for malignancy. Lesions detected sonographically should be investigated even if they do not correlate with a mammographically visible abnormality.

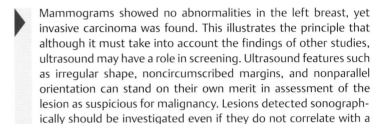

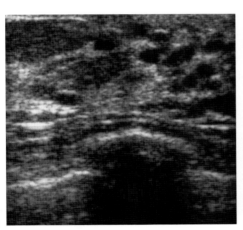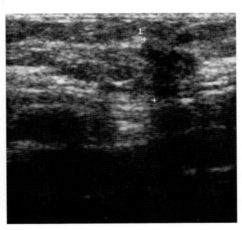

a, b

Fig. 6.24 a, b Mammograms in this 48-year-old premenopausal woman showed clustered microcalcifications in the right breast. Both breasts were dense with no other abnormalities (10-MHz transducer).
a Ultrasound in the right breast showed microcystic changes in the area of the microcalcifications.
b Scans through the lower inner quadrant of the left breast revealed a suspicious, hypoechoic, noncompressible mass 10 mm in diameter. Because of the unequivocal sonographic criteria, the lesion was excised. Histology identified the right lesion as fibrocystic change and the left lesion as invasive ductal carcinoma.

❗ Comment:
Equivocal ultrasound findings should be investigated even if mammograms are negative. If there is any doubt, a definitive diagnosis must be confirmed by guided interventional procedures. Without ultrasound, only the healthy side would have been operated.

	(a) right	(b) left
Shape	Round	Irregular
Orientation	Horizontal	Not parallel
Margins	Sharp	indistinct, angular
Lesion boundary	No echogenic halo	Echogenic halo
Echo pattern	Anechoic	Hypoechoic
Posterior acoustic features	Enhancement (at least some of the microcysts)	Shadowing
Surrounding tissue	None	Architectural distortion, Cooper ligament disruption
Calcifications	None	None
Vascularity	Not present	Present immediately adjacent to lesion
Ducts:		
Caliber	2–3 mm	–
Margins	Smooth	–
Echogenicity	Anechoic	–

Further Diagnostic Procedures

MRI and Color Doppler

A diagnostic dilemma can arise in "dense" breasts and in cases where a discrepancy exists between mammographic, sonographic, and clinical findings. The use of techniques for blood-flow analysis, such as dynamic contrast-enhanced MRI and color Doppler flow imaging, should be considered. The user must have considerable experience, since fibrocystic change and fibroadenomas may enhance on MRI and show flow with color or power Doppler. These and other false positives are associated with increased blood flow and may prompt a recommendation for percutaneous core biopsy. Open surgical biopsy is no longer recommended for diagnosis.

Case 3

A 59-year-old woman complained of recurring blue spots on her left breast. Mammograms and physical examination were normal. Ultrasound showed slight dilatation of the smooth-walled subareolar ducts. Sagittal scans revealed large, round cystic masses in the peripheral portion of the outer left breast (**Fig. 6.25a–d**). When the spatial extent of the lesions was analyzed by moving and rotating the transducer, they were defined as tubular structures that resembled grossly dilated ducts but could be traced into the axilla. The suspicion of a vascular anomaly was confirmed by color Doppler, which obviated the need for aspiration.

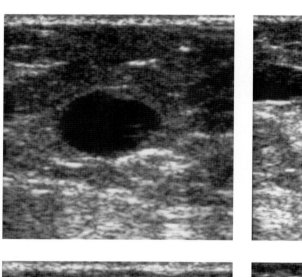
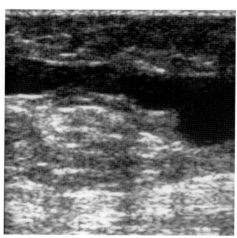

a, b

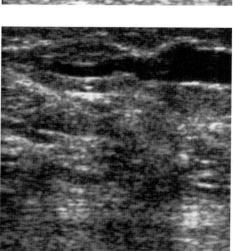

c, d

Fig. 6.25 a–d Ectatic veins in the left breast.
a Sagittal scan of the left breast at the 3 o'clock position shows a round lesion that could be traced laterally.
b Transverse scan shows a tubular structure resembling a dilated duct.
c Sagittal scan shows a round lesion in the left breast at the 4 o'clock position.
d Transverse scan defines its longitudinal course.

Shape	Oval
Orientation	Parallel
Margins	Circumscribed
Lesion boundary	Abrupt interface
Echo pattern	Anechoic
Posterior acoustic features	None
Surrounding tissue	No changes
Calcifications	None
Vascularity	High blood flow in large ectatic veins
Ducts:	
Caliber	1–2 mm
Margins	Circumscribed
Echogenicity	Anechoic

! Comment:
Before proceeding with aspiration or core biopsy, the examiner should consider the possible differential diagnoses to avoid complications due to inappropriate measures. The calibers observed at ultrasound would be unusual for ectatic ducts.

Aspiration and Core Biopsy

The diagnostic algorithm is straightforward in the case of focal sonographic breast lesions that can be evaluated by percutaneous biopsy, i. e., core biopsy or fine-needle aspiration, if expert cytopathology is available (**Figs. 6.26 a, b; 6.27 a, b**). The success of a percutaneous biopsy should be considered examiner-dependent. For large-needle core biopsy, the accuracy rate for those experienced in doing these procedures is over 90 %. Following all biopsy procedures, the imaging studies and clinical history should be reviewed with the histopathology or cytology interpretations for discordance. A negative result does not exclude carcinoma with absolute confidence, and when there is discordance, it is necessary to re-biopsy percutaneously or surgically. When the increased risk of breast cancer that is associated with certain forms of proliferative fibrocystic changes is taken into consideration, the importance of scheduling regular mammographic and sonographic follow-ups is evident.

Ductography

In a patient with a unilateral nipple discharge, smear cytology can be done to detect any ductal epithelial cells that are suspicious for proliferation, although efficacy of this test is currently in question. Care should be taken that discharge is sampled from the secreting duct orifice when the smear is obtained. The color of the material should also be documented: clear, serous, turbid, yellow, greenish, brown, bloody.

With a unilateral spontaneous discharge from one or few ducts, ductography should be done to identify possible intraluminal masses and to define the course, caliber, and branching pattern of the ducts.

Nonionic iodinated contrast material is instilled into the discharging duct using a 30- or 31-G ductography cannula. If the duct segment is not ectatic, 1 mL or less may be sufficient to opacify the duct segment. Lateral and craniocaudal mammographic images as well as magnification views are taken. Ultrasound can also be used to trace the course of the abnormal duct, but mammography is essential.

Ductography is not indicated for discharge from multiple ducts, and patients experiencing this type of discharge may be reassured that their discharge is benign. If necessary, they should be referred for gynecologic or endocrinologic evaluation. It may be helpful to check the patient's prolactin level. If it is normal, or if a goiter is present, thyroid hormone levels should also be tested since fibrocystic breast changes can be associated with thyroid dysfunction.

Role of Ultrasound

At mammography, the fibrocystic breast displays a patchy or more generalized increase in density and may show diverse radiographic features. This can diminish the accuracy of mammograms, particularly in heterogeneously and extremely dense breasts with and variable numbers of micro- and macrocalcifications. When these changes are present, it is becoming common practice in the United States to supplement mammograms with an ultrasound examination of both breasts to detect lesions that are clinically and mammographically occult. For screening of women with *BRCA* 1 and 2 or familial patterns suggesting these genetic abnormalities, especially those women with mammographically dense breast tissue, the American Cancer Society has recently changed its guidelines to advocate contrast-enhanced breast MRI in addition to mammography.

If a suspicious mammographic lesion correlates with an equivocal sonographic finding, it should be evaluated histologically. This particularly applies to clustered pleomorphic microcalcifications, where, if the calcifications are embedded in dense fibroglandular tissue, sonography may uncover a mass, possibly invasive, unsuspected clinically or on mammograms. A core or vacuum-assisted biopsy can then be done with either ultrasound or stereotactic guidance. Fibrocystic change can create conditions unfavorable for an accurate radiographic or sonographic breast examination. A suspicious finding in either modality requires definitive evaluation.

The problem of intraductal proliferation illustrates the practical limits of imaging procedures. Apparent foci of intraductal proliferation should always be correlated with mammographic findings. Mammograms may show grouped microcalcifications, in associa-

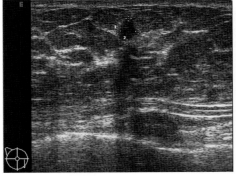 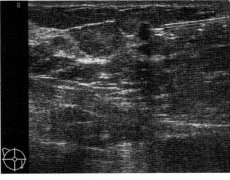

a, b

Fig. 6.26 a, b Ultrasound-guided aspiration of a fibrocystic nodule. Cytology revealed slight nuclear enlargement. Mild proliferation was suspected, and surgery was withheld. Follow-ups after 6, 12, and 24 months showed no change. Mammograms were also negative (13-MHz transducer).

❗ Comment:
Equivocal solid focal lesions or those with frankly suspicious mammographic or sonographic findings must be investigated. Percutaneous biopsy can provide a histological diagnosis in most cases.

Shape	Oval
Orientation	Not parallel
Margins	Indistinct
Lesion boundary	Echogenic halo
Echo pattern	Hypoechoic
Posterior acoustic features	Shadowing
Surrounding tissue	Architectural distortion
Calcifications	None
Vascularity	Adjacent to lesion

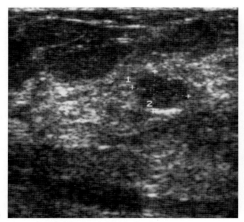
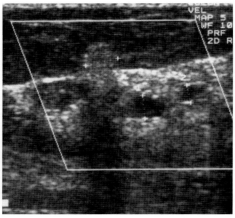

a, b

	(a)	(b)
Shape	Oval	Oval
Margins	Circum-scribed	Circum-scribed
Lesion boundary	Abrupt interface	Abrupt interface
Echo pattern	Hypoechoic	Hyperechoic
Posterior acoustic features	Enhanced	Attenuated
Surrounding tissue	No changes	Architectural distortion
Calcifica-tions	None	None
Vascularity	Not assessed	Not assessed

Fig. 6.27 a, b Suspicious ultrasound finding in sclerosing adenosis. A 49-year-old premeno-pausal women with a painful breast nodule was referred for mammography, which showed large patchy densities consistent with fibrocystic change (10-MHz transducer).
a Ultrasound scan through the upper outer quadrant of the right breast shows a hypoechoic, smoothly marginated nodule resembling a fibroadenoma.
b Farther laterally is a hypoechoic mass with an acoustic shadow. Fine-needle aspiration of both lesions revealed dyskaryosis and nuclear changes consistent with proliferative fibrocystic change. Following ultrasound localization, both lesions were excised. The lesion in **a** was identified as grade II fibrocystic change, the lesion in **b** as sclerosing adenosis.

 Comment:
In patients with mammograms that are not suspicious for malignancy, it is difficult to base the desicion to operate on sonographic findings. But if cytology raises suspicion of proliferative change or core biopsy shows atypia, surgery would be recommended.

tion with intraductal carcinoma. Although similar calcification patterns may be seen in benign proliferative disease, magnification mammography is important in patient selection. Stereotactic vacuum-assisted biopsy should be done whenever suspicious clustered microcalcifications are found if the calcifications are not recognized with ultrasound. If mammographic findings are not suspicious, the extent of sonographic changes will determine how best to proceed. There should be little hesitation in recommending ultrasound-guided core biopsy when it is felt that a lesion has more than a 2% likelihood of being malignant.

> Clustered microcalcifications seen on mammograms can often be demonstrated with ultrasound. This does not mean that ultrasound is as well suited for the primary workup or differentiation of calcifications. The role of ultrasound is to determine whether the microcalcifications correlate with a soft-tissue mass. Ultrasound can then be used as the imaging guide for biopsy. Mammography determines whether the particle and group morphology of the microcalcifications is suspicious.

Documentation

In Germany, where bilateral ultrasound breast surveys have been done for many years, the documentation of diffuse processes should include the central subareolar area and at least one peripheral scan from each breast. The central images cover most of the breast parenchyma and most accurately portray the extent of fibrosis and ductal changes. The fatty tissue component of the breast can be evaluated on both the central and peripheral scans. The interpretation is always based on the examination of both

breasts. Any conspicuous change should be documented and its location described. Because sound attenuation is an important factor in breasts with fibrocystic changes, appropriate labeling should be used to identify noncompression and compression scans. Every hypoechoic focal lesion should be documented in at least two and preferably four images, i.e., noncompression and compression views obtained in two mutually perpendicular planes (e.g., sagittal and transverse). This is important in assessing lesion compressibility, sound transmission, and spatial extent. Ductal abnormalities should be documented on radial scans to demonstrate variations in caliber. In patients with equivocal palpable or mammographic findings, the ultrasound appearance of these questionable areas should be described. Conversely, sonographic abnormalities should be compared with mammographic and physical findings to check for correlations (**Table 6.8**).

In the United States, protocols for screening the breasts with ultrasound are being developed, but there is as yet no universal acceptance.

> A dynamic examination with compression and supplemental radial scans is important in evaluating the ducts. It is essential to correlate the sonograms with palpable findings and with mammograms, especially when microcalcifications are present. This should be noted explicitly in the ultrasound report.

Table 6.8 Documentation of fibrocystic change

▸ Mammary ducts (radial scans)
▸ Central portion of breast parenchyma
▸ Peripheral scan
▸ Focal lesions documented on noncompression and compression scans in perpendicular planes
▸ Correlation with clinical and mammographic findings

Cysts and Intracystic Tumors

7

Clinical Significance

Breast cysts are usually the result of degenerative fibrocystic changes in the glandular breast tissue (**Table 7.1**). They are the most common palpable breast masses for which women seek medical attention (**Table 7.2**). In addition to fibrosis and intraductal proliferation, the pathogenesis involves an increase in secretory activity leading to fluid retention, ductal dilatation, and cyst formation. Cysts more than 2 mm in diameter are called *macrocysts* (**Fig. 7.1**), and those smaller than 2 mm are called *microcysts* (**Fig. 7.2**). Aspiration is warranted only in patients with clinical symptoms or suspected intracystic proliferation (**Table 7.3**).

Diagnostic Criteria

Simple Cysts

The correct interpretation of a sonogram often depends on the ultrasonographic technique, but when technique is optimal, most breast cysts can be confidently diagnosed (**Table 7.4**). The four criteria for diagnosis are round or oval shape, anechogenicity, circumscribed margins, and posterior acoustic enhancement (**Fig. 7.1**). Cysts do not augment sound transmission, although they may appear to do so; they merely attenuate the sound less than the solid surrounding tissues. Because the ultrasound system's time gain compensation (TGC) corrects for the attenuation of the tissues adjacent to the cyst, there is an apparent enhancement or brightening of echoes deep to the cyst.

The tangential incidence of the ultrasound beam on the smooth side walls of the cyst, along with the impedance mismatch between the cyst fluid and adjacent tissues, causes refractive effects that produce an edge shadow emanating from each side of the cyst.

With a low-frequency transducer (< 7 MHz) and poor lateral resolution, it can be difficult to confirm the sharp thin lateral walls of a simple cyst. Cysts may be solitary or multiple and may occur in one or both breasts (**Figs. 7.1–7.3 a–c**). They may be unilocular or have thin internal septations (**Fig. 7.4 a, b**). Numerous small cysts or microcysts may be closely aggregated in a bunch-of-grapes pattern (**Fig. 7.2**). Cysts often contain small calcifications, punctate echoes that fall to the dependent portion of cysts (**Fig. 7.5 a, b**). The surrounding breast parenchyma may show increased echogenicity and sound attenuation, correlating with fibrotic and chronic inflammatory changes. The increased density of the tissues surrounding a cyst may obscure it on mammograms.

Table 7.1 Causes of breast cysts

▸ Imbalance between secretion and reabsorption in the lactiferous ducts
▸ Duct obstruction with retained secretions due to stromal fibrosis or ductal proliferation, usually involving the terminal ducts and ductules
▸ Hormonal dysfunction as in fibrocystic change

Table 7.2 Clinical manifestations of cystic breast disease

Symptoms	Features
Pain	Usually focal
Firmness	Localized or diffuse with little cyclic variation
Nodules	Firm or rubbery, smooth, moderately mobile, occasionally painful, not always palpable, depending on size and consistency of surrounding tissues

Table 7.3 Treatment of breast cysts

▸ Simple cysts that are asymptomatic do not require treatment
▸ If a solid mass or inspissated material is suspected in a patient with focal pain or nodularity: percutaneous aspiration first followed by core biopsy if aspiration is ineffective
▸ With mural proliferation or an intracystic tumor (papilloma or carcinoma): ultrasound-guided core biopsy with placement of marker clip or excisional biopsy

Table 7.4 Criteria for the diagnosis of simple cysts

Shape	Oval or round
Orientation	Parallel
Margin	Circumscribed
Lesion boundary	Abrupt interface
Echo pattern	Anechoic
Posterior acoustic features	Enhancement
Surrounding tissue	No changes
Calcifications	Occasionally present
Vascularity	Not present *

* Assessment of vascularity not indicated.

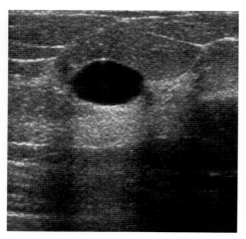

Shape	Oval
Size	11 mm diameter
Orientation	Parallel
Margin	Circumscribed
Lesion boundary	Abrupt interface
Echo pattern	Anechoic
Posterior acoustic features	Enhancement
Surrounding tissue	No changes
Calcifications	None
Vascularity	Not assessed

Fig. 7.1 Typical sonographic features of a cyst (13-MHz transducer).

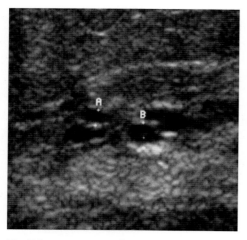

Shape	Oval
Orientation	Parallel
Margin	Circumscribed
Lesion boundary	Abrupt interface
Echo pattern	Anechoic
Posterior acoustic features	Enhancement
Surrounding tissue	No changes
Calcifications	None
Vascularity	Not assessed

Fig. 7.2 Microcystic disease. Magnified view of a 20 × 20-mm area (13-MHz transducer) demonstrates a focal lesion composed of several microcysts, each 1–2 mm in diameter.

Complicated Cysts

The diagnostic criteria for complicated cysts and complex cystic masses are summarized in **Table 7.5**.

Internal Echoes and Posterior Features

The high reflectivity of the anterior cyst wall often gives rise to *reverberations* (**Figs. 7.6 a, b; 7.7 a, b**), a band of echoes from the cyst wall that project into the interior of the cyst. These artifacts may be mistaken for solid areas of wall thickening. By moving the transducer and alternating compression and decompression, or by changing the angle of the transducer against the breast tissue or altering the patient's position somewhat, the examiner can cause the reverberations to shift their position within the cyst and confirm them as artifacts. In addition, reverberations can be reduced by lowering the gain or power settings. Because the focal zone setting represents the highest concentration of acoustic energy, shifting the focal zone to a deeper level may also diminish the reverberations.

Cysts occasionally contain low-level internal echoes if the cyst fluid is inspissated, if the fluid contains hemosiderin, or if the cellularity of the fluid is increased (**Fig. 7.8 a, b**). This type of cyst, a *complicated cyst* in BI-RADS nomenclature, may resemble a fibroadenoma, especially when a transducer of 10 MHz or higher frequency is used. If doubt exists, cyst/solid differentiation can be accomplished by ultrasound-guided aspiration (**Fig. 7.8 a, b**). Despite their internal echoes, these cysts usually show an enhanced pattern of sound transmission. The cyst contents may also cause sound attenuation, producing a posterior acoustic shadow that creates the impression of a suspicious solid mass (**Figs. 7.9 a, b; 7.10 a, b**). This effect is common in cysts that contain milk of calcium and inflammatory cysts. The shadowing is most conspicuous when a high-frequency transducer is used.

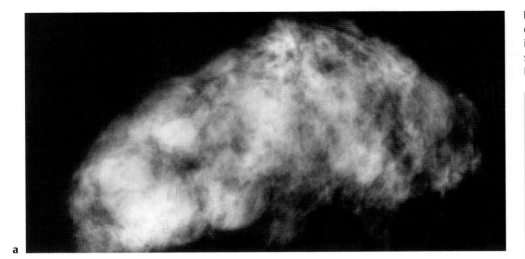

a

Fig. 7.3 a–c Macrocystic disease. **a** Mediolateral mammogram shows several rounded opacities in a dense breast. **b, c** Ultrasound reveals several macrocysts 4–20 mm in diameter (7.5-MHz transducer).

Shape	Oval
Orientation	Parallel
Margin	Circumscribed
Lesion boundary	Abrupt interface
Echo pattern	Anechoic
Posterior acoustic features	Enhancement
Surrounding tissue	No changes
Calcifications	None
Vascularity	Not assessed

! Comment:
The presence of multiple cysts does not signify increased proliferation. All focal lesions should be carefully examined, however, to ensure that solid tumors and subtle abnormalities are not missed. Mammography alone does not permit an adequate evaluation.

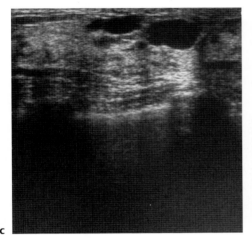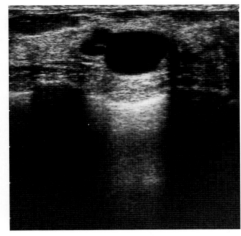

b, c

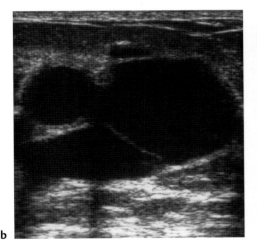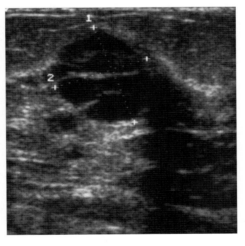

a, b

! Comment:
The large cysts (**a**) are clearly defined. The unilateral edge shadow (**b**) arises from a Cooper ligament that is oblique to the beam direction. Behind and to the left of the cyst is a smaller cyst (3 mm in diameter) cut off-center by the scanning plane. Because of this eccentricity, the cyst walls appears indistinct. Because of the multiple septa, the internal structure of the cyst is unclear (**b**). The fibrous changes in the surrounding tissue cause increased scattering and refraction, making it difficult to evaluate the septa and wall contours.

Fig. 7.4 a, b Cysts with multiple septations.
a Multiple septa within a cystic area 40 × 25 mm in size (7.5-MHz transducer).
b Two septa in a cyst measuring 16 × 17 mm.

Shape	Oval
Orientation	Parallel
Margin	Circumscribed
Lesion boundary	Abrupt interface
Echo pattern	Anechoic, septate
Posterior acoustic features	Enhancement
Surrounding tissue	No changes
Calcifications	None
Vascularity	Not assessed

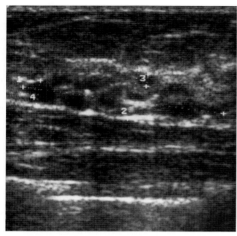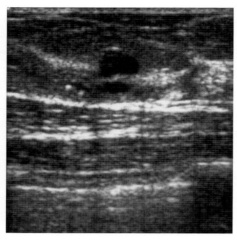

Shape	Oval
Orientation	Parallel
Margin	Circumscribed
Lesion boundary	Abrupt interface
Echo pattern	Anechoic
Posterior acoustic features	Enhancement
Surrounding tissue	No changes
Calcifications	Microcalcifications in mass
Vascularity	Not assessed

a, b

Fig. 7.5 a, b Microcystic lesions in a parenchymal area measuring 33 × 8 mm in the sagittal plane. The area contains multiple microcysts 1–4 mm in diameter (10-MHz transducer).

Because mammograms showed clustered pleomorphic microcalcifications, the lesion was excised. Histology revealed grade II fibrocystic change.

❗ Comment:
The scans show a somewhat lobular but circumscribed focal lesion composed of an aggregation of multiple microcysts. The axial orientation of the individual cysts and the overall complex is horizontal. There are several bright, punctate mural echoes that represent microcalcifications.

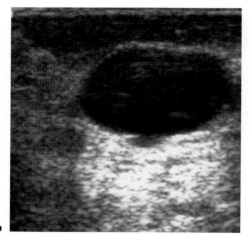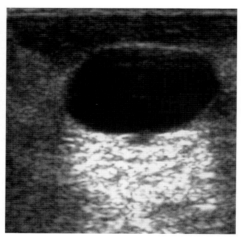

Shape	Oval
Orientation	Parallel
Margin	Circumscribed
Lesion boundary	Abrupt interface
Echo pattern	Anechoic
Posterior acoustic features	Enhancement
Surrounding tissue	No changes
Calcifications	None
Vascularity	Not assessed

a, b

Fig. 7.6 a, b Intracystic reverberations. **a** Focus in the near field at 7 mm, **b** Focus shifted 5 mm deeper (10-MHz transducer).

❗ Comment:
Focusing in the near field concentrates the sound energy in that region. Moving the focal zone distally diffuses the sound energy in the near field, reducing the intensity of the artifacts.

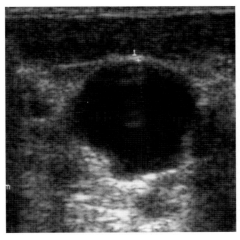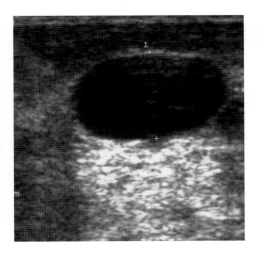

Shape	Oval
Orientation	Parallel (under compression)
Margin	Circumscribed
Lesion boundary	Abrupt interface
Echo pattern	Anechoic
Posterior acoustic features	Enhancement
Surrounding tissue	No changes
Calcifications	None
Vascularity	Not assessed

a, b

Fig. 7.7 a, b   Intracystic reverberations.
a Without compression, anteroposterior diameter 15 mm.
b Light compression with the transducer, anteroposterior diameter 11 mm (10-MHz transducer).

❗ Comment:
Reverberations appear under compression and in the noncompression scans. Real-time scanning with dynamic compression identifies the echoes as reverberations rather than intracystic structures. As pressure is applied and released, the echoes move up and down within the cyst as the transducer moves closer to and farther from the anterior cyst wall. As compression is increased, the layer of subcutaneous fat becomes thinner and the transducer moves closer to the cyst, causing the reverberations to appear closer together.

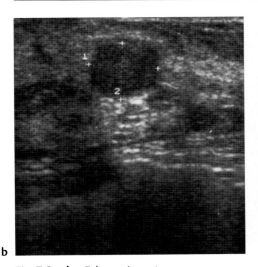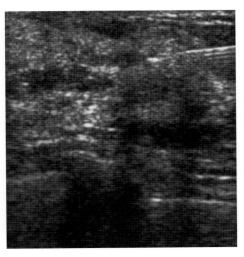

Shape	Oval
Orientation	Parallel
Margin	Circumscribed
Lesion boundary	Abrupt interface
Echo pattern	Hypoechoic
Posterior acoustic features	Enhancement
Surrounding tissue	No changes
Calcifications	None
Vascularity	Not present

a, b

Fig. 7.8 a, b   Echogenic cyst.
a Before aspiration.
b After aspiration, with the needle still in place (10-MHz transducer).

❗ Comment:
The ultrasonic image resembles a fibroadenoma. It cannot be classified as cystic or solid by its imaging features alone, and aspiration is necessary to exclude a solid, potentially proliferative tumor. Aspiration identified the lesion as an inspissated cyst.

 Aspiration can establish whether a lesion is cystic or solid and, in the case of a simple cyst, can avoid unnecessary surgery.

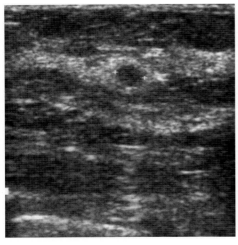 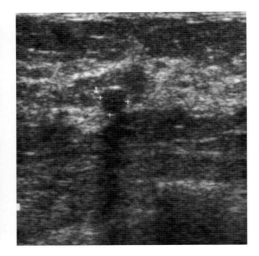

Shape	Round
Orientation	Not parallel
Margin	Circumscribed
Lesion boundary	Abrupt interface
Echo pattern	Hypoechoic
Posterior acoustic features	(a) none, (b) shadowing
Surrounding tissue	No changes
Calcifications	None
Vascularity	Not present

a, b

Fig. 7.9 a, b Hemosiderin-containing cyst.
a No shadowing or enhancement.
b Posterior acoustic shadow (10-MHz transducer).

⚠ Comment:
Screening mammograms in this 60-year-old woman showed two densities in the left breast. When ultrasound revealed internal echoes, the patient was hospitalized for surgery. Ultrasound-guided aspiration yielded hemosiderin-containing fluid with no evidence of proliferation.

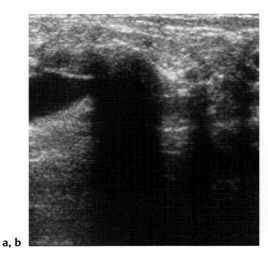 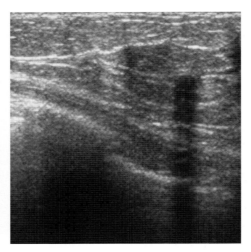

Shape	Oval
Orientation	–
Margin	Indistinct
Lesion boundary	Abrupt interface
Echo pattern	Hypoechoic
Posterior acoustic features	Shadowing
Surrounding tissue	Architectural distortion
Calcifications	None
Vascularity	Not present

a, b

Fig. 7.10 a, b Bilateral milk of calcium cysts with acoustic shadows.
a Upper outer quadrant of the right breast.
b Upper left breast (12-MHz transducer).

⚠ Comment:
The axial orientation of the lesions is indeterminate because of acoustic shadowing (only the horizontal dimension can be measured). Similarly, compressibility cannot be assessed because the posterior wall is not defined. The lack of sound transmission through the cysts makes it impossible to evaluate the surrounding structures, and so the architecture is uninterpretable.

 Sound absorption by the dense fluid gives rise to a suspicious ultrasound pattern, but aspiration promptly identified the lesions as cysts. If the mammograms were also suspicious, core biopsy or primary excision would have been indicated.

Table 7.5 Criteria for the diagnosis of complicated cysts and complex cystic masses

Shape	Oval, round or lobulated
Orientation	Parallel
Margin	Circumscribed
Lesion boundary	Abrupt interface
Echo pattern	Complicated: low-level internal echoes or fluid–fluid level Complex: cystic and solid components
Posterior acoustic features	Variable
Surrounding tissue	No changes
Calcifications	Microcalcifications may be present
Vascularity	Not present *

* Assessment of vascularity is not required if lesions show typical cystic characteristics and if proliferative changes are not suspected.

Fluid Levels and Oil Cysts

Fluid levels develop in cysts that contain liquids with different specific gravities (**Fig. 7.11**). Fluid levels often form when immiscible oily and watery fluid phases coexist in the same cyst. The oily phase, which is usually more echogenic, floats on top of the watery phase and creates a fluid–fluid level. This phenomenon is also seen in galactoceles, milk collections found in lactating women where the hyperechoic, high-fat cream layer is found anteriorly while the anechoic, watery component of milk occupies the deeper portion of the cystic lesion. When the patient is moved from the supine to a sitting position, the level will gradually shift in response to gravity. A layering effect also occurs when cyst fluid becomes inspissated and the more echogenic material settles to the cyst floor.

When the cysts contain only liquefied fat or oil (fat necrosis), the mass may appear anechoic or hypoechoic, and either posterior enhancement or shadowing may be associated with it. The clinical history of accidental or surgical trauma may support the diagnosis and correlating the sonographic finding with a circumscribed radiolucent mammographic mass will establish the benign etiology without need for intervention.

Clustered Microcysts

Multiple microcysts that are aggregated in a cluster may form a palpable mass with indistinct margins that is difficult to evaluate clinically. An area of increased soft tissue density, at times partially circumscribed, may be the only mammographic manifestation. The tiny individual cystic components are poorly resolved, and only an ill-defined hypoechoic mass may be seen using lower-frequency transducers or ultrasound systems of poor quality. High-resolution scanners can usually define the individual microcysts that comprise the lesion (see **Fig. 7.2**). Occasionally, these microcysts, dilated lobular acini, contain small, bright, punctate mural echoes that correlate with microcalcifications (see **Fig. 7.5 a, b**). Ultrasound is not a suitable modality for the primary detection of microcalcifications, but once microcalcifications have been identified on mammograms, ultrasound can help identify their source when they are located in microcysts. These microcystic conglomerations should be carefully interrogated sonographically to identify or exclude a solid component. If there is no solid component, clustered microcysts can be considered probably benign with two initial short interval follow-up visits (commonly at 6-month intervals) with annual follow-ups thereafter.

If a solid component is found, ultrasound should be used to guide core biopsy. If proliferative changes or atypical cells are reported from fine-needle aspiration cytology, core biopsy or excision of the lesion would be the next step.

The microcalcifications associated with microcysts are rounded, punctuate, and adenosic. If mammograms reveal pleomorphic or dot-dash microcalcifications suggestive of malignancy in an area where benign-appearing microcysts are found with ultrasound, the higher level of suspicion for malignancy associated with the microcalcifications will override the microcystic lesion's benign assessment. The microcalcifications will require a histologic diagnosis, most commonly obtained with stereotactic guidance.

Complex Cystic Masses

Intracystic Papillomas and Cyst Wall Proliferation

Ultrasound is ideally suited for its ability to evaluate intracystic structures and cyst walls (**Figs. 7.12, 7.13**). Thus, a thorough examination requires that every cyst be imaged in real-time in at least

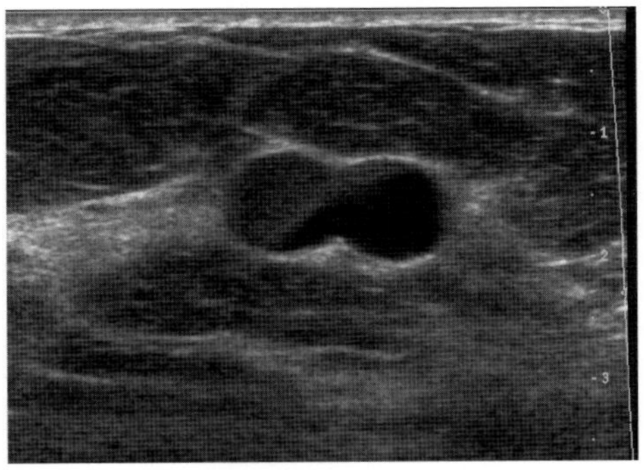

Fig. 7.11 Oil cyst with a fluid level between the aqueous and oily phases (12-MHz transducer).

Shape	Oval
Orientation	Parallel
Margin	Circumscribed
Lesion boundary	Abrupt interface
Echogenicity	Hypoechoic/anechoic
Posterior acoustic features	Enhancement
Surrounding tissue	No changes
Calcifications	None
Vascularity	Not assessed

❗ Comment:
Inspissated, hemosiderin-containing, fatty or cellular cyst fluid is more echogenic than water. Because fat is lighter than water and is immiscible with it, a fluid–fluid level is formed. Aspiration yielded a fatty, viscous fluid with no signs of proliferation.

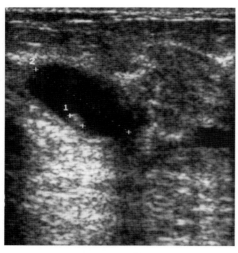

Shape	Oval
Orientation	Parallel
Margin	Circumscribed
Lesion boundary	Abrupt interface
Echo pattern	Anechoic/hyperechoic
Posterior acoustic features	Enhancement
Surrounding tissue	No changes
Calcifications	None
Vascularity	Present in lesion

■ Comment:
A small papilloma is visible at the base of the smooth marginated cyst. One single vessel with low flow velocity could be detected by color Doppler (see **Fig. 19.5**). The cyst casts an unilateral edge shadow, but the dominant effect is posterior acoustic enhancement.

▶ If core biopsy is done for histologic diagnosis, a marker clip should be placed with US guidance immediately after the biopsy so that the tumor can be localized if surgical excision is planned.

Fig. 7.12 Intracystic papilloma (10-MHz transducer).

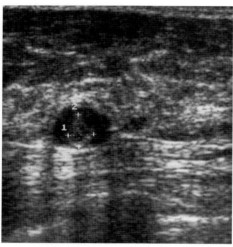

Shape	Oval
Orientation	Cyst parallel, papilloma not parallel
Margin	Circumscribed
Lesion boundary	Abrupt interface
Echo pattern	Anechoic/hyperechoic
Posterior acoustic features	Enhancement
Surrounding tissue	No changes
Calcifications	None
Vascularity	Not present

■ Comment:
This type of lesion may require excisional biopsy, even with a negative cytologic analysis.

Fig. 7.13 Intracystic papilloma (10-MHz transducer).

two perpendicular planes so that the curved cyst walls can be assessed completely (**Fig. 7.14**). Solid intracystic vegetations and focal wall thickening should be distinguished from debris and artifacts to ensure that an intracystic papilloma or carcinoma is not missed (**Fig. 7.15**). Color-flow Doppler or power Doppler depiction of blood flow within an intracystic nodule is confirmatory of a solid mass and useful to exclude artifact or intracystic detritus.

Until recently, if cyst wall proliferation or intracystic papilloma was suspected, surgical excision for diagnosis was the recommendation. Percutaneous aspiration was contraindicated due to difficulty of locating the lesion after the cyst fluid has been drained.

Currently, there are many marker clips available for placement with ultrasound guidance, and after a small amount of fluid has been aspirated from a large cyst, the intracystic mass can be examined by ultrasound-guided core biopsy. At the completion of the procedure, the marker clip can be placed, and its location at the site of biopsy confirmed on craniocaudal and 90° lateral mammograms. For papillomas, vacuum-assisted and single-speci-men basketing-type biopsy devices guided by ultrasound have been employed for removal of the lesion.

Juvenile Cysts

During menarche and the initial years of breast development, the mammary ducts arborize and elongate in a process that starts in the nipple area and proceeds deeper into the breast. During this time, abnormalities of ductal development or a transient increase in secretory activity will often cause palpable nodules to form in the nipple region. These nodules are often painful and may be associated with inflammation. Ultrasound in these cases demonstrates retro- or periareolar anechoic cysts (**Fig. 7.16**). Low-level internal echoes are occasionally seen due to inspissated secretions. Sedimentation of the inspissated cyst contents may cause a fluid–fluid level to form, separating the cyst's contents into two layers of different echogenicity (**Figs. 7.17, 7.18 a, b**).

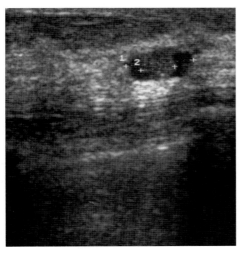

Shape	Oval
Orientation	Parallel
Margin	Circumscribed
Lesion boundary	Circumscribed
Echo pattern	Anechoic/hyperechoic
Posterior acoustic features	Enhancement
Surrounding tissue	No changes
Calcifications	None
Vascularity	Not present

! Comment:
This lesion, like all focal lesions, should be documented in at least two perpendicular planes so that the walls of the cyst and intracystic tumor can be accurately evaluated.

Fig. 7.14 Intracystic papilloma (10-MHz transducer)

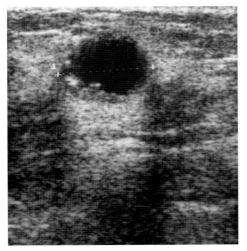

Shape	Oval
Orientation	Parallel
Margin	Outer wall circumscribed, inner wall microlobulated
Lesion boundary	Echogenic halo
Echo pattern	Anechoic/Hyperechoic
Posterior acoustic features	Enhancement
Surrounding tissue	No changes
Calcifications	Microcalcifications in lesion
Vascularity	Present immediately adjacent to lesion

! Comment:
The lesion has the external features of a smoothly marginated cyst, but there is irregular thickening of the inner cyst wall.

 The walls of a cyst should always be evaluated, even if the initial impression is of only a "simple" cyst.

Fig. 7.15 Intracystic carcinoma (10-MHz transducer)

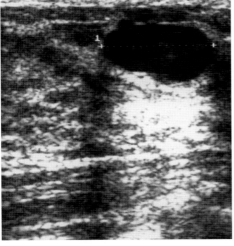

Shape	Oval
Orientation	Parallel
Margin	Circumscribed
Lesion boundary	Abrupt interface
Echo pattern	Anechoic (faint reverberations)
Posterior acoustic features	Enhancement
Surrounding tissue	No changes
Calcifications	None
Vascularity	Not assessed

! Comment:
Treatment is not required in most cases. The patient should be reassured that the lesion is harmless.

 Follow-up should precede invasive procedures. Aspiration would be indicated only in patients with severe symptoms or inflammation.

Fig. 7.16 Juvenile cyst in a 14-year-old girl with unilateral painful nodularity in the subareolar region of the left breast (10-MHz transducer).

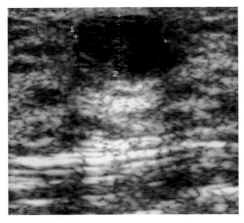

Shape	Oval
Orientation	Parallel
Margin	Circumscribed
Lesion boundary	Abrupt interface
Echo pattern	Anechoic, hypoechoic, 2 fluid phases
Posterior acoustic features	Enhancement
Surrounding tissue	No changes
Calcifications	None
Vascularity	Not assessed

◼ Comment:
This cyst contains two different fluid phases separated by an interface. The echogenic fluid is uppermost, so presumably it is lipomatous. There were no clinical signs of inflammation, and the lesion resolved spontaneously without percutaneous aspiration.

Fig. 7.17 Juvenile cyst with a fluid–fluid level (10-MHz transducer).

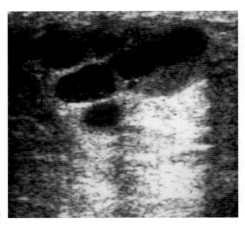 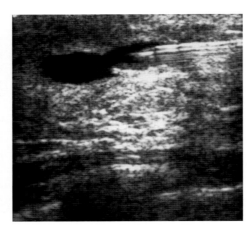

Shape	Oval
Orientation	Parallel
Margin	Circumscribed
Lesion boundary	Abrupt interface
Echo pattern	Anechoic, hypoechoic, 2 fluid phases
Posterior acoustic features	Enhancement
Surrounding tissue	No changes
Calcifications	None
Vascularity	Present immediately adjacent to lesion

a, b

Fig. 7.18 a, b Inflammatory aggregation of juvenile cysts with fluid levels.
a Sagittal scan prior to aspiration.
b Scan during the aspiration, with the needle in place.

◼ Comment:
The inflammation in this case definitely warrants aspiration. The purulent material forms a layer of sediment at the base of the cysts. Aspiration cytology can detect inflammatory cells and exclude proliferative changes. Bacteriologic analysis is also indicated, and antibiotic susceptibility testing may also be done.

Differential Diagnosis, Pitfalls

Echogenic Cysts Versus Solid Tumors

As described above, the properties of the cyst fluid may cause the cyst to resemble a homogeneous solid tumor (**Fig. 7.19 a, b**). This is not a serious problem, however, because benign-appearing solid tumors, typically fibroadenomas, can in any case be differentiated from fluid-containing lesions by aspiration. In addition, masses that are probably benign based on BI-RADS feature analysis (circumscribed, oval masses, long axis oriented parallel to the skin) may be managed by short interval follow-up.

If an intervention is planned for definitive diagnosis of these cysts vs. solid masses, aspiration should be attempted to ascertain whether or not the lesion is fluid-containing before a core biopsy is done. Aspiration cytology can also provide the diagnosis of some solid lesions, "naked nuclei" as the hallmark of fibroadenomas, for example.

Fluid Levels

Unless the mammographic appearance is definitive, aspiration is the method of choice even for oil cysts with fluid–fluid levels, because cytologic analysis can simultaneously exclude intracystic proliferation. Because cysts are often multiple and are a common

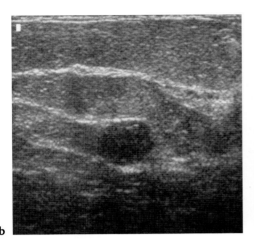
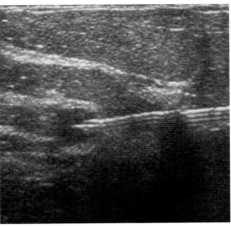

Shape	Oval
Orientation	Parallel
Margin	Circumscribed
Lesion boundary	Abrupt interface
Echo pattern	Hypoechoic
Posterior acoustic features	None
Surrounding tissue	No changes
Calcifications	None
Vascularity	Not present

! Comment:
Sonographic and mammographic findings are inconclusive for cystic/solid differentiation. Ultrasound-guided aspiration identified the lesion as a nonproliferative inspissated cyst.

a, b

Fig. 7.19 a, b Echogenic, solid-appearing cyst **a** before and **b** during aspiration (12-MHz transducer).

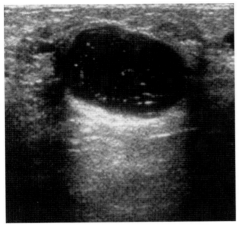

Shape	Oval
Orientation	Parallel
Margin	Circumscribed
Lesion boundary	Abrupt interface
Echo pattern	Hypoechoic (with moving echoes)
Posterior acoustic features	None
Surrounding tissue	No changes
Calcifications	None
Vascularity	Not assessed

! Comment:
This case illustrates another technique for identifying inspissated cyst fluid and distinguishing it from solid components. Shaking movements of the transducer or palpating finger can mobilize the inspissated particles and cause them to float around in the cyst fluid.

Fig. 7.20 Inspissated cyst fluid. The inspissated particles were mobilized by external manipulation (12-MHz transducer).

diagnosis, a meticulous examination is of prime importance. A shaking movement of the transducer or palpating finger will often help to distinguish inspissated cyst fluid from solid material (**Fig. 7.20**). This maneuver imparts a swirling motion to the inspissated particles that can be observed in the real-time image. Power Doppler at high intensity may also bring about motion of intracystic particles.

Reverberations

True internal echoes must be distinguished from the reverberation artifacts described above. This is done by watching for movement of the internal echoes in response to varying compression of the breast (see **Fig. 7.7a, b**) and by changing the focal depth of the transducer or switching from multiple to single focusing.

Malignant Tumors

It is as important to detect an intracystic tumor as any other focal lesion. Intracystic papillomas should be excised because they cannot be confidently distinguished from the less common intracystic carcinoma (**Fig. 7.21**). Carcinomas, moreover, may arise in proximity to cysts (**Fig. 7.22 a, b**) or in other breast regions (**Fig. 7.23 a–d**), and cystic structures may develop within carcinomas as a result of secretion, duct obstruction, or necrotic degeneration (**Fig. 7.24**).

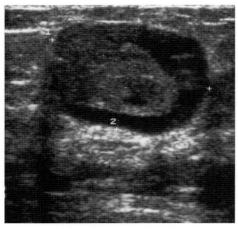

Shape	Oval
Orientation	Parallel
Margin	Circumscribed
Lesion boundary	Abrupt interface
Echo pattern	Anechoic/Hypoechoic
Posterior acoustic features	Enhancement
Surrounding tissue	No changes
Calcifications	None
Vascularity	Present in lesion

! Comment:
Every cyst should be carefully evaluated in two planes so that solid intracystic tumors are not missed.

Fig. 7.21 Intracystic carcinoma in a patient with known fibrocystic change, neglected for years (10-MHz transducer).

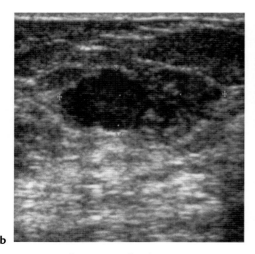 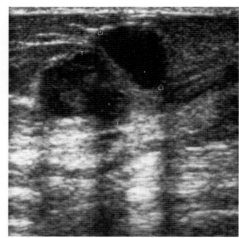

a, b

Shape	Oval
Orientation	Parallel
Margin	Microlobulated
Lesion boundary	Abrupt interface
Echo pattern	Anechoic/hypoechoic
Posterior acoustic features	Enhancement
Surrounding tissue	Architectural distortion
Calcifications	None
Vascularity	Present immediately adjacent to lesion

Fig. 7.22 a, b Cyst with adjacent carcinoma, neglected for years.
a Sagittal.
b Transverse (7.5-MHz transducer).

! Comment:
The area surrounding a cyst should also be scrutinized. The conspicuous cyst should not divert attention from a detailed analysis of the adjacent parenchyma.

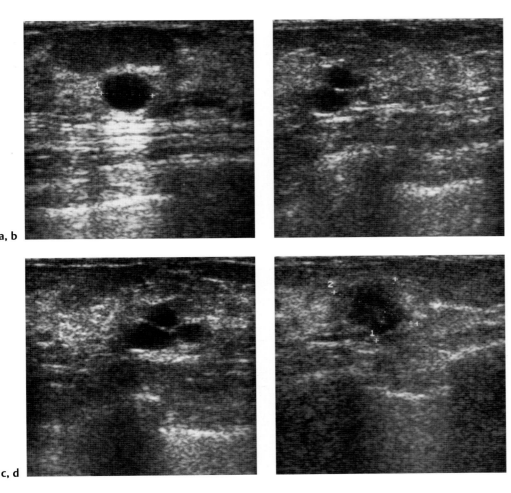

a, b

c, d

Fig. 7.23 a–d Invasive carcinoma in a setting of cystic breast disease. The scans show solitary and clustered simple cysts at various sites in the left breast (**a–c**). A carcinoma 15 × 11 mm in size is detectable at one site (**d**).

	Cysts	Tumor
Shape	Oval	Irregular
Orientation	Parallel	Not parallel
Margin	Circum-scribed	Angulated
Lesion boundary	Abrupt interface	Echogenic halo
Echo pattern	Anechoic	Hypo-echoic
Posterior acous-tic features	Enhance-ment	None
Surrounding tissue	No changes	Architec-tural dis-tortion
Calcifications	None	None
Vascularity	Not assessed	Present immedi-ately ad-jacent to lesion

❗ Comment:
It is all too easy for the sonologist to rely on negative mammograms. But cystic breast changes make mammograms difficult to interpret, and the transparency of these breasts to ultrasound should be utilized to detect nonpalpable and mammographically occult tumors.

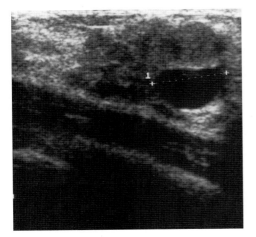

Fig. 7.24 Invasive carcinoma with a cystic internal structure (10-MHz transducer).

Shape	Oval
Orientation	Parallel
Margin	Circumscribed
Lesion boundary	Abrupt interface
Echo pattern	Anechoic/hypoechoic
Posterior acous-tic features	Shadowing (slight)
Surrounding tissue	Architectural distor-tion
Calcifications	None
Vascularity	Present immediately adjacent to lesion

❗ Comment:
Because the cyst is more conspicuous than the adjacent solid tumor, the latter is easily over-looked.

Case 1

A 40-year-old woman with a positive family history of breast cancer detected a lump in her left breast and consulted a gynecologist. Palpation revealed a smooth, rubbery nodule consistent with cystic breast disease. Mammography showed a rounded mass with smooth margins. The same mass had been seen on films taken 2 years before, but on this occasion clustered pleomorphic microcalcifications were also found directly adjacent to the mass. The patient was referred for breast ultrasound, which showed an ill-defined infiltrative tumor lining the entire cyst wall. Doppler scanning registered high flow velocities in that portion of the tumor (**Fig. 7.25 a–c**). Histopathology of core biopsies of the mural mass as well as the adjacent microcalcifications was invasive ductal carcinoma and ductal carcinoma in situ.

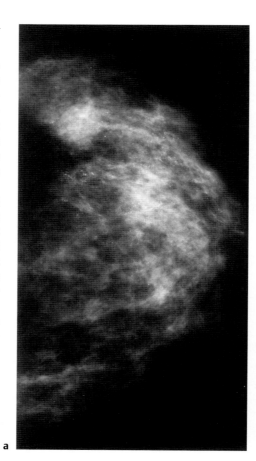

a

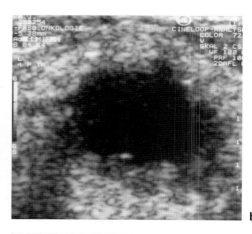

b

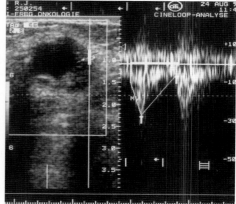

c

Fig. 7.25 Intracystic breast carcinoma in a 40-year-old woman.
a The mammogram shows a smoothly marginated round lesion and microcalcifications in the surrounding parenchyma.
b B-mode ultrasound.
c Color Doppler and duplex (triple mode). Flow analysis indicates high flow velocity of 27 cm/s (10-MHz transducer).

Shape	Oval
Orientation	Parallel
Margin	Microlobulated
Lesion boundary	Abrupt interface
Echo pattern	Anechoic/hypoechoic
Posterior acoustic features	Enhancement
Surrounding tissue	Architectural distortion
Calcifications	Microcalcifications present in lesion
Vascularity	Present immediately adjacent to lesion

█ Comment:
When the family history is positive, as in this case, special care should be taken in carrying out the ultrasound examination. Experience shows that high-risk patients often have pronounced fibrocystic changes. But these changes are also associated with an increased risk of breast cancer, emphasizing the importance of a thorough and meticulous breast examination.

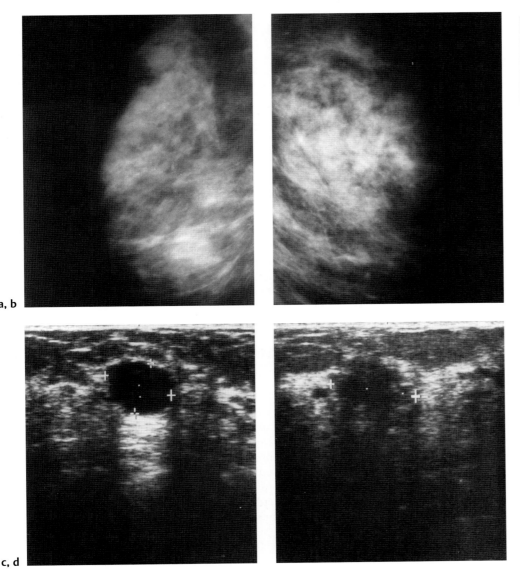

a, b

c, d

Fig. 7.26 a–d Cystic breast disease and multifocal breast carcinoma in a 50-year-old woman. Annual mammograms consistently revealed large round lesions with smooth outlines. Ultrasound now shows several cysts of varying size and a large, invasive tumor mass surrounded by multiple smaller foci. **a, b** Left and right mammograms, mediolateral views. Ultrasound demonstrates a large cyst in **c** and a large invasive tumor in **d** (7.5-MHz transducer).

Screening mammograms were obtained in a 50-year-old woman with a positive family history and no clinical abnormalities. Mammograms taken 1 year earlier had shown no abnormalities other than cystic breast changes. Findings on current mammograms were unchanged relative to prior films: multiple bilateral patchy densities, some rounded, with no spiculated masses or microcalcifications. An ultrasound examination showed multiple cysts in both breasts as well as an unsuspected 2.5-cm mass with irregular, ill-defined margins, posterior acoustic shadowing, and satellite nodules (**Fig. 7.26 a–d**). Histology identified the lesion as multifocal invasive ductal carcinoma (pT2). Axillary metastases were found in 12 of 40 lymph nodes.

▶ The conspicuity of cysts should not divert attention from detecting other coexisting lesions.

❗ Comment:
This case again illustrates that ultrasound is important in cystic breast disease for lesion characterization and is superior to mammography in the differentiation of soft-tissue changes.

	Cyst	Tumor
Shape	Oval	Irregular
Orientation	Parallel	Parallel
Margin	Circumscribed	Ill-defined
Lesion boundary	Abrupt interface	Abrupt interface
Echo pattern	Anechoic	Hypoechoic
Posterior acoustic features	Enhancement	Shadowing
Surrounding tissue	No changes	Architectural distortion
Calcifications	None	None
Vascularity	Not assessed	Present immediately adjacent to lesion

Case 3

A 12-year-old girl found a nodule in her left breast. Mammography showed an ill-defined subareolar density. A surgeon elected to excise the nodule, but because the nodule represented the developing breast bud, the surgery was tantamount to a mastectomy. The patient will have little or no breast development on the operated side. Two years later, her family doctor found a similar nodule on the right side and referred the patient for surgery, but an ultrasound examination was first carried out. On the basis of clinical and ultrasound findings of a cyst, we were able to reassure the girl and her worried mother (**Fig. 7.27**). Follow-up at several months showed spontaneous regression of the nodule.

This case illustrates how juvenile breast cysts, lack of imaging, and little understanding of pediatric and adolescent physiology can lead to inappropriate treatment. At birth and in early adolescence a subareolar "breast mass" may develop in response to circulating hormones and if it is removed, no breast will develop on that side. Ultrasound can usually establish the nature of the nodular lesions. In most cases it is sufficient to reassure the patient and her parents that these nodules are harmless.

A wait-and-see approach is advised, since many nodules will regress spontaneously within a few months. Aspiration is warranted only in patients who have severe pain. In rare cases, retained secretions can lead to inflammation. Most of these cases respond poorly to antibiotics alone because of the persistence of microorganisms in the secretions. The treatment of choice is ultrasound-guided aspiration followed by cytologic and bacteriologic analysis. The patient should also be treated with an antibiotic that is active against staphylococci. Treatment can be supported with a low-dose regimen of anti-inflammatory agents and dopamine agonists. Managed in this way, most cases of nonpuerperal mastitis will resolve without percutaneous or surgical intervention.

Interventional Procedures

Aspiration

Simple anechoic cysts with smooth margins do not require further investigation. If cysts are painful or present as a firm palpable mass that is distressing for the patient, they should be aspirated. If proliferative changes are suspected, or with an inspissated cyst that resembles a solid mass, it should be aspirated to establish a diagnosis. It may also be appropriate to aspirate larger cysts in an extremely dense or heterogeneously dense breast so that the breast can be more accurately evaluated by mammography.

Negative aspiration cytology may not be relied upon to exclude a significant abnormality, and if there is sonographic evidence of a solid mural intracystic component or mass, aspiration may be withheld in favor of excisional biopsy in practices where experience in percutaneous ultrasound-guided interventional procedures is limited. If a percutaneous core biopsy procedure is undertaken, a marker clip should be placed with ultrasound guidance immediately upon completion of the biopsy so that when excision is required, as it would be with an atypical papilloma or papillary carcinoma, the mass can be accurately localized preoperatively.

Pneumocystography

In years past, when ultrasound was little used in breast imaging, pneumocystography was frequently used in the investigation of palpable masses identified on mammograms. The principle was to aspirate the suspected cyst, fill the evacuated cavity with air, and then film the area to define the contours of the cyst wall (not possible mammographically without air insufflation). This decrease in localized breast density also made it easier to evaluate

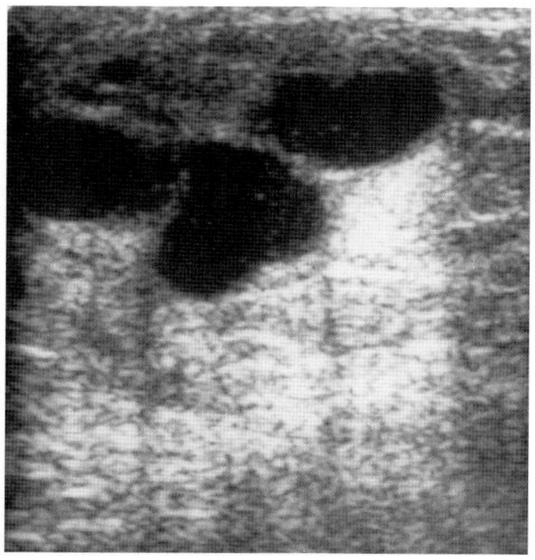

Fig. 7.27 Subareolar juvenile cysts in the right breast of a 14-year-old girl who underwent mastectomy at age 12 for similar lesions in the left breast (10-MHz transducer).

Shape	Oval
Orientation	Parallel
Margin	Circumscribed
Lesion boundary	Abrupt interface
Echo pattern	Anechoic
Posterior acoustic features	Enhancement
Surrounding tissue	No changes
Calcifications	None
Vascularity	Not assessed

! Comment:
This case serves as a cautionary example that cystic changes should be considered in the differential diagnosis of adolescent breast disease (p. 106).

other breast areas. Thus, pneumocystography was used diagnostically to allow the mammographic confirmation of cysts. It has also been proposed but not confirmed that pneumocytography may have therapeutic value, based on a theory that instilling air in a cyst could dry out the cyst wall and reduce the likelihood that the cyst would refill. Ultrasound is so reliable in the characterization and diagnosis of cysts, however, that pneumocystography, with its additional radiation, is no longer needed.

Role of Ultrasound

The advantage of ultrasound is that it is generally successful in differentiating cystic and solid masses. Mammography alone may be limited in detecting the presence of cysts and solid masses, because many patients with cystic breasts have radiographically dense breasts. Cysts in involuted breasts are clearly visible on mammograms, where they appear as light gray or white circumscribed masses against a background of dark gray fatty tissue. Nevertheless, ultrasound is still required for characterization of these masses.

In recent decades, the use of ultrasound has changed the management of breast masses. At one time surgery was routinely recommended for palpable breast cysts that presented as mammographic densities. In the 1970 s, before the advent of breast ultrasound, a triple diagnostic approach based on palpation, mammography, and aspiration cytology was widely practiced. However, many cysts were incompletely drained by manually guided needle aspiration, and often these lesions soon refilled with fluid. Faulty placement of the aspirating needle was also a common problem when manual guidance was used. Failure to aspirate fluid prompted a recommendation for excisional biopsy, since an unsuccessful aspiration could not exclude a solid tumor or intracystic carcinoma. Some practices, citing the economy of using the same intervention for diagnosis and therapy, will still attempt to aspirate a palpable mass prior to any imaging.

Intracystic hemorrhage is a common problem in patients who are referred for breast ultrasound following an unsuccessful aspiration. Because of the postprocedural hematoma, what was originally a simple cyst will frequently appear on ultrasound as a complex cystic or solid heterogeneous mass with indistinct margins. For this reason, breast ultrasound should be done before any interventional procedure, and since ultrasound permits the reliable diagnosis of simple cysts, commonly there will be no need to proceed with aspiration. If aspiration is necessary based on ultrasound findings or for clinical reasons, ultrasound-guided aspiration is more reliable than manual guidance. This strategy will obviate the need for many additional invasive procedures.

Documentation

Cysts, like all masses, should be scanned in at least two perpendicular planes to ensure the detection of proliferative wall changes and intracystic masses. When multiple cysts are present, it may not be feasible to document or measure each one individually. It is important, however, to list the locations of the lesions or record them on a line drawing, measuring the dimensions of the largest and most conspicuous lesions, and documenting these lesions on hard-copy images or PACS. Dilated or beaded mammary ducts should be imaged on radial scans to document caliber changes along the course of the ducts. Clock-face notation should be used to record the location of the ducts, and the labeling for cysts and other masses should include their distance in centimeters from the nipple.

Breast Implants 8

Clinical Significance

Breast implants are used for cosmetic augmentation or for breast reconstruction after mastectomy (**Tables 8.1, 8.2**). There are many different types of breast prostheses, each purporting to minimize complications such as fibrous encapsulation or rupture (**Table 8.3**). For imaging purposes, most of these may be regarded as large artificial cysts filled with either silicone gel or saline. Because implants strongly absorb X-rays, the surrounding breast tissue is compressed and difficult to evaluate with mammography until implant displacement techniques reported by G.W. Eklund in 1988 became widely adopted as the standard of care for radiographing augmented breasts (**Figs. 8.1, 8.2**).

Recognition of some of the limitations of X-ray mammography combined with the fear, most often unfounded, of causing implant rupture, led to other techniques being sought for breast cancer screening and the detection of rupture of silicone implants. MRI is currently acknowledged as the most sensitive imaging technique for confirming or excluding both intra- and extracapsular rupture in patients with breast implants (**Fig. 8.3**). However, the sequences

Table 8.1 Indications for breast implants

▸ Augmentation of hypoplastic breasts
▸ Cosmetic breast enlargement
▸ Symmetrization of unequal breasts
▸ Postmastectomy reconstruction
▸ Inlays for replacement of tissue defects

Table 8.2 Sites of implant placement

▸ Subglandular, prepectoral
▸ Subpectoral, submuscular
▸ Prepectoral (subcutaneous), subglandular
▸ Intramammary (inlays)

Table 8.3 Types of breast implants

▸ Smooth-walled silicone implants
▸ Polyurethane-coated or textured silicone implants
▸ Free silicone injection (obsolete)
▸ Saline-filled implants
▸ Expanders (for postmastectomy reconstruction)
▸ Autologous tissue (myocutaneous transfers)
▸ Heterologous tissue (fat allograft)

Fig. 8.1 Mammogram of a silicone breast implant used for primary reconstruction after mastectomy.

❗ Comment:
The implant absorbs X-rays, and consequently the tissue cannot be evaluated.

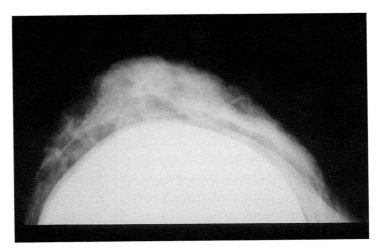

Fig. 8.2 Mammogram following breast augmentation with a silicone implant. This view was obtained by extending as much breast tissue as possible between the compression plates while pushing the implant back against the chest wall. Some of the breast tissue is visible, but a portion is obscured.

❗ Comment:
The implant-displaced view can improve mammographic imaging of the breast, but the implant still obscures some of the breast parenchyma.

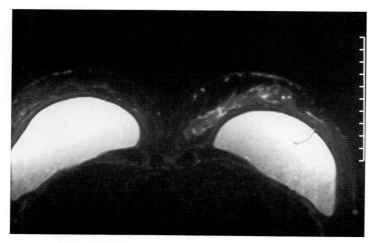

MRI is more sensitive than mammography in detecting breast parenchymal abnormalities in women with silicone breast implants, but MRI is a more technically demanding and costly procedure that requires intravenous administration of contrast material. Its sensitivity is high, but false positives are common.

Fig. 8.3 MRI scan following bilateral augmentation with silicone implants.

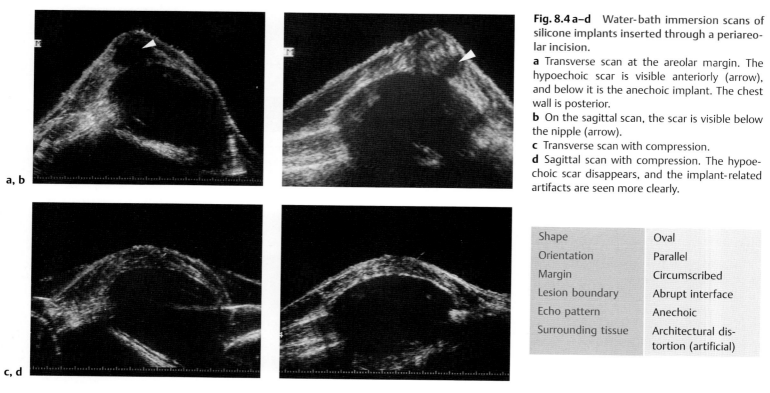

a, b

c, d

Fig. 8.4 a–d Water-bath immersion scans of silicone implants inserted through a periareolar incision.
a Transverse scan at the areolar margin. The hypoechoic scar is visible anteriorly (arrow), and below it is the anechoic implant. The chest wall is posterior.
b On the sagittal scan, the scar is visible below the nipple (arrow).
c Transverse scan with compression.
d Sagittal scan with compression. The hypoechoic scar disappears, and the implant-related artifacts are seen more clearly.

Shape	Oval
Orientation	Parallel
Margin	Circumscribed
Lesion boundary	Abrupt interface
Echo pattern	Anechoic
Surrounding tissue	Architectural distortion (artificial)

! Comment:
Two findings are noteworthy. The hypoechoic scar mimics a mass but disappears when compression is applied and is therefore not further described as a lesion. The implant appears as a large cystic structure that causes image distortion along the chest wall. This is common with silicone implants.

used for MRI evaluation of possible rupture are carried out without the injection of gadolinium contrast agents, and they are therefore unsuitable and inadequate for breast cancer detection. With the 1992 restrictions on silicone implants recently being relaxed by the United States Food and Drug Administration (FDA), there is interest in broadening utilization of MRI techniques so that breast cancer screening as well as diagnosis of rupture might be accomplished at the same examination. In general, the cost of MRI and the requirement for an intravenously administered contrast agent are deterrents to using MRI for screening women whose risk of breast cancer is average and for whom mammography may or may not be significantly reduced in sensitivity.

Breast ultrasound provides an important option, particularly for detecting rupture of silicone implants through the fibrous capsule or lymph nodal uptake of gel bleed, the ooze of silicone gel through micropores of the silicone polymer envelopes. Familiarity with the

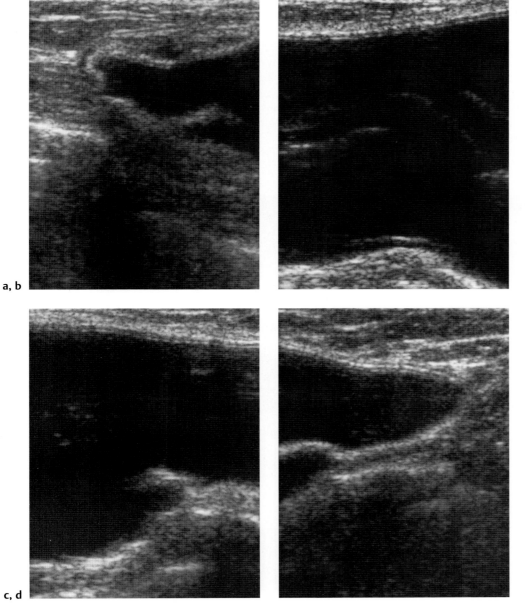

a, b

c, d

Fig. 8.5 a–d Real-time sagittal scans of a silicone implant. **a** Superior extension of breast. **b, c** Center of breast. **d** Inferior extension. Because of the small field of view, multiple scans are needed to cover the whole implant. Again, reverberations and projection artifacts are seen.

Shape	Oval
Orientation	Parallel
Margin	Circumscribed
Lesion boundary	Abrupt interface
Echo pattern	Anechoic
Surrounding tissue	Architectural distortion (artificial)

⚠ Comment:
The real-time transducer provides better acoustic coupling at the periphery of the breast. The field of view is small, but sharper lateral definition is obtained.

ultrasound findings, which may be confusing initially, will help to increase specificity in attributing the origin of a mass or other ultrasound abnormality to an implant-related phenomenon or to the breast tissue itself. Water-immersion images, which provide a broader perspective, and real-time scanning examples, can familiarize the ultrasound practitioner with the variety of sonographic manifestations. (**Figs. 8.4 a–d, 8.5 a–d**).

Sonographic Findings

Breast implants resemble large cysts and do not significantly attenuate ultrasound (**Table 8.4**). As in other types of examination, the instrument settings should be adjusted to eliminate reverberations and optimize image quality. It is particularly important to achieve complete breast coverage by scanning in contiguous planes. Silicone-filled implants transmit sound at a lower sound velocity than aqueous cysts or tissue, resulting in distortion of the ultrasound image and causing the implant to appear larger in an anterior–posterior dimension than its actual size (**Fig. 8.4 a–d**). This effect, the magnitude of which depends on the material properties of the implant, creates an apparent discontinuity at sites where the implant overlies normal tissues. In particular, the chest wall appears shifted to a deeper level. This is most apparent

Table 8.4 Sonographic features of breast implants

Shape	Oval
Orientation	Parallel
Margin	Circumscribed
Lesion boundary	Abrupt interface
Echo pattern	Anechoic
Posterior acoustic features	Enhancement
Surrounding tissue	Architectural distortion (artificial)

when the pectoralis major muscle is traced from the periphery to the implant. For real-time scanning, the field of view should be deepened, although visualization of the back wall of a silicone implant may still not be possible with the high-resolution linear broadband transducers commonly used for breast ultrasound.

Different types of implants transmit sound at different velocities, resulting in varying degrees of image distortion (**Figs. 8.4 a–d–8.6 a, b**). Because implant placement is either subpectoral or prepectoral (subglandular), and the relationship of the implant to the muscle is easy to identify with ultrasound, the breast tissue to be examined is anterior to the implant. This is important particularly in breast cancer patients treated with mastectomy, because tumors that recur after reconstruction will develop between the implant and the skin, at skin incision sites, and for some, at the chest wall. Most of the tissue region at risk is accessible to ultrasound imaging. The significance of sonographic findings will vary according to the reason for cosmetic surgery: postmastectomy reconstruction, reconstruction after skin-sparing mastectomy, or primary augmentation for mammary hypoplasia (**Figs. 8.6 a, b, 8.7 a, b**).

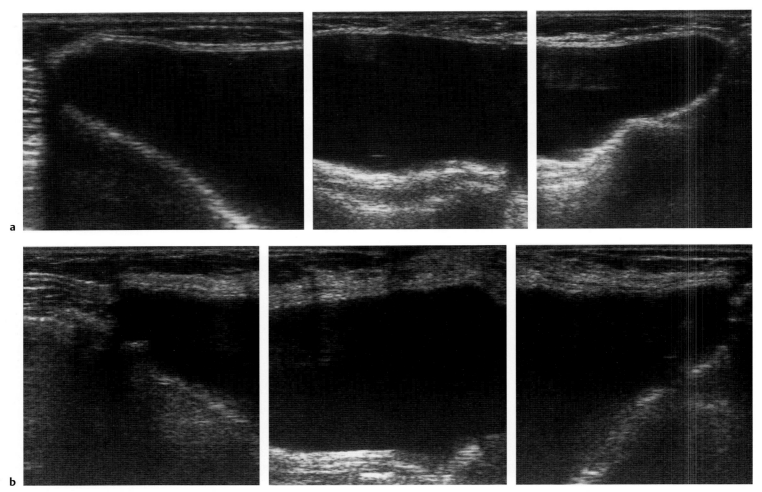

Fig. 8.6 a, b Evaluation of the breast tissue around a silicone implant.
a Postmastectomy reconstruction. The implant, covered by a thin layer of subcutaneous tissue, appears to extend past the bottom of the left scan because of image distortion. A smaller scale is used for the central and lower images in order to define the chest wall.

b Reconstruction following a partial subcutaneous mastectomy with nipple-conserving technique. A small layer of breast parenchyma is still visible between the skin and implant.

Shape	Oval
Orientation	Parallel
Margin	Circumscribed
Lesion boundary	Abrupt interface
Echo pattern	Anechoic
Surrounding tissue	Architectural distortion (artificial)

! Comment:
Sound transmission in these scans is slower than in **Fig. 8.5**, as indicated by the greater parallel shift of the chest wall. Reverberations are less pronounced.

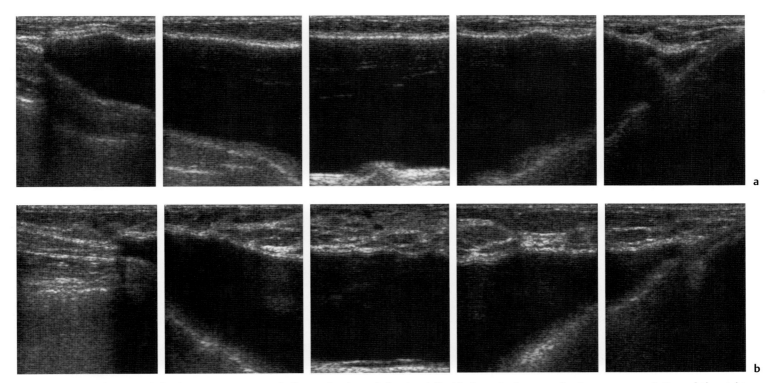

a

b

Fig. 8.7 a, b Evaluation of the breast tissue around silicone implants following left-sided mastectomy and primary augmentation of the right breast.
a Following mastectomy, a thin layer of subcutaneous fat can be seen anterior to the implant.
b Augmented breast with a thin anterior layer of breast parenchyma.

Shape	Oval
Orientation	Parallel
Margin	Circumscribed
Lesion boundary	Abrupt interface
Echo pattern	Anechoic
Surrounding tissue	Architectural distortion (artificial)

❗ Comment:
The subcutaneous tissue and breast parenchyma between the skin and implant are clearly visualized.

Testing Ultrasound Properties of Different Implant Types

Technical problems often arise in the ultrasound examination of patients with silicone breast implants. Different materials transmit sound at different speeds, resulting in varying degrees of image distortion. Ultrasound instrument settings must be adjusted accordingly. The following test set-up is useful for learning how instrument settings affect the imaging of breast implants: the prosthesis is placed into a vessel of appropriate height and its surface wetted with water or ultrasound gel. To keep the transducer from sinking into the soft surface of the implant, the mouth of the vessel is covered with a Plexiglas or lucite disk. The transducer is placed on to the disk, and the thickness of the implant is measured using the digital calipers of the scanner. This measurement is compared with the known implant thickness to determine the degree of image distortion, which is proportional to the speed of sound transmission through the implant.

If this model is tested with standard instrument settings, it will be found that the internal structure of the implant is not uniformly anechoic, as one might expect (**Fig. 8.8 a–d**). As the sound waves enter and leave the implant shell, they give rise to strong reverberations. The gain setting, and especially the TGC, should be reduced accordingly. Particularly in the region of the anterior wall, the TGC should be adjusted to produce very little amplification of the received signals. Because the sound energy is most concentrated in the focal zone and this energy concentration accentuates artifacts, the focal zone should be moved to a somewhat deeper level. This principle applies equally to examination of breast implants in the clinical setting (**Fig. 8.9 a, b**). If the purpose of the examination is to detect or exclude implant rupture, it is important to make an accurate evaluation of the implant itself. As the examination moves from the superficial subcutaneous region to the deeper structures of the chest wall, the focal zone placement should be adjusted accordingly.

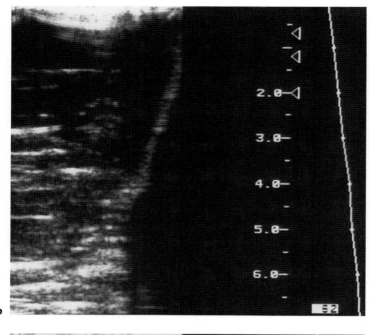
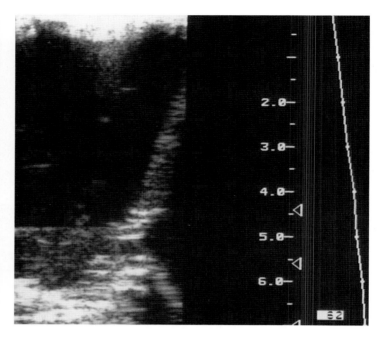

a, b

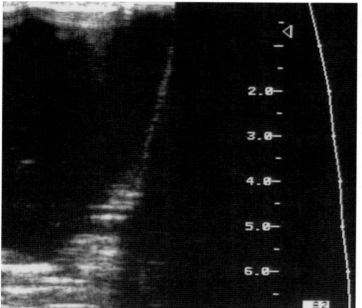
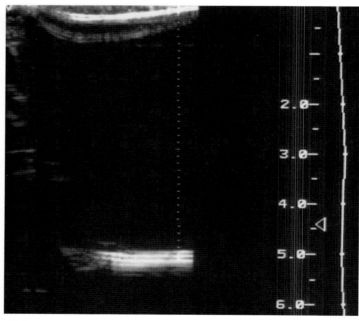

c, d

Fig. 8.8 a–d Silicone implant imaged by direct transducer contact.
a Triple focus in the near field, normal TGC.
b Triple focus at a depth of 5 cm, normal TGC.
c Single focus in the near field with normal TGC.
d Optimum setting: single focus at 4.5 cm, optimized TGC.

ℹ Comment:
Moving the focal zone decreases reverberations in the implant (**a, b**). Switching to a single focus further reduces this artifact (**c, d**). The most significant effect of silicone is to slow sound transmission. It causes minimal attenuation, and therefore a lower TGC setting should be used than in normal breast tissue (**d**).

Implant Abnormalities: Fibrous Encapsulation, Capsular Contracture, Extra- and Intracapsular Implant Rupture

Abnormalities that can be diagnosed with ultrasound are summarized in **Table 8.5** and are described below. Fibrous encapsulation of a breast implant is usually diagnosed clinically. In most cases the fibrous capsule is not visualized with ultrasound because the implant shell itself is highly reflective. Fibrous encapsulation is frequently accompanied by capsular contracture, however. This causes the formation of irregularities or wrinkles in the normally smooth surface of a silicone implant (**Fig. 8.10**). Deep implant wrinkles are common and not abnormal with saline implants, and they are not a definite sign of capsular contracture associated with silicone gel implants, because the implant may have been inserted into an inadequately dissected pocket or the elastomeric envelope may have been incompletely filled. Fibrous encapsulation is not considered a significant problem unless clinical symptoms develop, such as immobilization of the implant and pain.

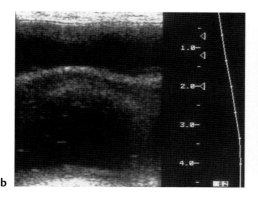 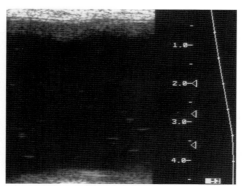

a, b

Fig. 8.9 a, b Equipment settings for imaging a silicone implant used for primary postmastectomy reconstruction.
a Triple focus in the near field, normal TGC. The image is washed out in the near and far fields, and reverberations are present.
b Triple focus at 2–4 cm, normal TGC. When the focal zone is placed more distally, the reverberations disappear.

! Comment:
Even with a normal implant, it is important to check the instrument settings. Reverberation artifacts may be misinterpreted as implant rupture. Optimum settings are equally important for evaluating the breast tissue and detecting tumor recurrence.

Fig. 8.10 Implant wrinkles due to capsular contracture.

Shape	Oval
Orientation	Parallel
Margin	Circumscribed, lobulated (wrinkles)
Lesion boundary	Abrupt interface
Echo pattern	Anechoic
Surrounding tissue	Architectural distortion (artificial)

! Comment:
Fibrous capsular contracture is a clinical diagnosis. In most cases the thick fibrous capsule cannot be seen, but generally ultrasound will show implant wrinkling caused by the contracture.

Table 8.5 Atypical findings in and around breast implants

▸ Fibrous encapsulation, capsular contracture, implant wrinkles
▸ Implant rupture
▸ Silicone migration
▸ Granulomas, siliconomas
▸ Tumors, including recurrent tumors

Extra- and Intracapsular Implant Rupture, Silicone Migration, Granulomas, Siliconomas

No matter whether the implant is subglandular or retropectoral, a fibrous capsule will form, said to encase the implant less if the implant is placed behind the muscle. Muscular contractions are postulated to lyse the adhesions that form around the prosthesis, a foreign body. Closed capsulotomy, a vigorous manual massage of the encapsulated implant (no longer done) was the most common cause of silicone implant rupture.

A distinction is made between intra- and extracapsular rupture. Intracapsular rupture involves the disintegration of the silicone polymeric envelope in which the silicone gel is contained. Many women, now in their 40 s, 50 s, or 60 s, have had implants inserted 20 or more years ago. When these women arrive for breast cancer screening, the implant contours, including implant diverticula (the rounded protrusions of silicone still contained within the implant, most often seen in the axillary tail portion of the breast), are unchanged on their mammograms, with no radiographic evidence of silicone extravasation into the soft tissue of the breast. Although the clinical significance of intracapsular rupture is still discussed, if a diagnosis of this type of rupture is made, surgical explantation including capsulectomy will commonly be scheduled. Anecdotally and in my own breast imaging practice, many women who have refused removal and replacement of these implants have had stable mammograms over the years with no radiographic (or sonographic) findings to suggest that the intracapsular rupture has progressed to allow silicone to escape through a rent in the tough fibrous capsule, to enter the breast where it can migrate through tissue planes and be picked up by lymphatics. Nevertheless it is important to detect implant rupture so that the device can be explanted before the silicone disseminates within the tissues, Confirmatory imaging should be done so that unnecessary surgery is avoided. MRI and ultrasound are superfluous in confirming rupture of saline implants, which is evident on clinical examination as deflation and collapse of the implant.

Several reliable ultrasound findings are recognized for diagnosing both extracapsular implant failure and intracapsular rupture (**Table 8.6**). In intracapsular and combined intra- and extracapsular rupture, one such finding is increased echogenicity caused by mixing of the silicone with tissue fluids. Cystic areas are present within the implant, no longer anechoic but now hypoechoic and of heterogeneous echogenicity, and sometimes the rupture site itself is visible. As the implant leaks, some of the semi-liquid silicone extravasates. A thin anechoic fluid layer surrounding the implant envelope can be seen with ultrasound and MRI. It is sometimes seen with normal implants as a solitary finding (**Figs. 8.11–8.14**). If doubt exists, MRI should be the next imaging examination. Ultrasound signs of extracapsular rupture include an often amorphous

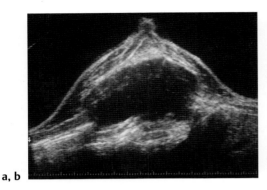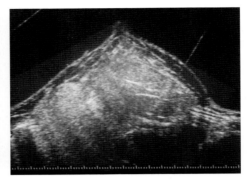

a, b

Fig. 8.11 a, b Comparison of intact and ruptured silicone implants on water-bath immersion scans.
a Intact implant in the right breast.
b Ruptured implant in the left breast.

	a	b
Shape	Oval	Oval
Orientation	Parallel	Parallel
Margin	Circumscribed	Indistinct
Lesion boundary	Abrupt interface	Abrupt interface
Echo pattern	Anechoic	Hyperechoic, heterogeneous
Surrounding tissue	Architectural distortion (artificial)	Architectural distortion

! Comment:
The evaluation of a normal implant is difficult in itself, and a ruptured implant compounds the difficulties. Comparison with the opposite side is always very helpful.

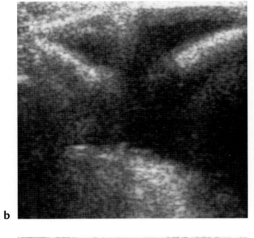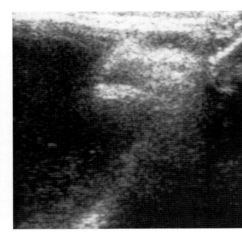

a, b

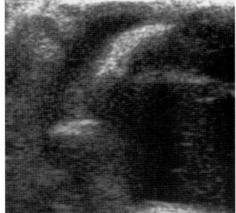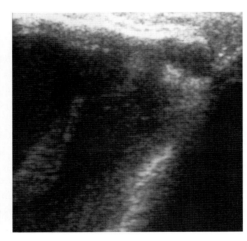

c, d

Fig. 8.12 a–d Misdiagnosis of a confined implant rupture. Ultrasound shows prominent artifacts.
a Wrinkles in the upper part of the implant (due to capsular contracture) cause strong reverberations.
b Infolding at the lower edge of the implant was misinterpreted as a rupture.
c Another scan at the upper edge of the implant.
d Lower edge of the implant.

Shape	Oval
Orientation	Parallel
Margin	Indistinct
Lesion boundary	Abrupt interface
Echo pattern	Hypoechoic, heterogeneous
Surrounding tissue	Architectural distortion (artificial)

! Comment:
Capsular contracture causes heavy wrinkling of the implant, giving rise to artifacts that make it difficult to evaluate the implant contours. If silicone leaks through a rupture into the surrounding tissue, the implant becomes soft. The moderate compressibility of this implant suggested an intracapsular rupture, but in fact the "abnormality" consisted of a simple infolding of the implant shell.

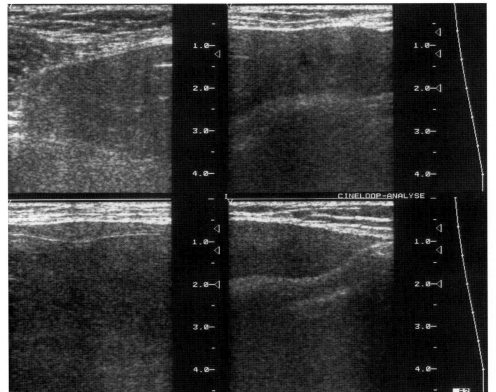

a

b

Fig. 8.13 a, b Comparison of a ruptured and unruptured implant in the same patient.
a The ruptured implant shows increased echogenicity, and the shell is seen floating in the silicone.
b With faulty instrument settings (images at left), the intact implant shows strong reverberations and increased echogenicity, making it difficult to distinguish from implant rupture. When the settings are corrected (images at right), the largely anechoic silicone can be seen.

	a	**b**
Shape	Oval	Oval
Orientation	Parallel	Parallel
Margin	Circumscribed	Circumscribed
Lesion boundary	Abrupt interface	Abrupt interface
Echo pattern	Isoechoic	Anechoic, reverberations
Surrounding tissue	Architectural distortion (artificial)	Architectural distortion (artificial)

! Comment:
This implant rupture is relatively easy to diagnose. But when faulty instrument settings are used, the intact implant will have findings that suggest implant rupture.

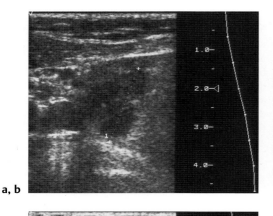
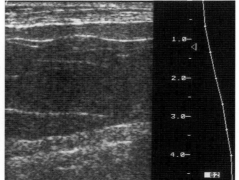
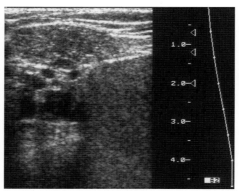

a, b

c, d

Fig. 8.14 a–d Various signs of implant rupture.
a Visible rupture site.
b Increased echogenicity and floating shell.
c Heterogeneous structures in the silicone.
d Silicone cysts (granulomas) outside the implant.

Shape	Oval
Orientation	Parallel
Margin	Predominantly circumscribed, indistinct laterally
Lesion boundary	Abrupt interface
Echo pattern	Hyperechoic, complex
Surrounding tissue	Architectural distortion—projection artifacts caused by the ruptured implant and extravasated silicone

 Comment:
Silicone cysts and granulomas may form even when the implant is intact. When combined with increased echogenicity and a floating shell, they are highly suggestive of implant rupture.

Table 8.6 Criteria for a ruptured silicone implant

Shape	Flattened oval, collapsed
Orientation	Parallel
Margin	Circumscribed; visible rupture site with adjacent silicone cysts or granulomas
Lesion boundary	Abrupt interface
Echo pattern	Isoechoic or complex; shell floating in silicone
Surrounding tissue	Architectural distortion (artificial)

focus of echogenicity that trails off gradually posterior to the rupture site. This echogenic focus can be seen in the soft tissues adjacent to the implant, sometimes adjacent to the point of rupture, and sometimes in a distant location, not uncommonly in the axilla where the same "silicone signature," the "snowstorm" pattern or echogenic noise, can be seen in lymph nodes, obscuring both the nodal hilum and its cortex.

Other ultrasound findings in extracapsular rupture include silicone granulomas: sharply outlined, cuboidal cystic lesions with central areas of anechogenicity or hypoechogenicity (**Fig. 8.15 a, b**). Small rents may be sealed by the surrounding fibrous capsule, allowing very little silicone to escape into the tissue. In other cases there may be gradual seepage causing small cystic accumulations of silicone or granulomas to form in nearby tissues.

If these granulomas have been present for many years, calcifications may form in their margins. The small focal collections of silicone indicate a long-standing leak or gel bleed, and they are encountered far less often than the echogenic noise associated with areas of free silicone in tissue.

Implant rupture is sometimes difficult to detect because of the artifacts that between the shell and tissue boundary, and the shell can be seen floating in the silicone as the transducer is moved. A ruptured implant is easily compressible, and applied pressure will push the extravasated gel along tissue planes far into the periphery. As a result, free silicone cysts, or silicone granulomas may be found distant from the implant.

▶ Implant rupture can be difficult to diagnose, even with MRI, and false-positive and false-negative diagnoses may occur. Given the need for surgical explantation of ruptured silicone prostheses, clinical understanding and multimodal imaging experience are necessary in recognizing this complication.

Primary and Recurrent Tumors

Breast carcinoma may develop following breast augmentation. Breast augmentation alone does not increase the cancer risk in these patients, but women with reconstructions following mastectomy have elevated breast cancer risk because of their personal history of breast malignancy. Although for some women with breast implants the presence of the prostheses may limit mammographic depiction of the breast tissue, mammography screening recommendations hold. Double the number of views is standard for breasts with silicone or saline prostheses, the routine views (mediolateral oblique and craniocaudal) with the implants in place supplemented by views with implant displacement.

With both subglandular and retropectoral implantations, all of the diagnostically relevant breast tissue lies anterior to the implants and easily accessible to ultrasound evaluation and to phys-

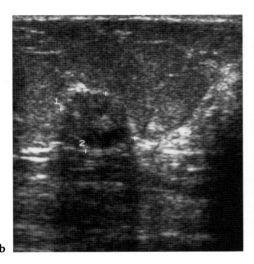 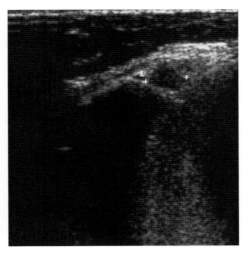

a, b

Fig. 8.15 a, b Focal abnormalities near an intact implant following mastectomy and primary reconstruction. The surgery was done for a suspected recurrence based on mammographic and MRI findings.
a Granuloma.
b Silicone cyst.

Shape	Oval
Size	**a** 13 mm, **b** 7 mm
Orientation	Parallel
Margin	Partially indistinct
Lesion boundary	Abrupt interface
Echo pattern	**a** Hyperechoic, **b** hypoechoic
Posterior acoustic features	**a** Shadowing, **b** no posterior acoustic features
Surrounding tissue	No changes
Calcifications	None
Vascularity	Not present

! Comment:
Silicone leakage from an unruptured implant can incite the formation of cysts and granulomas. If doubt exists, the lesions can be identified by ultrasound-guided fine-needle aspiration biopsy.

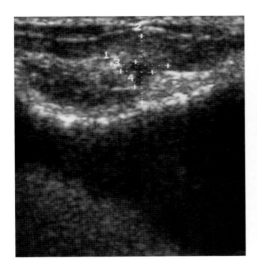 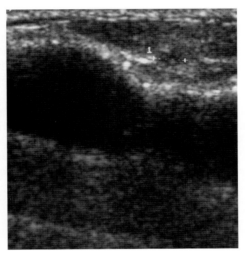

Fig. 8.16 Recurrence after subcutaneous mastectomy. Scans taken 7 months postoperatively show a recurrent tumor anterior to the implant in the upper inner quadrant of the left breast, along with echogenic residual parenchyma.

Shape	Irregular
Size	4 × 3 mm
Orientation	Parallel
Margin	Indistinct
Lesion boundary	Echogenic halo
Echo pattern	Hypoechoic
Posterior acoustic features	None
Surrounding tissue	Architectural distortion
Calcifications	None
Vascularity	Present immediately adjacent to lesion (not visible here)

! Comment:
The primary tumor and the recurrence display typical malignant criteria. Note that the residual parenchyma following subcutaneous mastectomy is easily evaluated with ultrasound. The sonograms were used to plan the subsequent mastectomy, in which the tumor and all detectable parenchymal remnants were removed. The breast was again reconstructed by prosthetic implantation.

ical examination. In breast reconstructions, the same accessibility of tissue applies to detection of recurrent tumors following skin-sparing or modified radical mastectomy (**Fig. 8.16**). The appearance of these tumors following augmentation or reconstructions follows the same interpretive criteria as in breasts without implants. A potential diagnostic problem is that silicone granulomas may be palpable and present as hypoechoic masses with irregular margins, mimicking carcinoma. But the diagnosis can still be established, and surgery avoided, by fine-needle aspiration of the thick silicone gel or ultrasound-guided core biopsy of the lesion under sonographic guidance (**Fig. 8.17 a, b**).

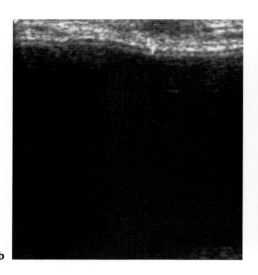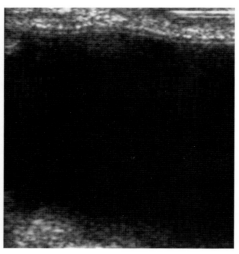

a, b

Fig. 8.17 a, b Tumor recurrence after mastectomy with primary reconstruction.
a Recurrent tumor between the skin and implant.
b Ultrasound-guided fine-needle aspiration. The needle, visible at upper right, has been inserted into the lesion. It is directed parallel to the skin and implant.

Shape	Oval
Size	4 × 5 mm (**a**)
Orientation	Parallel
Margin	Indistinct
Lesion boundary	Abrupt interface*
Echo pattern	Hypoechoic
Posterior acoustic features	None
Surrounding tissue	Architectural distortion*
Calcifications	None
Vascularity	Not present*

* Difficult to evaluate because of the small size of the lesion.

! Comment:

The diagnostic criteria for primary surgical planning are difficult to evaluate in this small tumor, and therefore fine-needle aspiration was done under ultrasound guidance. Caution: only an experienced examiner should attempt to aspirate a lesion in such a confined space.

Differential Diagnosis, Pitfalls

Implant wrinkles may form a peculiar palpable mass that is worrisome to the patient and to many physicians. Ultrasound can allay these concerns in most cases by identifying the cause of the mass. Difficulties sometimes arise in the exclusion of recurrent disease. Recurrent carcinoma typically appears as a small, hypoechoic lesion in the tissue between the implant and skin, or just beneath the skin. The diagnosis is established by core or fine-needle aspiration biopsy with ultrasound guidance to avoid puncture of the implant. Implant wrinkles may occasionally bulge far out into surrounding tissues, appearing as hypoechoic nodules adjacent to the implant with ultrasound mimicking a breast parenchymal mass. Aspiration is contraindicated in these cases, as it would destroy the implant. In ultrasound-guided procedures for diagnosis of recurrent tumor, the shaft of the needle must be kept in view above the implant envelope at all times (**Figs. 8.16, 8.17 a, b**).

A postmastectomy seroma or hematoma can resemble a breast implant (**Fig. 8.18 a, b**), but the history (taken before every breast examination) will indicate the correct diagnosis.

Further Diagnostic Procedures

We noted earlier that, for technical reasons, mammography without implant displaced views is of limited value following cosmetic breast augmentation and probably unnecessary after mastectomy with saline or silicone implant reconstruction. In most practices MRI cannot be recommended for routine screening and follow-up because its availabity is limited by high cost and insufficient available magnet time. But this does not diminish the importance of follow-up in mastectomy patients for the early detection of tumor

recurrence. Many recurrences are found on clinical examination, but high-resolution ultrasound is excellent as a detection method, since most recurrent lesions develop in the thin tissue layer between the skin and breast implant or at the chest wall. PET scanning may be of benefit when recurrence is suspected.

Considerable ultrasound experience is required, however, in interpreting the special conditions that are encountered in the implanted breast. If this experience is lacking, at present we would recommend that all equivocal cases be evaluated by MRI. At the same time, the follow-up patient, who is often under emotional stress, should be spared the ordeal of a false-positive diagnosis. Thus, the need for biopsy in this setting should be carefully weighed by an experienced diagnostician.

Role of Ultrasound

Fibrous encapsulation is a purely clinical diagnosis. Next to clinical evaluation, ultrasound is the method of choice in cases that require further investigation. Although mammography may be of limited value because of the superimposition of breast structures, it should always be done with and without implant displaced views. Even when masses are hidden in dense fibroglandular tissue or obscured by compressed, superimposed tissues, mammography remains the best imaging technique to see microcalcifications, possibly the first sign of recurrence or new tumor. For masses perceived on clinical examination or for masses suspected on mammography or MRI, the standard of care and imaging modality of choice is ultrasound. MRI also has established its value in the diagnosis of primary and recurrent tumors and implant rupture. Although it is not as cost-effective as a routine study, patients should be referred for MRI in selected cases where other studies have yielded equivocal or discordant findings.

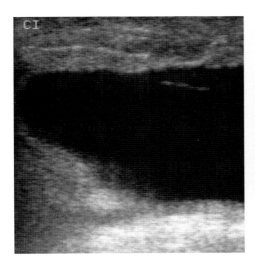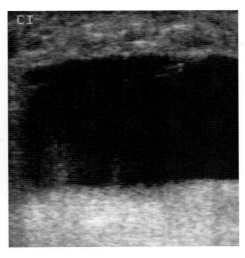

Fig. 8.18 a, b   Postmastectomy seroma.

Shape	Oval
Size	100 × 35 mm
Orientation	Parallel
Margin	Circumscribed
Lesion boundary	Abrupt interface
Echo pattern	Anechoic with re-verberations
Posterior acoustic features	Enhancement
Surrounding tissue	No changes
Calcifications	None
Vascularity	Not assessed

❗ Comment:
The mass resembles an implant, but the history suggests the correct diagnosis. Note that the fluid accumulation does not cause projection artifacts.

Case 1

A 68-year-old woman underwent mastectomy with axillary lymphadenectomy for a carcinoma in the left breast. The chest-wall and axillary drains were removed on postoperative days 4 and 6. Within 48 hours fluid began to re-accumulate in the wound bed around the mastectomy scar. **Fig. 8.18** shows the appearance of the seromatous collection at 1 week. The collection was large enough to warrant ultrasound-guided aspiration. Two aspirations were carried out, and the collection did not recur. The ultrasound appearance of the seroma closely resembled that of a breast implant.

Documentation

In patients with bilateral implants, the same minimum documentation should be obtained for each side. One scan of each axillary breast extension is needed to document subglandular or retropectoral placement. Most leaks or fluid collections (e. g., seromas) are found inferior to the implant, and so the caudal breast extension should also be insonated and its appearance recorded. Because scars may appear as hypoechoic lesions that are difficult to distinguish from tumors, the mastectomy or implantation scar and its relationship to the overlying skin should be captured and archived as well. Thus a minimum of three scans should be documented for each implant. In addition, every focal abnormality should be measured and documented in at least two planes. Hypoechoic scar tissue is documented with and without external pressure to show compressibility. This is necessary to differentiate the scars from noncompressible hypoechoic tumors.

▶ Hypoechoic lesions near breast implants should be evaluated by an experienced breast diagnostician. It is easy to misdirect a biopsy needle, resulting in potentially severe consequences and a very angry patient. No one should attempt these procedures unless they have had considerable experience with ultrasound-guided breast interventional procedures and are confident they can do them safely. For those with long experience, accurate percutaneous sampling of lesions near the implant with ultrasound guidance should not be a challenge.

Clinical Significance

Lactational Abscesses

Mastitis can be classified according to whether or not it occurs during the special hormonal environment of pregnancy or lactation (**Table 9.1**). The mammary ducts provide a hospitable environment for microorganisms, which enter most commonly through a fissured nipple, and bacterial inflammation is particularly common during lactation. The majority of these infections are staphylococcal.

Bacterial mastitis, a breast cellulitis, can be further characterized as an acute inflammation or as a more advanced process that has matured to abscess formation. The time of diagnosis has major clinical implications for treatment. A florid inflammatory process marked by redness and breast edema without liquefaction responds well to antibiotic therapy, especially when supported by antibiotics such as amoxicillin or clindamycin, anti-inflammatory drugs, analgesics, and frequent breast-feeding or pumping to keep the breast empty. If the symptoms are communicated to the obstetrician as soon as they become evident, antibiotic therapy may

forestall development of an abscess. Ultrasound is indicated for evaluation of patients with mastitis to confirm or exclude an underlying abscess. Once abscess formation has occurred, the lesion must be drained. The drainage procedure, which may be done with ultrasound guidance or surgically, may be preceded by heat application to promote liquefaction and demarcation of the suppurative focus (**Table 9.2**).

Nonpuerperal Abscesses

Mastitis and abscess can occur at any age. Inflammatory processes may involve the entire breast or only a small segment. Cysts are sometimes affected by inflammation, which usually resolve following aspiration and complete drainage of the purulent material Although many cysts that contain low-level internal echoes are clinically insignificant, infected cysts are symptomatic with pain and sometimes redness and warmth to the touch. If they are accompanied by systemic signs such as leukocytosis, fever, or an elevated C reactive protein (CRP), antibiotics should be administered, although ultrasound-guided aspiration of the cyst contents may bring prompt relief.

Women of any age who are immunosuppressed, diabetic, or have had significant trauma or previous breast surgery including major duct excisions, may develop abscesses or infected hematomas or seromas. Mastitis and abscess in these women are diagnosed and treated as for puerperal inflammatory processes. Additional sites of inflammatory processes are in the axilla, where infected hair follicles or sebaceous glands can result in drainable collections, or the areola where small infected pockets may involve the glands of Montgomery. In men inflammatory processes occur less commonly, but infected epidermal inclusion cysts near the nipple may result in a cancer-mimicking breast mass.

In older women, or any adult woman, particularly if the inflammatory process is nonlactational, the most important distinction to be made is mastitis and abscess vs. inflammatory carcinoma. The first step in the management sequence is antibiotic therapy (although inflammatory carcinoma also may show some response initially). Once abscess has been excluded and, if present, treated, and if there is incomplete resolution after the entire antibiotic course, mammography and ultrasound should be performed, with core biopsy of any solid masses found with ultrasound for histology—most often poorly differentiated invasive ductal carcinoma—and a punch biopsy of the thickened skin expecting to find tumor emboli in the subdermal lymphatics. The primary treatment of inflammatory carcinoma is chemotherapy, and if a tumor

Table 9.1 Forms of mastitis

▸ Puerperal	▸ Nonpuerperal
▸ Bacterial	▸ Abacterial
▸ Specific	– Granulating
– e. g., tuberculosis	– Immunologic
▸ Acute	▸ Suppurative, chronic recurring
▸ Diffuse	▸ Focal
	– Granulomas
	– Cysts, ducts, or wound area

Table 9.2 Treatment of mastitis

Acute inflammation	Liquefaction
Antibiotics	Surgical percutaneous drainage*
Anti-inflammatory agents (local or systemic)	Aspiration (if appropriate), with or without catheter insertion for drainage and irrigation
Dopamine agonists Specialized treatment as in granulomatous sarcoidosis (cortisone)	

* Gram stain, bacterial culture and antibiotic sensitivity

infiltrate is not found in the lymphatics, treatment will still be for inflammatory carcinoma based on the clinical presentation.

The nipple area may become acutely inflamed as a result of infected *juvenile cysts* with retained secretions in the ducts. A careful, tissue-conserving approach is warranted in these cases to avoid damage to the breast bud by spreading inflammation or excessive surgical manipulation. With the abundant blood supply to juvenile tissue, it is generally sufficient to do a single aspiration and provide supportive antibiotics. In older women, inflamed or ulcerated nipples (not areolae) can signify Paget disease, ductal carcinoma in situ involving the large ducts nearing and in the nipple. Invasive carcinoma may also be present.

Immune responses can also lead to chronic mastitis conditions, which may be diffuse or may take the form of focal inflammatory nodules and granulomas as in erythema nodosum or sarcoidosis (Boeck disease). Chronic granulomatous mastitis, of noninfectious but unclear etiology, can mimic invasive lobular carcinoma on ultrasound. Ultrasound-guided core needle biopsy can provide the diagnosis, and biopsy is indicated. Foreign-body reactions (e.g., to implantation of a prosthesis) can also incite mastitis.

Diagnostic Criteria

Edema

Acute mastitis is initially characterized by increased fluid accumulation in the breast tissue. Initially, the parenchyma becomes more diffusely hypoechoic, but the glandular structures can still be discerned. With the onset of abscess formation, the tissue becomes increasingly hypoechoic toward the center of the focus (**Fig. 9.1**), and as the surrounding tissue becomes more edematous, the area appears more echogenic, the overlying skin is thickened, and a hypoechoic network representing interstitial fluid can be seen.

Mass

Once an abscess has formed, the glandular tissue undergoes necrotic liquefaction and generally appears as a heterogeneous, doughy, complex cystic irregularly shaped mass with sharp marginal definition in some areas of the lesion and indistinct or angular margins in other areas (**Figs. 9.2–9.5, Table 9.3**). There is relatively little sound attenuation by the purulent material, as evidenced by posterior acoustic enhancement.

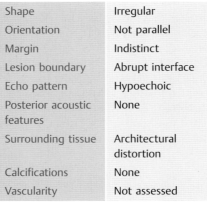

Shape	Irregular
Orientation	Not parallel
Margin	Indistinct
Lesion boundary	Abrupt interface
Echo pattern	Hypoechoic
Posterior acoustic features	None
Surrounding tissue	Architectural distortion
Calcifications	None
Vascularity	Not assessed

! Comment:
Artifactual attenuation in a noncompression scan can create the appearance of a hypoechoic mass. Compression is necessary to confirm the lesion.

Fig. 9.1 Water-bath compound scan in suppurative mastitis.

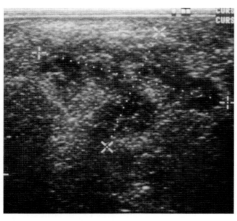

Shape	Irregular
Orientation	Parallel
Margin	Indistinct
Lesion boundary	Echogenic halo
Echo pattern	Complex
Posterior acoustic features	None
Surrounding tissue	Architectural distortion
Calcifications	None
Vascularity	Diffusely increased in surrounding tissue

! Comment:
The parenchymal structure can still be recognized within the edematous, hypoechoic lesion. Antibiotic treatment is indicated.

Fig. 9.2 Acute mastitis with an edematous tissue pattern.

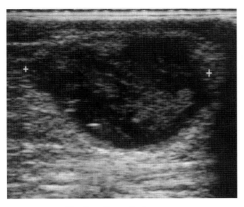

Shape	Oval
Orientation	Parallel
Margin	Circumscribed
Lesion boundary	Echogenic halo
Echo pattern	Hypoechoic
Posterior acoustic features	Enhancement
Surrounding tissue	Architectural distortion
Calcifications	None
Vascularity	Present immediately adjacent to lesion

! Comment:
Systemic antibiotics are of no benefit at this stage. Surgical treatment is required.

Fig. 9.3 Fully developed abscess.

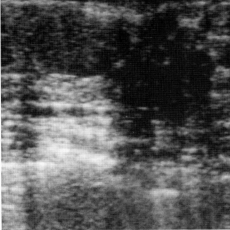

Shape	Complex, irregular
Orientation	Not parallel
Margin	Microlobulated
Lesion boundary	Abrupt interface
Echo pattern	Hypoechoic
Posterior acoustic features	Combined pattern
Surrounding tissue	Architectural distortion, skin irregularity
Calcifications	None
Vascularity	Present immediately adjacent to lesion

! Comment:
This focus is on the verge of spontaneous perforation. The scan shows cutaneous involvement.

Fig. 9.4 Superficial breast abscess.

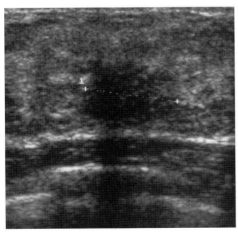

Shape	Complex, irregular
Orientation	Parallel
Margin	Indistinct
Lesion boundary	Abrupt interface
Echo pattern	Hypoechoic
Posterior acoustic features	None
Surrounding tissue	Architectural distortion
Calcifications	None
Vascularity	Not present

! Comment:
Sonographically, this lesion resembles a carcinoma. Clinical signs of inflammation suggest the correct diagnosis, but cytologic or histologic confirmation is still required. A negative Doppler examination does not exclude malignancy.

Fig. 9.5 Inflammatory focus in the liquefaction stage.

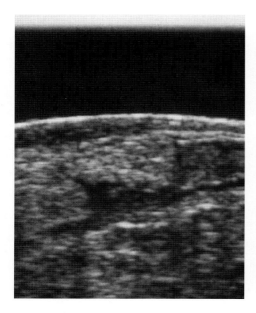 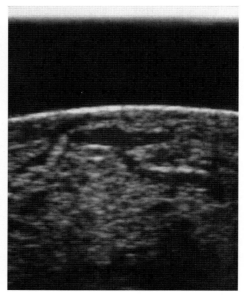

Fig. 9.6 Confluent, interconnecting breast abscesses.

Shape	Complex
Orientation	Parallel
Margin	Indistinct
Lesion boundary	Abrupt interface
Echo pattern	Hypoechoic
Posterior acoustic features	None
Surrounding tissue	Architectural distortion
Calcifications	None
Vascularity	Diffusely increased vascularity in surrounding tissue

❗ Comment:
To prevent recurrence, it is important to identify all the abscesses and interconnecting tracks prior to surgical intervention.

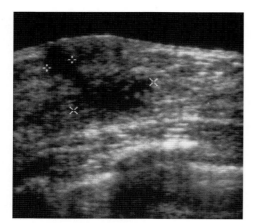

Fig. 9.7 Deep abscess with skin perforation.

Shape	Complex
Orientation	Parallel
Margin	Indistinct
Lesion boundary	Abrupt interface
Echo pattern	Hypoechoic
Posterior acoustic features	Enhancement
Surrounding tissue	Architectural distortion, skin irregularity
Calcifications	None
Vascularity	Not present

❗ Comment:
This patient had had recurring episodes of mastitis with spontaneous perforation for several years. The opening of the sinus tract is at the areolar margin. The abscess cavity and sinus tract were localized with ultrasound and surgically evacuated.

Table 9.3 Criteria for the diagnosis of abscesses

Shape	Variable
Orientation	Parallel
Margin	Circumscribed or indistinct
Lesion boundary	Abrupt interface
Echo pattern	Hypoechoic
Posterior acoustic features	Enhancement
Surrounding tissue	Architectural distortion
Calcifications	None
Vascularity	Diffusely increased in surrounding tissue or immediately adjacent to lesion

Diagnosing the presence, stage, and extent of abscess formation is important for planning treatment. Location and spread must be evaluated before percutaneous drainage or surgical treatment is provided. Occasionally the abscesses are multiple and are interconnected by tracks (**Fig. 9.6**), and a broad area around the symptomatic focus should be scanned. Unless most of the purulent material is evacuated, the abscesses will recur and lead to progressive destruction of the breast tissue. Sometimes an abscess will spontaneously track upward and discharge its contents through a break in the overlying skin. If the main focus is deep within the breast, the sinus tract can be demonstrated with ultrasound and utilized for surgical access (**Fig. 9.7**).

Additional Diagnostic Considerations

Exclude Malignancy

Occasionally, purulent material obtained at operation or aspirated percutaneously is found to be bacteriologically sterile. With the possibility of a necrotic tumor kept in mind, tissue specimens from the walls of the abscess cavity should be submitted for histologic analysis. This may indicate a nonspecific immunologic inflamma-tion or a granulomatous process directing attention to a systemic disease (**Figs. 9.8–9.10 a, b**). The main purpose of histology, how-ever, is to differentiate an abscess from a necrotic carcinoma, sarcoma, or lymphoma.

Most important differentiation of mastitis from inflammatory carcinoma (**Fig. 9.11 a, b**). Some malignant tumors, frequently those that are grade 3, are nearly anechoic, or have very low-level internal echoes and posterior acoustic enhancement, bear a par-ticularly strong resemblance to abscesses. Doppler scans contrib-ute little to the differential diagnosis, because blood flow is in-

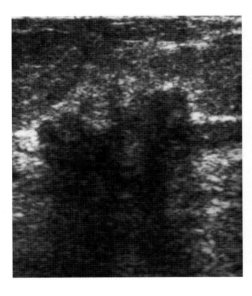 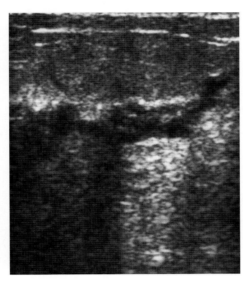

Fig. 9.8 Lymphoplasmacytic periductal mas-titis.

Shape	Complex
Orientation	–
Margin	Indistinct
Lesion boundary	Abrupt interface
Echo pattern	Hypoechoic
Posterior acous-tic features	Shadowing
Surrounding tissue	Architectural distor-tion
Calcifications	None
Vascularity	Not assessed

❗ Comment:
This 38-year-old woman presented with acute pain in the upper outer quadrant of the right breast. Mammograms showed an ill-defined density, and ultrasound showed a suspicious shadowing lesion. There were mild clinical signs of inflammation. Smears taken at operation did not contain detectable microorganisms. Orientation cannot be described because of strong shadowing.

a, b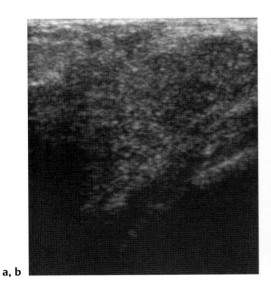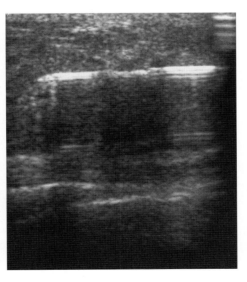

Fig. 9.9 a, b Granulomatous inflammation in a patient with sarcoidosis. The primary mani-festation of the disease in this 37-year-old woman was a large nodule in the right breast, palpable as a tense, painful mass. Slight skin redness was apparent clinically but no cutaneous edema. **a** Lesion, **b** core biopsy.

Shape	Oval
Orientation	Parallel
Margin	Indistinct
Lesion boundary	Abrupt interface
Echo pattern	Hypoechoic
Posterior acous-tic features	Combined pattern
Surrounding tissue	Architectural distor-tion
Calcifications	None
Vascularity	Present immediately adjacent to lesion

❗ Comment:
Core biopsy was done because the mass was indeterminate by clinical and ultrasound findings. The lesion gradually resolved in response to antibiotic coverage and cortisone therapy.

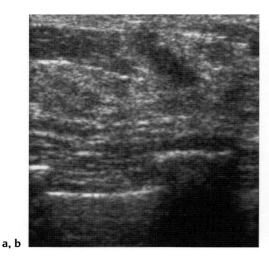
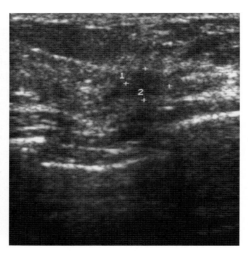

Fig. 9.10 a, b Granulomatous inflammation. The 35-year-old patient presented with a painful nodule in her left breast. **a** Sagittal, **b** transverse scan.

Shape	Irregular
Orientation	Nonparallel
Margin	Indistinct
Lesion boundary	Echogenic halo
Echo pattern	Hypoechoic
Posterior acoustic features	Combined pattern
Surrounding tissue	Architectural distortion
Calcifications	None
Vascularity	Present immediately adjacent to lesion

❗ Comment:
Aspiration was done because the lesion was sonographically indeterminate. Cytology revealed giant cells consistent with a granulomatous process. Surgery was withheld, and the lesion underwent spontaneous perforation and resolved completely within a few months.

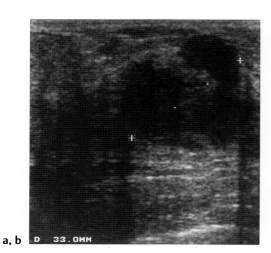
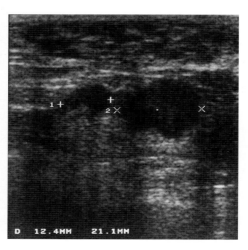

Fig. 9.11 a, b Inflammatory carcinoma with axillary metastases. The patient had a 2-week history of breast pain and redness.
a Transverse scan in the upper outer quadrant of the left breast.
b Transverse scan of the axilla (level I).

Shape	Complex
Orientation	Horizontal
Margin	Indistinct
Lesion boundary	Abrupt interface
Echo pattern	Hypoechoic
Posterior acoustic features	Shadowing
Surrounding tissue	Architectural distortion
Calcifications	None
Vascularity	Present in lesion and diffusely increased vascularity in surrounding tissue

❗ Comment:
The patient had been treated with antibiotics for suspected mastitis. The breast mass resembles an abscess, but the lymph nodes show signs of metastatic involvement.

creased both in malignancies and in mastitis (Chapter 19). Monitoring the response to antibiotic therapy is the only noninvasive means of distinguishing mastitis from inflammatory carcinoma. An accurate interpretation requires experience, however, since antibiotics can suppress the inflammatory reaction associated with an inflammatory carcinoma.

Long-standing Lesions

Unless adequately treated, an abscess will usually cause progressive tissue destruction that may culminate in the loss of the entire breast. In other cases the abscess may become encapsulated and resolve by draining spontaneously through the skin. With the passage of time, the residual abscess cavity may form a calcific shell that mimics the sonographic appearance of carcinoma (**Fig. 9.12 a, b**).

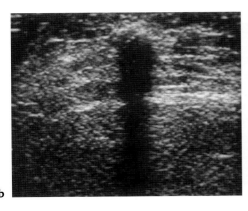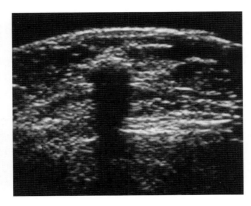

a, b

Fig. 9.12 a, b Calcified abscess cavity. There were no visible signs of inflammation, and the skin was not thickened.
a Real-time scan with direct transducer contact.
b Scan with a standoff pad, providing better delineation of the skin.

Shape	Complex
Orientation	–
Margin	Indistinct
Lesion boundary	Echogenic halo
Echo pattern	Anechoic
Posterior acoustic features	Shadowing
Surrounding tissue	Architectural distortion
Calcifications	Macrocalcification out of mass
Vascularity	Not present

❗ Comment:
This type of lesion is difficult to distinguish from carcinoma by ultrasound. Mammography reveals patchy calcifications, which account for the acoustic shadow.

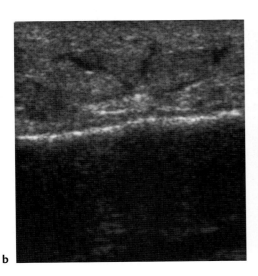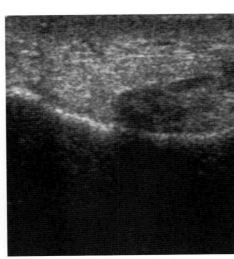

a, b

Fig. 9.13 a, b Mastitis following the insertion of a silicone implant.
a Expanded lymphatics in the subcutaneous fat.
b Hypoechoic edematous focus anterior to the implant.

Shape	Oval
Orientation	Parallel
Margin	Circumscribed
Lesion boundary	Abrupt interface
Echo pattern	Hypoechoic
Posterior acoustic features	Shadowing
Surrounding tissue	No changes
Calcifications	None
Vascularity	Diffusely increased vascularity in surrounding tissue

❗ Comment:
There is no abscess formation, and the parenchymal architecture in **b** is intact. Surgery was withheld, and the mastitis resolved with antibiotic treatment.

Peri-implant Inflammatory Processes

Although small fluid collections surrounding an implant, often seen on MRI, can be a normal finding, the early detection of an inflammatory focus is particularly important in women with breast augmentation or reconstruction with an implant (**Fig. 9.13 a, b**). If the inflammatory process advances to involve the entire surgical cavity, surgical removal of the implant will be required.

Skin Thickening: Other Causes

Keloids, superficial skin inflammations, eczema, and fungal infections show no abnormalities in the underlying tissue at ultrasound examination. Massive staphyloderma (cutaneous pyogenic infection caused by staphylococci), however, can lead to marked skin thickening. Ulceration, weeping or eczematous changes involving the nipple itself should always raise suspicion of Paget disease and underlying ductal carcinoma, confirmed by biopsy.

Management Procedures

Needle aspiration of a sample of the lesion comes first in the sequence of diagnostic procedures. Cytologic analysis of the aspirate can detect inflammatory cells, and a concurrent bacteriologic smear is examined for infectious microorganisms. Culture and antibiotic sensitivity of the purulent material is standard, but these patients should be receiving antibiotics expectantly at the time of the aspiration and drainage procedures. If the mass is solid, as in granulomatous mastitis, core biopsy for histology would be the next diagnostic procedure.

As discussed earlier, core biopsy of the lesion's walls is indicated if there is suspicion of carcinoma (**Fig. 9.14 a, b**). Once histologic confirmation is secured, primary (neoadjuvant) chemotherapy can be initiated to downstage the tumor in preparation for surgical excision or palliative mastectomy.

Unilocular abscesses and those with discrete pockets can be aspirated percutaneously with ultrasound guidance, which will allow assessment of completeness of evacuation, presence of inflammatory extensions, and in complex, multiloculated collections, recommendation for surgical incision and drainage. Good results have been achieved, at least in puerperal mastitis, by ultrasound aspirations repeated every few days until only no abscess remains, but only residual mastitis that will clear with antibiotic therapy. Ultrasound-guided insertion of a drainage catheter can be effective for larger abscesses (more than 3–4 cm in diameter) and those abscesses treated initially with repetitive aspirations that refill with a large volume of material in a day or two.

With circumscribed inflammatory changes due to an infected cyst, it is appropriate to do ultrasound-guided aspiration and evacuation (**Fig. 9.15 a, b**).

Role of Imaging

Physical examination can detect erythema and cutaneous edema but cannot reveal the cause or stage of the inflammation. Older surgical textbooks recommend checking for palpable fluctuation to distinguish acute mastitis from breast abscess. However, the breast is usually too tender to allow effective palpation, and in any case only large abscesses can be detected by this method.

Ultrasound has a leading role to play in the evaluation of mastitis and should be the first imaging study. The examination requires little compression and can be tolerated by the patient during the acute stage of the inflammation. Ultrasound can differentiate diffuse inflammatory edema, treated medically, from abscess formation requiring drainage. In addition, in inflammatory carcinoma masquerading as mastitis, malignant-appearing solid masses obscured mammographically and undetectable at clinical examination can be sometimes seen during sonography and biopsied with ultrasound guidance.

Mammography is impossible in acute mastitis because of severe pain, and its use is also limited in inflammatory cancer by the high X-ray absorption of the edematous and poorly compressible breast. Mammography should be deferred until there is sufficient resolution of the inflammatory process and the pain has largely subsided. Adequate compression then can be applied.

For young women with puerperal mastitis or abscesses, mammography can be done, possibly as a baseline study, when the patient returns for follow-up, but if antibiotics have not effected adequate resolution and inflammatory carcinoma remains a concern, mammography must be done as soon as possible. If microcalcifications are present as the sign of cancer, they should be visible if the radiographic exposure factors are appropriate and compression can be applied. If much edema remains, masses will be poorly depicted, if at all, with mammography, and ultrasound can be relied upon.

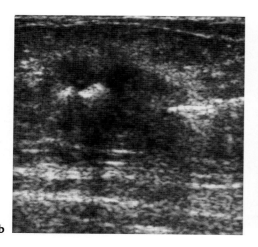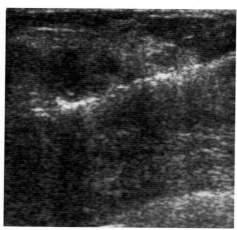

a, b

Fig. 9.14 a, b Invasive ductal carcinoma with an inflammatory reaction.
a Sagittal scan of the tumor.
b Core biopsy for histologic confirmation.

Shape	Complex
Orientation	Parallel
Margin	Indistinct
Lesion boundary	Echogenic halo
Echo pattern	Complex
Posterior acoustic features	Combined pattern
Surrounding tissue	Architectural distortion
Calcifications	None (bright echoes caused by entrapped air after core biopsy)
Vascularity	Present immediately adjacent to lesion

! Comment:
When histologic confirmation was secured, it was possible to institute primary chemotherapy.

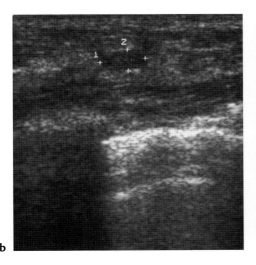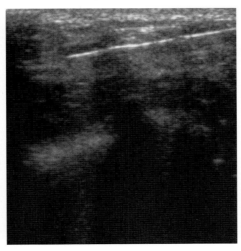

a, b

Fig. 9.15 a, b Infected cyst treated by aspiration.
a Hypoechoic focal lesion.
b Aspirating needle within the lesion.

Shape	Oval
Orientation	Parallel
Margin	Indistinct
Lesion boundary	Abrupt interface
Echo pattern	Hypoechoic
Posterior acoustic features	No posterior acoustic features
Surrounding tissue	No changes
Calcifications	None
Vascularity	Not present

! Comment:

Image **a** shows low-level internal echoes and an absence of posterior enhancement. This lesion cannot be identified as a cyst. There is an associated inflammatory reaction with cutaneous edema. Aspiration was done to establish the diagnosis and to direct treatment. The lesion resolved under antibiotic therapy.

MRI is unnecessary in the initial evaluation of mastitis and abscess. Both tumors and abscesses will enhance after administration of gadolinium contrast agents, and ultrasound is a less costly and more direct method of diagnosing and, in many cases, treating abscesses. If inflammatory breast cancer is suspected sufficiently to occasion a punch biopsy of the thickened skin, and carcinoma is confirmed in the subdermal lymphatics, malignant masses, which also may be seen with ultrasound, can be depicted on contrast-enhanced MRI examinations. MRI will also show enhancement of the thickened, edematous skin involved in inflammatory carcinoma.

Documentation

As with all focal lesions, the images should be documented in two planes. Because abscesses may be very large, several sectional images spliced together are sometimes needed to cover the entire lesion. If the ultrasound system offers wide field of view or panoramic imaging, the entire lesion may be depicted in one frame.

If the inflammatory process is limited to mastitis or cellulitis without abscess, the affected area should be scanned completely and documented on PACS or hard copy. The extent of the inflammatory area should be defined to provide a baseline for monitoring response to medical treatment. Similarly, thickness of the skin should also be recorded for comparison in follow-up visits.

Because the echogenicity of this tissue differs markedly from that of normal breast tissue, and because edema may result from noninflammatory causes, the corresponding region of the healthy breast should be scanned and an image recorded for comparison.

Lymphadenopathy may occur in reaction to the inflammatory process or may reflect metastatic involvement in inflammatory carcinoma. The axilla should be scanned and any lymphadenopathy noted. It may be difficult to distinguish reactive lymph nodes from those associated with carcinoma. Uniformly thickened cortices, greater than the normal 3 mm thickness, suggest benign reactivity. Cortical bulges or focal nodular areas, hypoechoic or hyperechoic, are associated with metastases. Nevertheless, the specific etiology of the lymphadenopathy may not be identifiable with ultrasound or clinical examination, and biopsy may needed.

Benign Solid Tumors 10

Clinical Significance

The most common benign breast tumors are fibroadenomas. They develop earlier than other breast tumors, beginning at puberty, and predominantly affecting women between 20 and 40 years of age. They respond to circulating estrogen and may increase in size during pregnancy and lactation. Fibroadenomas rarely develop after menopause, but screening examinations at that stage of life often detect lesions that were clinically occult in previous years. Fibroadenomas appear encapsulated, have well-defined boundaries, and show a mixed epithelial–mesenchymal histology.

Although fibroadenomas are by far the most common benign breast tumor, there are many other benign tumors that may be encountered incidentally. Some, like lipomas and hamartomas, have unique mammographic and/or ultrasound findings that allow confident assessment of the lesions as benign, whereas others have features that may not be distinctive enough to permit a specific diagnosis. The ultrasound feature analysis, however, will suggest a benign etiology. Breast physicians should be aware of these lesions and able to recommend appropriate management. These benign lesions are listed in **Table 10.1**.

Histologically, the fibroadenoma is a mixed neoplasm. Pathologists sometimes distinguish different types based on the proportion of different tissue elements. If there is a preponderance of connective tissue, as in most cases, the tumor is called a *fibroadenoma*. If glandular rather than mesenchymal tissue predominates, it is called an *adenofibroma*. If the lesion consists entirely of glandular elements, it is termed an *adenosis tumor*.

Although fibrous tissue is a common mesenchymal component of breast lesions, fat is a also major component of the adult breast itself. A benign mass entirely of mesenchymal origin is the *lipoma*, a circumscribed, encapsulated mass of fat density, or radiolucent on mammograms and with ultrasound, slightly more echogenic than fat lobules. The lipoma is a "leave me alone lesion" unless it is growing in an inconvenient location.

Other masses contain more than one type of mesenchymal tissue in varying proportions, such as *lipofibromas* or *fibrolipomas*. Some tumors consist of a combination of fibrous, glandular, and fatty tissues, reflected in the designation of the neoplasm, the dominant component named first: fibroadenolipoma, for example. Mammographically, such masses have a unique appearance: encapsulated, with the three tissue components mixed together within the mass. With ultrasound, these masses show benign features—circumscribed, oval masses, long axis parallel to the skin—and echogenic and hypoechoic elements in the heterogeneous matrix. As in the normal tissues of the breast, cysts can arise in hamartomas. The management of this "leave me alone lesion," as with lipomas, is to recognize its identity and to recommend routine imaging follow-up. Tumors with a large fatty tissue component are highly compressible.

Diagnostic Criteria

Typical Findings of Fibroadenomas

Fibroadenomas usually present clinically as firm, mobile masses with circumscribed margins. Mammographically, fibroadenomas appears as well-defined oval masses that are indistinguishable from cysts, as both lesions show similar X-ray absorption (**Fig. 10.1 a**). Sonographically, the fibroadenoma typically appears as an oval or macrolobulated lesion, round in short axis view, with circumscribed margins. Fibroadenomas are hypoechoic or isoechoic compared with the echogenicity of fat and generally contain some internal echoes (**Fig. 10.1 b**). Ordinarily there is either posterior acoustic enhancement (**Table 10.2**) or no change in the echogenicity posterior to the mass. Some noncalcified fibroadenomas, presumably with a predominant fibrous component, will attenuate the sound transmission and shadowing will be seen deep to the mass. Bilateral refraction shadows, or edge shadows, are frequently seen at the lateral edges of the mass, commonly encountered with fat lobules and other round or oval masses, benign and malignant, or masses or anatomic structures with curved borders or tapered edges. Refraction shadowing has no diagnostic or clinical significance. On compression or sonopalpation, these tumors are relatively firm, poorly compressible, and very mobile.

The acoustic characteristics of a typical fibroadenoma in a waterbath immersion scan are illustrated in **Fig. 10.2**. The interior of the

Table 10.1 Benign solid breast tumors

- Fibroadenoma
- Juvenile adenoma
- Tubular adenoma
- Giant fibroadenoma
- Lipoma
- Fibroma (focal fibrosis)
- Sclerosing adenosis
- Phylloides tumor
- Hamartoma
- Galactocele

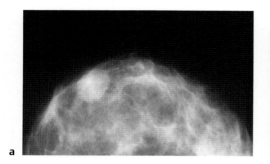

a

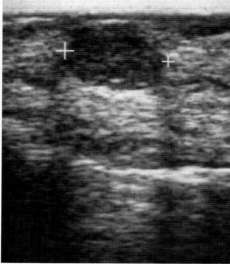

b

Fig. 10.1 Typical fibroadenoma in a 45-year-old woman.
a Mammography.
b Ultrasound (5-MHz transducer).

Shape	Oval
Orientation	Parallel
Margin	Circumscribed
Lesion boundary	Abrupt interface
Echo pattern	Hypoechoic
Posterior acoustic features	Enhancement
Surrounding tissue	No changes
Calcifications	None
Vascularity	Not present

Table 10.2 Criteria for the diagnosis of fibroadenoma

Shape	Round, oval
Orientation	Parallel
Margin	Circumscribed
Lesion boundary	Abrupt interface
Echo pattern	Hypoechoic
Posterior acoustic features	Enhancement or no posterior acoustic features
Surrounding tissue	No changes
Calcifications	None, or macrocalcifications
Vascularity	Not present

tumor is markedly hypoechoic to the surrounding tissues. Additionally, the echoes behind the tumor appear slightly enhanced. As with other lesions, equipment performance critically affects the quality of the diagnosis. A low-frequency transducer (5 MHz) is useful only for larger tumors, and the limited resolution makes it more difficult to evaluate lesion boundaries and margins. Because

lower-frequency transducers are usually focused at a greater depth, the near-field image quality can often be improved by using a standoff pad. By contrast, when a high-frequency transducer is used in a system with good image processing, the diagnostic criteria can easily be evaluated, even if the lesion is quite small (**Fig. 10.3**).

Fibroadenomas are isoechoic or hypoechoic compared with fat lobules; lipomas are more echogenic than fat lobules. Although lipomas are encapsulated, fat-containing benign lesions, they have reflective, connective tissue structures within them that increase their echogenicity. They are more compressible than fibroadenomas.

Fibromas are predominantly fibrous tumors that range from hypoechoic to very echogenic. When they are is iso- or hypoechoic to fat, their benign ultrasound features are indistinguishable from those of fibroadenomas.

As noted above, many benign breast tumors consist of a combination of the three breast components: glandular (epithelial), connective tissue, fat. Tumors composed chiefly of connective tissue are called fibromas, stromal fibrosis, and fibrolipomas. With the addition of the glandular component, fibroadenomas or fibroadenolipomas (hamartomas) are the most likely diagnosis.

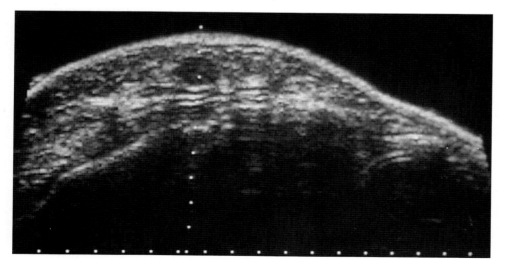

Fig. 10.2 Water-bath immersion scan of a fibroadenoma in a 44-year-old woman. Survey image.

Shape	Oval
Orientation	Parallel
Margin	Circumscribed
Lesion boundary	Abrupt interface
Echo pattern	Hypoechoic
Posterior acoustic features	Enhancement
Surrounding tissue	No changes
Calcifications	None
Vascularity	Not assessed

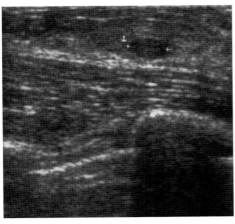

Shape	Oval
Orientation	Parallel
Margin	Circumscribed
Lesion boundary	Abrupt interface
Echo pattern	Hypoechoic
Posterior acoustic features	No posterior acoustic features
Surrounding tissue	No changes
Calcifications	None
Vascularity	Not present

■ Comment:
Even in this small tumor, the high resolution permits accurate interpretation of the diagnostic criteria. The surrounding dense parenchyma may restrict the mobility of a deeply situated tumor.

Fig. 10.3 Typical small fibroadenoma in a 34-year-old woman, imaged with a high-resolution transducer (10 MHz).

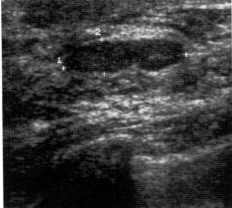

Shape	Oval
Orientation	Parallel
Margin	Circumscribed, lobulated
Lesion boundary	Abrupt interface
Echo pattern	Hypoechoic
Posterior acoustic features	Enhancement (weak)
Surrounding tissue	No changes
Calcifications	None
Vascularity	Not present

■ Comment:
Fibroadenomas may enlarge during pregnancy and often acquire a heterogeneous echo pattern, increasing the difficulty of differential diagnosis. In this case the tumor was followed for 6 years and showed no changes during that period.

Fig. 10.4 Lobulated fibroadenoma in a 32-year-old woman in her 28th week of pregnancy.

The fibroadenolipomas, soft tumors on palpation, can be quite large and their sonographic appearance is nonspecific. Their heterogeneity causes enough uncertainty in the diagnosis for a biopsy to be recommended in spite of benign features: encasement in a visibly thin capsule which defines an abrupt border with the surrounding tissue, which is unaffected by the lesion's presence. The posterior features are also mixed; frequently, both shadowing and enhancement are seen.

Although ultrasound can be definitive in characterizing a benign-appearing soft-tissue density mass as a simple cyst, mammography can be definitive in the diagnosis of a hamartoma or hamartoma variant in visualizing the encapsulated mass containing an admixture of fat and soft tissue components. Ultrasound-guided core biopsies of these masses may be rewarded only with a nonspecific diagnosis of "benign breast tissue," the components of the lesion. Only if the capsule is identified microscopically can a pathologist report a fibroadenolipoma.

A basic goal of breast ultrasound is to differentiate benign from malignant disease so that patients are spared unnecessary interventions. Once a mass has been assessed with ultrasound as benign or probably benign, management consists of serial observation. If the diagnosis is based on valid criteria and there is no evidence of proliferative change, the follow-up examinations will generally show no change in the lesion over time (**Fig. 10.4**).

Although most fibroadenomas can be recognized by the typical appearance described above, it is not uncommon for larger tumors to have a heterogeneous internal structure. Although heterogeneous areas may represent foci of proliferation, this sign is not always reliable (**Fig. 10.5**).

Although in the United States targeted sonography directed to characterization of a palpable mass or mammographic finding is standard in many practices, the ultrasound exam will include a complete survey of each breast. The rationale for the bilateral survey is the expected 15% likelihood of finding coexisting nodules at other sites in the breast or contralaterally. It is important to include these lesions in the baseline documentation so that change can be detected if and when it occurs. It is also important to detect and document all other abnormalities. The ultrasound examination should be thorough enough to ensure that subsequent examinations do not reveal "new" tumors that were present previously but undetected. It is also important to appreciate additional abnormalities. Given the prevalence of fibrocystic breast changes, it is common to find coexisting cysts, duct ectasia, and fibrotic changes in patients with fibroadenomas (**Fig. 10.6**). Occasionally, an unsuspected cancer will be detected.

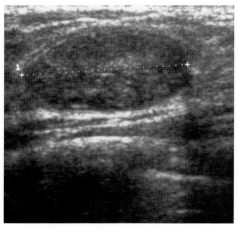

Shape	Oval
Orientation	Parallel
Margin	Circumscribed
Lesion boundary	Abrupt interface
Echo pattern	Hypoechoic
Posterior acoustic features	Enhancement
Surrounding tissue	No changes
Calcifications	None
Vascularity	Present immediately adjacent to lesion

! Comment:
Nonhomogeneity may signify proliferation, and therefore cytologic or histologic evaluation is definitely required. In this case the lesion was excised because of its large size. Histology showed no evidence of proliferation.

Fig. 10.5 Large fibroadenoma with no histologic signs of proliferation (25-year-old patient).

Fig. 10.6 Bilateral fibroadenomas in a cystic breast (35-year-old patient).

Shape	Oval
Orientation	Parallel
Margin	Circumscribed
Lesion boundary	Abrupt interface
Echo pattern	Hypoechoic
Posterior acoustic features	No posterior acoustic features
Surrounding tissue	No changes
Calcifications	None
Vascularity	Not present

! Comment:
Ultrasound was done to investigate a palpable nodule in the left breast. The tumor in the right breast was detected incidentally. This emphasizes the importance of a thorough examination of both breasts.

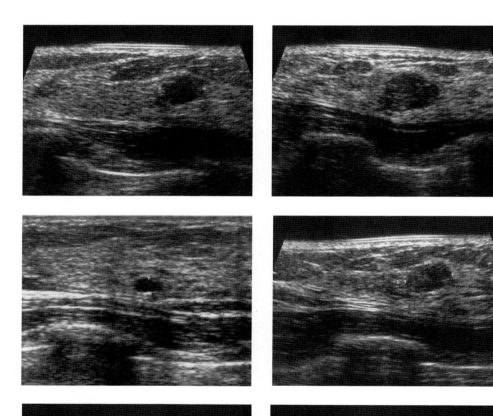

Less Common Findings of Fibroadenomas

Some fibroadenomas have a heterogeneous internal echo pattern as a result of proliferative changes, regressive changes, or calcification (**Figs. 10.7 a, b–10.10 a, b**). Proliferative fibroadenomas and those occurring in association with other benign histologies such as sclerosing adenosis will increase the woman's relative risk of breast cancer by approximately 3 times. Isolated proliferative fibroadenomas are relatively easy to diagnose. But when multiple tumors with proliferative features coexist in the same breast, diagnostic and therapeutic decision-making can become difficult issues. Standard guidelines cannot be offered, and each case must be evaluated on an individual basis, because the sonographic features are variable and can be difficult to interpret (**Table 10.3**).

Other Benign Tumors

Fibrocystic change is usually a diffuse process (see Chapter 6), but occasionally it takes the form of focal nodules that produce clinical, mammographic, and sonographic abnormalities. Fibrocystic nodules feel as circumscribed and firm as fibroadenomas when pal-

Table 10.3 Criteria for evaluating atypical fibroadenomas

Shape	Oval or complex
Orientation	Parallel
Margin	Circumscribed or partly indistinct
Surrounding tissue	No changes
Calcifications	None or macrocalcifications
Vascularity	Present in lesion or immediately adjacent to lesion

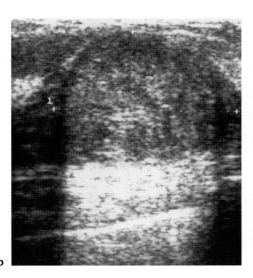
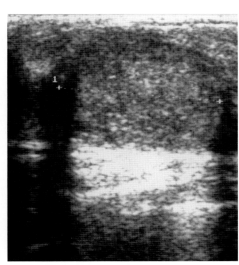

a, b

Fig. 10.7 a, b Proliferative fibroadenoma in a 49-year-old woman.
a Sagittal scan.
b Transverse scan.

Shape	Oval
Orientation	Parallel
Margin	Circumscribed
Lesion boundary	Abrupt interface
Echo pattern	Hyperechoic
Posterior acoustic features	Enhancement
Surrounding tissue	No changes
Calcifications	None
Vascularity	Present in lesion

! Comment:
The tumor was observed for 1 year following aspiration cytology. Despite cytologic evidence of proliferation, initially the tumor was not excised for medical reasons. Subsequent enlargement of the tumor prompted surgery, which confirmed proliferative fibroadenoma.

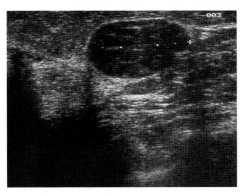
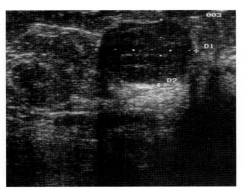

a, b

Fig. 10.8 a, b Proliferative fibroadenoma in a 50-year-old woman.
a Sagittal scan.
b Transverse scan.

Shape	Oval
Orientation	Parallel
Margin	Circumscribed
Lesion boundary	Abrupt interface
Echo pattern	Hypoechoic
Posterior acoustic features	Enhancement
Surrounding tissue	No changes
Calcifications	None
Vascularity	Present in lesion (weak)

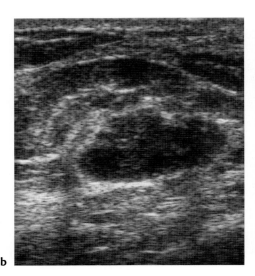

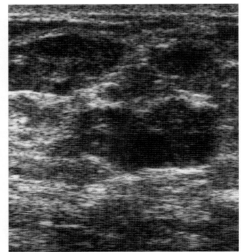

Fig. 10.9 a, b Proliferative fibroadenoma in a 29-year-old woman.
a Sagittal scan.
b Transverse scan

Shape	Oval
Orientation	Parallel
Margin	Microlobulated
Lesion boundary	Abrupt interface
Echo pattern	Hypoechoic
Posterior acoustic features	No posterior acoustic features
Surrounding tissue	No changes
Calcifications	None
Vascularity	Present in lesion (weak)

a, b

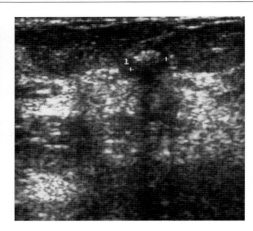

Fig. 10.10 a, b Calcified fibroadenoma in a 31-year-old woman.
a Mammography.
b Ultrasound.

Shape	Complex
Orientation	Not parallel
Margin	Indistinct
Lesion boundary	Abrupt interface
Echo pattern	Hypoechoic
Posterior acoustic features	Shadowing
Surrounding tissue	No changes
Calcifications	Macrocalcifications
Vascularity	Not present

a, b

❗ Comment:
The mammogram shows a typical calcified fibroadenoma. Often these degenerative changes are not seen until menopause, when the tumor is detected incidentally. The macrocalcifications in the tumor refract and attenuate ultrasound, creating a suspicious pattern. However, correlation of the mammographic and sonographic findings indicates that the lesion is benign.

pated, but they are less mobile. They usually resemble fibroadenomas in their mammographic and sonographic features and are often mistaken for them (**Figs. 10.11, 10.12**). These nodules may be solitary or multiple and are variable in size. Because they are indistinguishable from fibroadenomas, the diagnosis is usually established by percutaneous or surgical biopsy. The nodules usually represent simple, nonproliferative fibrocystic changes, but some lesions are associated with focal proliferative changes and therefore require surveillance. Other less common lesions must also be considered in the differential diagnosis (**Fig. 10.13 a, b**).

Inspissated cysts and milk of calcium cysts can also mimic fibroadenomas (Chapter 7). Solitary cysts with internal echoes are very easy to diagnose by aspiration, which will allay the patient's concerns.

Milk of calcium in small cysts can be diagnosed definitively with mammography. On a 90° lateral view, the calcifications fall to the bottom of the cysts where they conform to the rounded shape of the cyst as a curvilinear or "teacup" density On the craniocaudal view, the greatest density is present in the center of the nodule where the calcifications congregate in the deepest part of the cyst,

The borders of the cyst are blurred in the periphery, the thinnest portion of the cyst. Milk of calcium calcifications are benign, as are the cysts within which the calcium is precipitating. The management is mammographic follow-up appropriate for the patient's age.

Lipomas, fibrolipomas and adenofibromas are circumscribed masses that may resemble fibroadenomas or, in the case of the lipoma, show increased echogenicity compared with fat. Compressibility is a helpful diagnostic criterion for these tumors (**Figs. 10.14; 10.15 a, b; 10.16**). Lipomas, encapsulated masses of fat density, can be diagnosed on mammograms. The relatively increased echogenicity of the fatty components is another clue, although similar changes in echogenicity may develop after trauma due to the secondary fibrosis of hemorrhagic areas in fatty breast tissue. The key diagnostic feature in the latter case, however, is that the margins of an area of injury will not be circumscribed.

Another uncommon breast mass is the hamartoma or fibroadenolipoma, palpable as a soft rubbery mass with smooth borders. Ultrasound demonstrates a predominantly hypoechoic, heteroge-

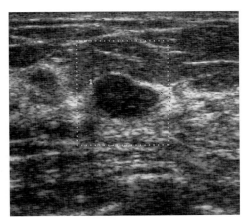

Shape	Oval
Orientation	Parallel
Margin	Circumscribed
Lesion boundary	Abrupt interface
Echo pattern	Hypoechoic
Posterior acoustic features	Enhancement
Surrounding tissue	No changes
Calcifications	None
Vascularity	Not present

❗ Comment:
Fibrocystic change can produce focal abnormalities that are indistinguishable from fibroadenoma by ultrasound but are plainly distinguishable by their cytologic and histologic features.

Fig. 10.11 Fibrocystic nodules in a 39-year-old woman who presented clinically with a moderately mobile mass 1.5×2 cm in size. Mammograms showed an asymmetric density that was indeterminate because of superimposed structures.

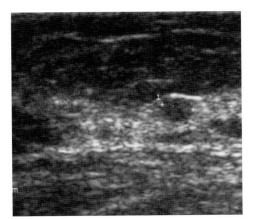

Shape	Oval
Orientation	Parallel
Margin	Circumscribed
Lesion boundary	Abrupt interface
Echo pattern	Hypoechoic
Posterior acoustic features	No posterior acoustic features
Surrounding tissue	No changes
Calcifications	None
Vascularity	Not present

❗ Comment:
This nonpalpable lesion was detected in a fibrocystic breast. The diagnosis of a cyst was established by aspiration and complete drainage of the lesion.

Fig. 10.12 Echogenic cyst in a 55-year old woman.

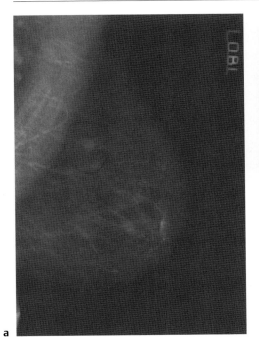

a

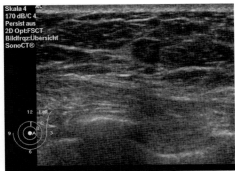

Fig. 10.13 a, b Granular cell tumor.

Shape	Oval
Orientation	Not parallel
Margin	Angular
Lesion boundary	Abrupt interface
Echo pattern	Hypoechoic
Posterior acoustic features	No posterior acoustic features
Surrounding tissue	Architectural distortion
Calcifications	None
Vascularity	Not present

❗ Comment:
This 7×7 mm lesion was detected by screening mammography in an unsymptomatic menopausal patient. Because of doubtful mammographic and sonographic signs, core biopsy and excision biopsy were recommended. Both histopathologies showed a benign granular cell tumor.

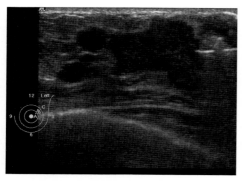

Fig. 10.14 Adenofibroma in a 15 year-old patient.

Shape	Complex, irregular
Orientation	Parallel
Margin	Circumscribed, lobulated
Lesion boundary	Abrupt interface
Echo pattern	Hypoechoic
Posterior acoustic features	No posterior acoustic features
Surrounding tissue	No changes
Calcifications	None
Vascularity	Present in lesion

! Comment:
Within 1 year the patient felt a growing firm nodule in her left breast. Sonomorphology was doubtful. Core biopsy revealed a lesion with adenofibrosis combined with papillary components and proliferative activity. Excision was recommended and a proliferative lesion with mixed tissue components was confirmed. After 3 years of follow-up the patient was free of recurrence.

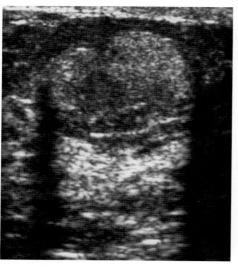 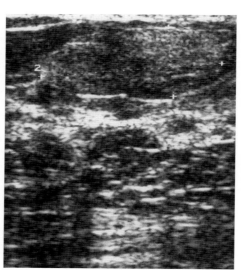

a, b

Shape	Oval
Orientation	Parallel
Margin	Circumscribed
Lesion boundary	Abrupt interface
Echo pattern	Hyperechoic
Posterior acoustic features	Enhancement
Surrounding tissue	No changes
Calcifications	None
Vascularity	Not present

! Comment:
This case illustrates the typically high echogenicity of lipomas. A significant feature of the lesion is its high compressibility.

Fig. 10.15 a, b Fibrolipoma in a 65-year-old woman.
a Without compression.
b With compression.

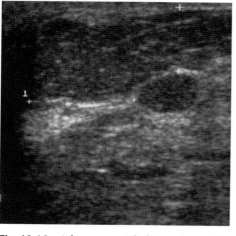

Fig. 10.16 Adenomyoepithelioma in a 53-year-old woman with a smooth palpable breast mass. Mammography showed an oval mass with smooth margins.

Shape	Oval
Orientation	Parallel
Margin	Circumscribed
Lesion boundary	Abrupt interface
Echo pattern	Hypoechoic
Posterior acoustic features	Enhancement
Surrounding tissue	No changes
Calcifications	None
Vascularity	Not present

! Comment:
Despite its histological differences, this lesion resembles a typical fibroadenoma in its ultrasonic features.

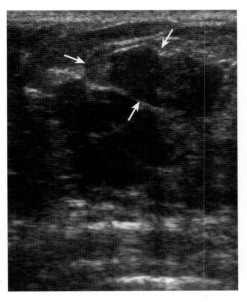
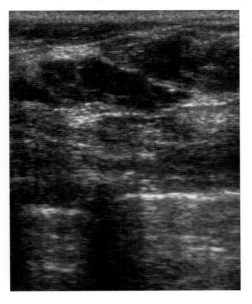

a, b

Fig. 10.17 a, b Hamartoma in a 27-year-old woman with a smooth, rubbery, slightly mobile mass in the outer right breast. Mammography showed slight asymmetry and increased lucency in the outer breast. Ultrasound demonstrates a compressible, heterogeneous, encapsulated mass (arrows).
a Sagittal noncompression scan.
b Compression scan.

Shape	Oval, complex
Orientation	Parallel
Margin	Circumscribed, lobulations
Lesion boundary	Abrupt interface
Echo pattern	Hypoechoic
Posterior acoustic features	No posterior acoustic features
Surrounding tissue	No changes
Calcifications	None
Vascularity	Not present

! Comment:
The ultrasound impression of hamartoma is supported by the fact that the heterogeneous, hypoechoic lesion contains structures that resemble glandular tissue. Additionally, ultrasound does not show architectural disruption. However, in the uncompressed scan the lesion is difficult to evaluate. Compression improves sound penetration and allows for better interpretation of the boundaries and the inner structures.

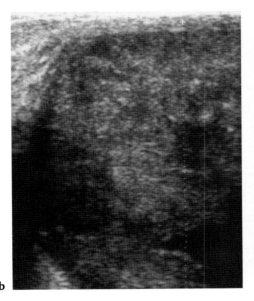
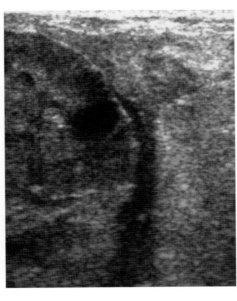

a, b

Fig. 10.18 a, b Phyllodes tumor in a 17-year-old girl.
a Cranial.
b Caudal portion.

Shape	Oval
Size	60 × 50 mm
Orientation	Parallel
Margin	Circumscribed
Lesion boundary	Abrupt
Echo pattern	Isoechoic
Posterior acoustic features	Enhancement
Surrounding tissue	No changes
Calcifications	None
Vascularity	Present in lesion

! Comment:
This lesion is typical of phyllodes (or phylloides) tumor. The size of the tumor makes it difficult to evaluate the whole lesion within the small field of view of the transducer.

neous septate, easily compressible mass. Closer scrutiny reveals intratumoral structures similar in appearance to the three tissue components of the breast, histologically fat, glandular, and connective tissue, forming a "breast within a breast." The tumor is oval or lobulated and displays a thin capsule-like border (**Fig. 10.17 a,b**).

In addition to the usual breast components, cells of other origins may form tumorlike nodules. Hemangiomas, neurofibromas, and myoepitheliomas occasionally develop in the breast as in other body regions (see **Fig. 10.16 a, b**).

Another rare breast tumor is the phyllodes tumor (formerly called cystosarcoma phyllodes), which tends to grow very rapidly. Average age at diagnosis is 45 years although it has occurred at ages ranging from 10 to over 80 years. Most of these tumors are benign, but because of tendency to recur locally, they should be surgically excised with wide margins. The margins of these masses are circumscribed and their internal echo pattern is heterogeneous, often with cystic elements (**Figs. 10.18, 10.19**).

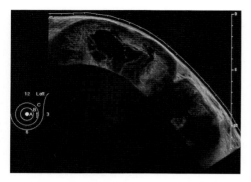

Shape	Oval
Orientation	Parallel
Margin	Circumscribed
Lesion boundary	Abrupt interface
Echo pattern	Complex
Posterior acoustic features	No posterior acoustic features
Surrounding tissue	No changes
Calcifications	None
Vascularity	Present in lesion

❗ Comment:
This lesion had grown within 5 years. Core biopsy revealed phyllodes tumor. Tumor excision confirmed this diagnosis and additionally small foci of invasive carcinoma were found in the center.

Fig. 10.19 Phyllodes tumor in a 65-year-old patient. Ultrasound shows a 20-cm lesion. Using panoramic view technology, the whole lesion could be displayed on one image (12-MHz transducer).

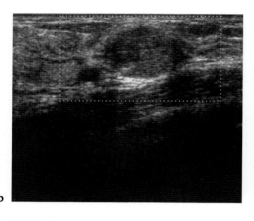 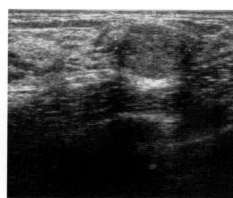

a, b

Fig. 10.20 a, b Mucinous carcinoma with the sonographic features of fibroadenoma in a 52-year-old woman.
a Sagittal scan.
b Transverse scan.

Shape	Oval
Orientation	Parallel
Margin	Circumscribed
Lesion boundary	Thin echogenic halo (a)
Echo pattern	Hypoechoic
Posterior acoustic features	Enhancement
Surrounding tissue	No changes
Calcifications	None
Vascularity	Present immediately adjacent to lesion

❗ Comment:
This case illustrates a common source of misinterpretation. The patient had detected the nodule by self-examination. Mammograms and ultrasound (done elsewhere) showed a benign round lesion. Follow-ups were scheduled and showed no change in the size of the lesion over time. When the patient came to us, we felt strongly that the lesion should be evaluated by percutaneous biopsy. Needle biopsy followed by surgical excision revealed mucinous carcinoma.

Differential Diagnosis, Considerations, and Pitfalls

The goal of feature analysis is to determine a lesion's likelihood of malignancy on a spectrum ranging from benign to varying degrees of indeterminate to near certainty of malignancy. Benign features are oval shape, circumscribed margins, and long axis parallel to the skin with no malignant characteristics such as microcalcifications. Most benign tumors and especially fibroadenomas have these typical features that can help differentiate them from carcinoma. It should be noted, however, that approximately 2 % of carcinomas have fibroadenoma-like benign features, including invasive ductal carcinoma. Other carcinomas that may at first glance appear circumscribed are mucinous and medullary. Metastases to the breast from lung and other organs can rarely have a bland, benign appearance, as can lymphoma. Length of observation is no guarantee, for even a tumor that has been followed for years may be a slow-growing carcinoma. Real-time scanning may reveal marginal microlobulation or angularity not observed initially. Previously un-appreciated architectural distortion or an echogenic rim around the mass or increased vascularity can be a tip-off to a malignant lesion originally thought to be benign, and biopsy rather than follow-up will be the recommendation (**Figs. 10.20 a, b, 10.21 a–d**).

A common source of difficulty, particularly for beginners, is distinguishing fat lobules from hypoechoic tumors (**Figs. 10.22 a, b, 10.23 a, b**). Hypoechoic fat lobules are encased in hyperechoic connective tissue and may be difficult to distinguish from fibroadenomas. Imaging in perpendicular planes can help; in one view the fat lobule resembles an oval mass, a fibroadenoma, but as the transducer is rotated to the orthogonal view, the fat lobule will elongate. An isoechoic fibroadenoma may be oriented in a slightly different direction than the interlocking fat lobules in which the lesion is hiding. In addition, one can distinguish circumscribed lesions from normal anatomic components, such as the subcutaneous fat layer by scanning the breast in perpendicular planes to determine their compressibility, moving the transducer in short anterior–posterior excursions to apply compression and release. These techniques are detailed in Chapter 2.

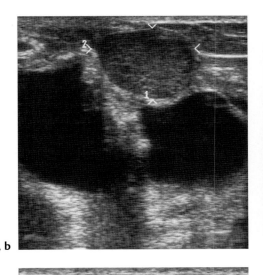
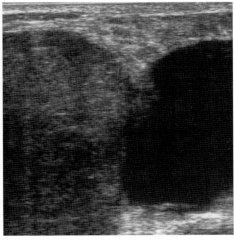

a, b

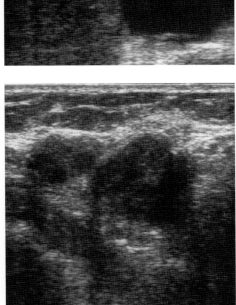

c, d

Fig. 10.21 a–d Extensive multicentric invasive ductal carcinoma in a 44-year-old woman. The clinical impression was fibroadenoma, which the patient had neglected for over a year. Multiple cysts are also present.

Shape	Oval
Orientation	Parallel
Margin	Circumscribed
Lesion boundary	Abrupt interface
Echo pattern	Hypoechoic
Posterior acoustic features	Combined pattern
Surrounding tissue	No changes
Calcifications	None
Vascularity	Present in lesions

❗ Comment:
Multiple, predominantly circumscribed nodules and cysts are found throughout the breast, consistent with the clinical impression of fibroadenoma. Histology revealed invasive ductal carcinoma in all foci.

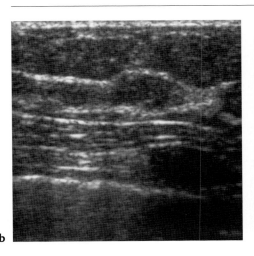
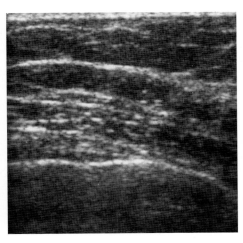

a, b

Fig. 10.22 a, b Fatty infiltration in a 42-year-old woman.
a Sagittal scan.
b Transverse scan.

❗ Comment:
The sagittal scan (**a**) creates the impression of a hypoechoic mass with smooth margins. Rotating the transducer 90° shows, however, that the lesion consists of fatty infiltration. This case serves as a reminder that all focal lesions should be examined in mutually perpendicular planes to avoid misinterpretation.

Another serious but fairly common error for the novice is to misinterpret the transverse sections of ribs as oval tumors with posterior acoustic shadowing. The anatomic setting of this pseudolesion behind the pectoral muscle is the initial piece of evidence, and the orthogonal view in which the rib elongates confirms the diagnosis. The rib is not a good target for a core biopsy (**Fig. 10.24 a, b**)! We review these points under *Differential Diagnosis: Considerations and Pitfalls*, because experience with testing and accreditation has shown that even fully trained examiners can be trapped by misinterpretations of this kind.

Post-traumatic changes are discussed in Chapter 11. They include scar formation, which typically produces irregularly shaped, spiculated focal lesions, and occasional areas of fat necrosis or circumscribed masses that can have a variety of sonographic features. Fat necrosis may be seen as a complex cystic and solid mass. Less commonly, fat necrosis may also appear as a solid, homogeneous mass that closely resembles fibroadenoma (**Fig. 10.25 a, b**).

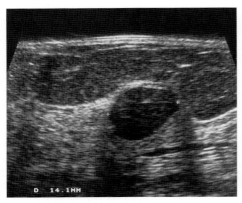 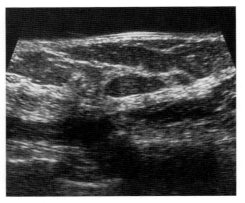

Shape	Oval
Orientation	Parallel
Margin	Circumscribed
Lesion boundary	Abrupt interface
Echo pattern	Hypoechoic
Posterior acoustic features	No posterior acoustic rfeatures
Surrounding tissue	No changes
Calcifications	None
Vascularity	Not present

a, b

Fig. 10.23 a, b   Fibroadenoma and lipoma in a 61-year-old woman.
a Fibroadenoma in the upper right breast.
b Lipoma in the lower right breast.

❗ Comment:
The fibroadenoma and lipoma have the same echogenicity and are also isoechoic to the subcutaneous fat. Examination in mutually perpendicular planes defines each lesion as a circumscribed tumor. However, the lipoma was easily compressible, while the fibroadenoma was not.

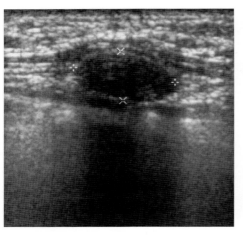 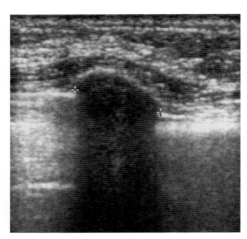

❗ Comment:
Ribs in cross section resemble tumors with circumscribed margins. The bony distal ribs cast strong shadowing, which can be a source of misinterpretation.

a, b

Fig. 10.24 a, b   A rib displayed in cross section may be misinterpreted as a breast tumor.
a Parasternal scan (cartilaginous part of rib).
b More distal scan (bony part of rib) with a strong acoustic shadow.

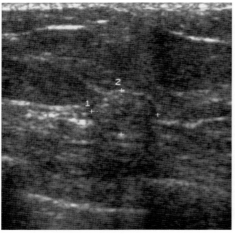 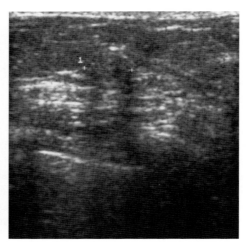

Shape	Oval
Orientation	Parallel
Margin	Circumscribed
Lesion boundary	Abrupt interface
Echo pattern	Hypoechoic
Posterior acoustic features	Combined pattern
Surrounding tissue	No changes
Calcifications	None
Vascularity	Not present

a, b

Fig. 10.25 a, b   Fat necrosis in a 57-year-old woman who had undergone prior breast surgery for fibrocystic change.

Further Diagnostic Procedures

Ultrasound

Every solid breast mass merits careful sonographic evaluation. This does not mean that every solid benign breast lesion should be percutaneously biopsied or removed. This would lead to a large number of unnecessary interventions, with the attendant financial costs and needless physical and emotional trauma.

The use of ultrasound is the standard of care in evaluating palpable and mammographically depicted breast masses. Mammography and ultrasound are not competitive imaging techniques—they complement each other. If breast density is not the limiting factor, mammography can depict a circumscribed, oval mass to be assessed mammographically as benign or probably benign, but mammography cannot be used to characterize the mass as cystic or solid. Here ultrasound can be definitive in identifying a benign simple cyst or a probably benign solid mass, most likely a fibroadenoma, on baseline mammography. Should there be doubt about the diagnosis, an ultrasound-guided biopsy can be done in real time, keeping the target in sight, to provide an accurate diagnosis in the great majority of cases.

Ultrasound is also important for planning and directing surgical treatment, particularly If multiple tumors are detected. An area of current research and debate in the United States is the management of multiple benign solid masses. Common practice, somewhat illogical if all of the lesions have the same sonographic characteristics, is to do core biopsy on the palpable one or the largest lesion. Logic would have it that either all would be sampled or none, with short-interval follow-up or even routine follow-up as the management plan. As more survey ultrasound is being done, finding a solution to this problem has become urgent.

The German approach is somewhat different. Following bilateral sonography and documentation of multiple uni- or bilateral lesions, fine-needle aspiration or core biopsy is done, and every lesion is considered potentially suspicious for proliferation or malignancy until proven otherwise. Thus, if cytology raises suspicion of proliferative change in a breast with multiple fibroadenomas, an attempt should be made to remove all the nodules, which is not done in the United States. This can be extremely difficult unless the surgeon has detailed information on the spatial distribution of the lesions. Ultrasound has a unique role in this regard, as it enables the surgeon to analyze without time pressure the route of approach, the best incision site, and the location and removal of the individual lesions (**Fig. 10.26**).

Pregnancy can cause special problems in breast imaging. Because of the hormonal changes, the breast becomes radiographically dense and difficult to evaluate by mammography. Palpable breast lesions in younger women are common, and particularly so in pregnancy where fibroadenomas and lactating adenomas respond to circulating estrogens by enlarging.

Most masses encountered in pregnancy are benign, but breast cancer remains an important concern, particularly as women increasingly defer having children until their mid-to-late 30 s and early 40 s. Unless the disease is detected early, the rich blood supply and proliferative changes may enable these tumors to progress swiftly. The difficulty is that fibroadenomas may also respond to hormonal stimulation with rapid growth and frequently develop a heterogeneous echo pattern and irregular borders. Much experience is needed to differentiate these tumors by cytology, because the hormonal changes activate the epithelial cells of the fibroadenoma as well as normal glandular cells, making them very difficult to interpret.

Very similar conditions are encountered in the lactating breast, in which galactoceles also may develop. Unlike simple, aqueous cysts, these milk-filled lesions are frequently heterogeneous and resemble hamartomas, are hyperechoic, or have fat-fluid layers as might be seen in complicated cysts (**Fig. 10.27 a, b**). The diagnosis is easily established, however, by simple percutaneous aspiration of the milky contents of the lesion.

For completeness, it should be noted that lymph nodes can occur within the breast as well as in the more typical areas of lymphatic drainage. Intramammary lymph nodes located superficially or peripherally in the breast often present clinically as smooth, mobile nodules with a soft, rubbery consistency. They appear mammographically as smoothly marginated round or oval lesions with fatty hilar areas. Sonographically, they resemble miniature kidneys and generally can be identified without difficulty (**Fig. 10.28 a, b**).

Mammography

Except in young women, mammograms should be available for correlation. In women under 30 years of age, if sonography shows a mass with indeterminate features or if there is no sonographic abnormality that might explain a palpable finding, mammography is recommended in the American College of Radiology's Appropriateness Criteria scenario of "palpable breast mass, woman under 30 years." When ultrasound shows a mass highly likely to be a fibroadenoma, mammography is not necessary.

MRI

MRI of the breast should be reserved for carefully selected cases. MRI with contrast enhancement is not recommended as the definitive imaging method for characterization of a palpable or mammographically visible mass. Most fibroadenomas enhance on MRI and have variable enhancement patterns, none of them specific. Many fibroadenomas exhibit dark internal septations which confirms their identity; but on MRI over half of fibroadenomas do not have this finding, and biopsy would then be performed.

If the mass is assessed as *probably benign* (BI-RADS category 3), to be managed with short-interval follow-up, and the patient is unwilling to wait, a more reasonable approach than MRI would be to evaluate the mass by fine-needle aspiration or core biopsy. Contrast-enhanced MRI is itself a minimally invasive study that requires the injection of a contrast agent, and so the percutaneous aspiration of a breast mass should not be dismissed as a more invasive procedure. Ultrasound-guided aspiration generally yields sufficient cellular material to make an accurate diagnosis. Most fibroadenomas and other benign tumors show a bland cytologic pattern that obviates the need for further evaluation other than follow-up. If cytology shows marked signs of proliferation, ultrasound-guided core biopsy or excisional biopsy is done (**Figs. 10.29, 10.30**).

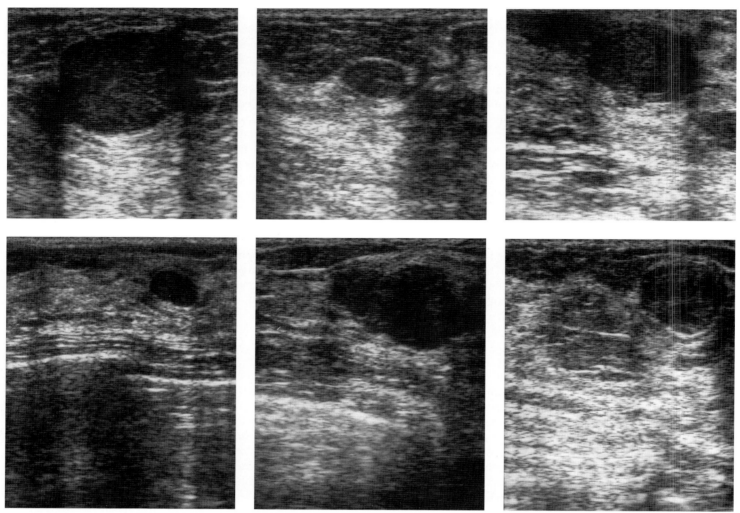

Fig. 10.26 Multiple fibroadenomas in the breast of a 23-year-old woman. Follow-up showed a gradual size increase, prompting recommendation for surgery.

❗ Comment:
Ultrasound is very important in the evaluation of complex findings such as these, which require the cosmetically acceptable removal of all foci. Ultrasound can direct surgical planning and presurgical localization, and ensure the reliable removal of the lesions.

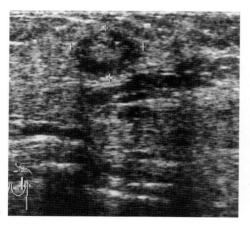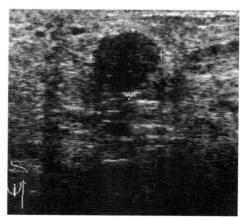

a, b

Fig. 10.27 a, b Focal lesion in a lactating patient 36 years of age.
a Galactocele in the upper left breast.
b Fibroadenoma in the lower left breast.

❗ Comment:
Ultrasound examination of a palpable nodule in the lower left breast revealed two lesions. Because the upper lesion also appeared solid, aspiration cytology was done. The upper lesion yielded a milky aspirate consistent with a galactocele. The lower lesion was firm and solid and showed the typical cellular features of fibroadenoma.

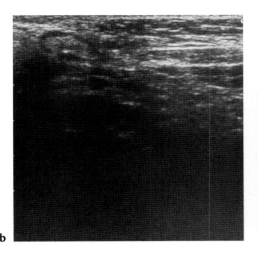
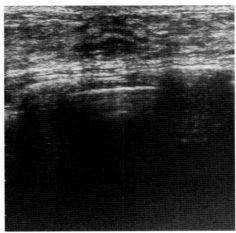

a, b

Fig. 10.28 a, b Intramammary lymph nodes. Lymph nodes may occur within the breast and produce clinically palpable and mammographically visible masses. If doubt exists, cytologic confirmation can be obtained.
a Transverse scan.
b Sagittal scan.

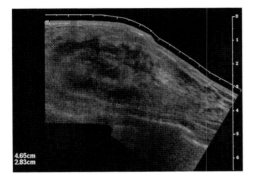

4.65cm
2.83cm

Fig. 10.29 Granulomatous tumor in a patient with sarcoidosis. Features suggest malignant etiology, and biopsy is required.

Shape	Oval
Orientation	Parallel
Margin	Circumscribed, lobulated
Lesion boundary	Abrupt interface
Echo pattern	Complex
Posterior acoustic features	No posterior acoustic features
Surrounding tissue	No changes
Calcifications	None
Vascularity	Present in lesion (weak signals)

❗ Comment:
This lesion has benign characteristics. However size and complex echo pattern require histologic confirmation. Core biopsy revealed a granulomatous tumor which disappeared under cortisol.

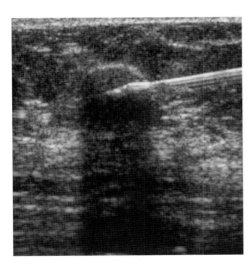

Fig. 10.30 Confirmation of fibroadenoma by core biopsy in a 50-year-old woman with a new breast nodule not seen on previous examination.

Shape	Oval
Orientation	Parallel
Margin	Circumscribed
Lesion boundary	Abrupt interface
Echo pattern	Hypoechoic
Posterior acoustic features	Shadowing
Surrounding tissue	No changes
Calcifications	None
Vascularity	Not present

❗ Comment:
Besides the prevalent benign characteristics this lesion showed shadowing. In addition, this tumor was not described in the previous examination. Therefore histologic confirmation was mandatory.

Fully automated vacuum-assisted biopsy systems have recently been developed that enable breast lesions (e. g., benign tumors) to be removed piecemeal through a small stab incision. There are other devices available commercially that can be used with ultrasound or stereotactic guidance to remove the lesion in one specimen. These minimally invasive techniques are definitely more elegant than open biopsy, certainly less costly, and presumably leave a smaller scar.

Documentation

It is particularly important for solid breast tumors to be documented in two planes. This permits a reliable assessment of the tumor margins in all three planes and the accurate estimation of tumor size and volume. Since many benign lesions are compressible, it is important also to obtain compression and noncompression scans.

A solid tumor should not be reported without a direct recommendation for its management. The final recommendation is based on the clinical evaluation and findings on all of the imaging modalities used and should be included in the written interpretation. The breast imaging physician is obliged to give the patient all the necessary information and note in the written documentation that this obligation has been fulfilled.

Clinical Significance, Diagnostic Problems

Scars can challenge the goal of accurate imaging interpretation. Scars and malignancies share many of the breast findings on which diagnosis hinges: architectural distortion, focal asymmetries, calcifications, and at times, masses (**Table 11.1**) Additional signs of advanced cancer—skin thickening and breast edema—are also hallmarks of the irradiated breast. Application of clinical history, review of imaging findings correlated with the chronology of surgical alteration and trauma, and knowledge of the specifics of the procedure will help to minimize the false-positive diagnosis of benign lesions and reduce the number of unnecessary biopsies, while at the same time avoiding a false-negative diagnosis of breast cancer.

Without having reviewed a sequence of previous examinations including preoperative studies, if available, the use of mammography alone can pose problems in differentiating spiculated scars from tumor. In using ultrasound, to distinguish scar from tumor—new or locally recurrent—considerable experience is often needed

Table 11.1 Problems associated with surgical scars

▸ Subjective complaints
  – Pain
  – Sensory disturbance
  – Cosmetic disfigurement
  – Breast lumps
▸ Interference with follow-up
  – Inspection: skin retraction
  – Palpation: indeterminate mass
  – Mammography: spiculated density
  – Ultrasound: indeterminate hypoechoic lesion
▸ Consequences: morbidity and costs due to repeat surgery, or costly additional diagnostic procedures

(**Fig. 11.1 a, b**). The greatest difficulties are encountered in women who have undergone breast-conserving cancer surgery. An adequate local excision of a carcinoma usually leaves a relatively large surgical cavity with a correspondingly extensive scar. The tumor bed fills with fluid, ordinarily not drained as the slow resorption is thought to promote cosmesis. The picture is further

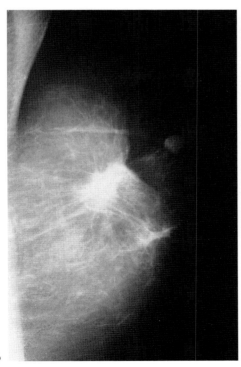 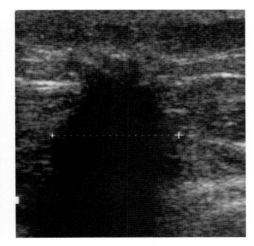

Fig. 11.1 a, b Typical findings 2 years after breast-conserving surgery.
a The mediolateral mammogram shows a spiculated density in the original tumor bed.
b The ultrasound appearance of the lesion is also suspicious.

Shape	Irregular
Orientation	Not parallel
Margin	Indistinct, spiculated
Lesion boundary	Abrupt interface
Echo pattern	Anechoic
Posterior acoustic features	Shadowing
Surrounding tissue	Architectural distortion
Calcifications	None
Vascularity	Not present

❗ Comment:
This case illustrates the difficulty of evaluating a scar. At physical examination, the lesion was palpable as a firm mass. Core biopsy excluded tumor recurrence. Orientation cannot be reliably assessed because of strong shadowing

a, b

157

complicated by breast edema and skin thickening caused by postoperative irradiation of the breast and a boost dose to the tumor bed. Contrasted with the near-complete resolution of findings related to benign surgical excisions, for many women in a year or 18 months, radiation therapy prolongs the resolution time of post-treatment changes to 2 years or more, and for some findings, there is never a return to the pretreatment appearance (**Fig. 11.2**). Initially the radiation mastitis obscures the scar, which then becomes increasingly conspicuous as the edema recedes in the same 3-year time frame that a local recurrence might be found at or near the lumpectomy site (**Fig. 11.3 a–e**). Unfortunately, this can start a chain reaction of unnecessary diagnostic procedures, including core needle or surgical biopsy, that causes a great deal of anguish that is frequently avoidable.

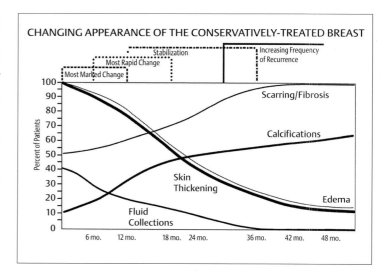

Fig. 11.2 Changing appearance of the conservatively treated breast. With permission from Elsevier, 1992.

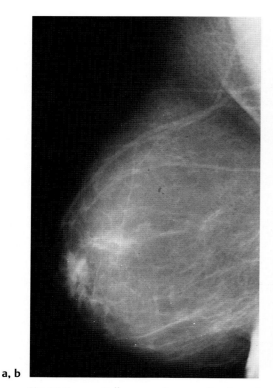
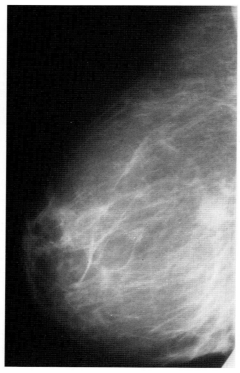
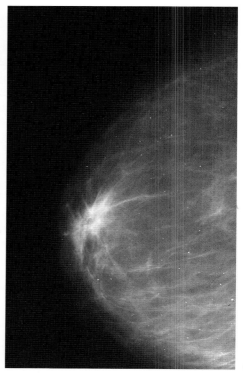

a, b

c

Fig. 11.3 a–e Follow-up of a scar after breast-conserving surgery and radiotherapy.
a Preoperative mammogram shows a typical carcinoma.
b 1 year after breast-conserving surgery and postoperative radiotherapy, increased density is seen throughout the whole breast.
c 2 years after surgery and irradiation, the breast appears less dense but the scar is more conspicuous and resembles a local recurrence.

Fig. 11.3 d, e ▷

Shape	Irregular
Orientation	Parallel
Margin	Indistinct
Lesion boundary	Abrupt interface
Echo pattern	Anechoic without compression, hypoechoic with compression
Posterior acoustic features	Strong shadowing without compression, moderate shadowing with compression
Surrounding tissue	Architectural distortion
Calcifications	None
Vascularity	Not present

❗ Comment:
Periodic follow-up is important in cancer management. This case illustrates typical postsurgical and postirradiation breast changes. Contrast-enhanced MRI was also done and yielded no suspicious findings.

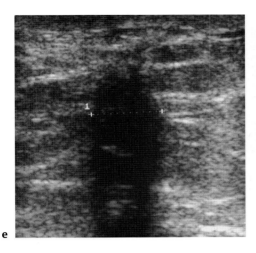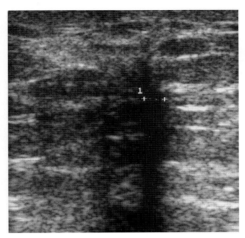

d, e

Fig. 11.3 d, e
d Ultrasound without compression at 2 years appears suspicious.
e Scanning with breast compression shows increased structural details, resulting in a lower index of suspicion.

Mammographic follow-up is essential, particularly in identifying and analyzing calcifications. Special views and careful sequential review of these mammograms, sonograms, and, when they are done, MRI scans can help to overcome some of the limitations imposed by conservative cancer treatment. Ultrasound can be a very valuable adjunct in differentiating postsurgical and postirradiation changes from malignancy. In difficult cases, when the lumpectomy scar is mature after approximately 2 years, contrast-enhanced MRI may be able to resolve the ambiguity between benign post-treatment changes and recurrence.

Diagnostic Criteria, Postoperative Follow-Up

A mammographic view tangential to the scar, best with spot compression and magnification, with a thin wire taped to the skin along the length of the scar, can separate the thickened skin at the entry site from the tumor bed itself, eliminating the extra density projected on to the lumpectomy site by the skin scar that at times suggests possibility of recurrence. But by the nature of the imaging modality, intramammary post-treatment changes can be visualized clearly and directly with ultrasound. One advantage of ultrasound is that it is tomographic, each image representing a thin slice of tissue, thus eliminating superimposed structures. Ultrasound also presents an opportunity to evaluate the compressibility of lesions during real-time scanning. Experience is needed, however, to correctly interpret the variety of changes that may be found.

Typical Findings

Intramammary scars often appear hypoechoic on ultrasound due to the refractive effects caused by the diffuse, regenerative proliferation of connective tissue (**Table 11.2**). The lesion has indistinct margins and often casts an acoustic shadow. The connective tissue fibers in scars are compressible, however. Pressure from the transducer flattens the fibers, frequently causing the hypoechoic lesion and posterior acoustic shadow to disappear (**Figs. 11.4 a, b, 11.5**), as may also happen in areas of native fibrotic tissue with no antecedent trauma or surgery. This alteration in sonographic appear-

Table 11.2 Criteria for the evaluation of scars

Shape	Irregular
Orientation	Not parallel
Margin	Indistinct
Lesion boundary	Abrupt interface
Echo pattern	Anechoic without compression*
Posterior acoustic features	Shadowing*
Surrounding tissue	Architectural distortion
Calcifications	None
Vascularity	Not present

* Because of strong sound attenuation the lesion shows almost no internal echo structures and appears anechoic with shadowing. Under compression the echogenicity increases and shadowing is less pronounced. The axial orientation of the lesion depends on the resection cavity. Frequently it appears not parallel because its posterior margin is obscured by a dense posterior shadow.

ance is helpful in the differential diagnosis, especially in attempting to distinguish a scar from recurrent tumor following breast-conserving surgery.

Besides evaluating compressibility, it is very important to examine the lesion in two planes. In imaging follow-up with both mammography and ultrasound after lumpectomy and radiation therapy, the scar can look entirely different in two projections: elongated in one view and more round and mass-like in the orthogonal view. The scalpel's path defines a tract from the skin incision to the tumor bed. The skin at the incision site is focally thickened in a "V" shape. As the transducer is moved along the course of the scar, the linear extent of the defect can be appreciated. Scanning perpendicular to the scar often shows only a narrow discontinuity in the breast architecture (**Fig. 11.6 a, b**).

Another important consideration is the time factor or age of the scar, keeping in mind that radiation therapy puts the healing process into slow motion. Benign surgical biopsy changes resolve relative rapidly. Fresh scars often appear as extensive hypoechoic lesions, circumscribed and with posterior acoustic enhancement if a fluid collection is present with indistinct and spiculated margins and posterior shadowing as the fluid is resorbed and fibrosis develops over a variable period of time 6–12 months or longer if

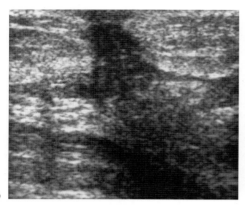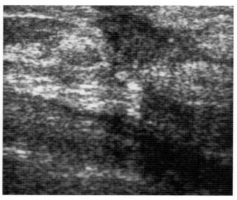

a, b

Shape	Irregular
Orientation	Not parallel
Margin	Indistinct
Lesion boundary	Abrupt interface
Echo pattern	Hypoechoic without compression, slightly more hyperechoic with compression
Posterior acoustic features	Shadowing without compression, no posterior acoustic features with compression
Surrounding tissue	Architectural distortion
Calcifications	None
Vascularity	Not present

Fig. 11.4 a, b Typical scar 3 months after breast-conserving surgery and chemotherapy (no postoperative radiation).
a Without compression ultrasound shows a suspicious lesion with marked architectural distortion.
b The echogenicity of the lesion increases markedly after compression.

■ Comment:
The shadowing and architectural distortion associated with a fresh scar decrease markedly when compression is applied. This excludes a recurrent tumor with reasonable confidence.

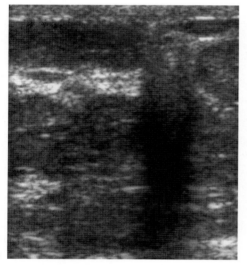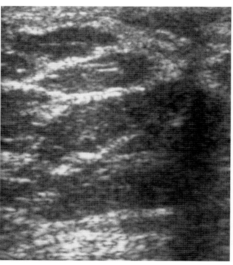

a, b

Shape	Irregular
Orientation	Not parallel
Margin	Indistinct
Lesion boundary	Abrupt interface
Echo pattern	Hypoechoic without compression, slightly more hyperechoic with compression
Posterior acoustic features	Shadowing without compression, less pronounced with compression
Surrounding tissue	Architectural distortion
Calcifications	None
Vascularity	Not present

Fig. 11.5 a, b Ultrasound findings 6 months after breast-conserving surgery and radiotherapy.
a Without compression.
b With compression.

■ Comment:
The fibrotic scar tissue causes marked sound attenuation on the noncompression scan. Applying compression greatly reduces the attenuation, and the parenchymal structure, now almost completely regenerated, can be seen.

the breast is irradiated (**Figs. 11.7 a, b and 11.8 a, b**). By 1–2 years after benign excisions, or if the breast is not irradiated, many scar defects are no longer visible with ultrasound, although a slightly hypoechoic area of subtle architectural distortion usually persists.

Less Common Findings

Hypertrophic scar formation can result in a firm lesion that, even in long-standing cases, cannot be adequately evaluated on biplane scans (**Fig. 11.9 a, b**) or by means of compression (**Fig. 11.10 a, b, Table 11.3**). These lesions display suspicious features and create problems of differential diagnosis. Even if the echogenicity of the lesion increases slightly when compression is applied, there is

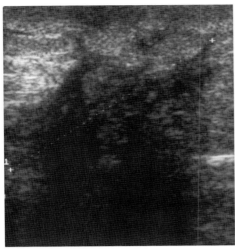 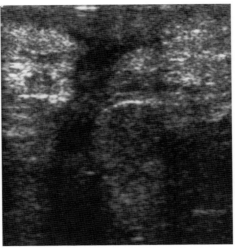

Shape	Irregular
Orientation	Not parallel
Margin	Indistinct
Lesion boundary	Abrupt interface
Echo pattern	Hypoechoic
Posterior acoustic features	Shadowing
Surrounding tissue	Architectural distortion
Calcifications	None
Vascularity	Not present

ⓘ Comment:
This case illustrates that the spatial extent of the scar conforms to the surgical incision. Examination in two planes is therefore necessary to identify the lesion as a scar.

a, b

Fig. 11.6 a, b Surgical scar 1 year after breast-conserving surgery and postoperative radiotherapy. **a** Transverse scan along the scar, **b** sagittal scan (10-MHz transducer).

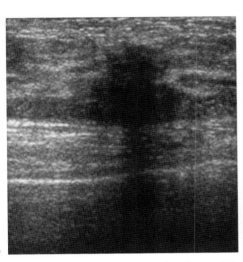 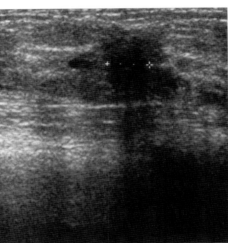

Shape	Irregular
Orientation	Parallel
Margin	Indistinct
Lesion boundary	Abrupt interface
Echo pattern	Hypoechoic
Posterior acoustic features	Shadowing
Surrounding tissue	Architectural distortion
Calcifications	None
Vascularity	Not present

ⓘ Comment:
This case illustrates the difficulty of evaluating a fresh scar. Even compression is not helpful, since the anatomic structures have not had time to regenerate. Thus, even the compression scan shows a hypoechoic, poorly marginated focal lesion with a structural discontinuity.

a, b

Fig. 11.7 a, b Fresh scar 4 weeks after excision of a fibroadenoma.
a Without compression.
b With compression.

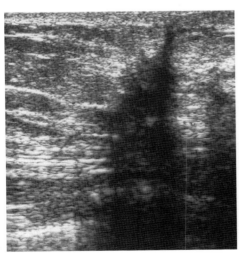 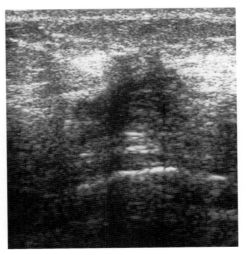

Shape	Irregular
Orientation	Not parallel
Margin	Indistinct
Lesion boundary	Echogenic halo
Echo pattern	Hypoechoic
Posterior acoustic features	Shadowing
Surrounding tissue	Architectural distortion
Calcifications	None
Vascularity	Not present

ⓘ Comment:
Comparison with the fresh scar in Fig. 11.6 shows that some degree of regeneration has taken place in this case.

a, b

Fig. 11.8 a, b Ultrasound findings 1 year after breast-conserving surgery and postoperative radiotherapy. **a** Sagittal scan, **b** transverse scan.

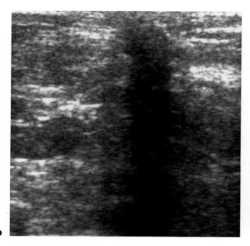
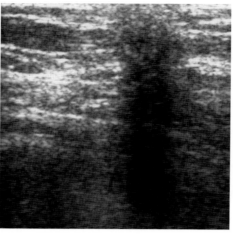

Shape	Irregular
Orientation	Not parallel
Margin	Indistinct
Lesion boundary	Echogenic halo
Echo pattern	Hypoechoic
Posterior acoustic features	Shadowing
Surrounding tissue	Architectural distortion
Calcifications	None
Vascularity	Not present

a, b

Fig. 11.9 a, b Hypertrophic scar formation 3 years after breast-conserving surgery and radiotherapy.
a Without compression.
b With compression.

❗ Comment:
Excessive collagen formation can lead to strong sound attenuation that does not decrease when compression is applied.

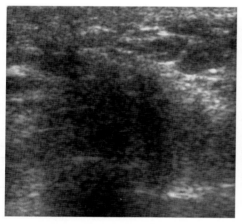
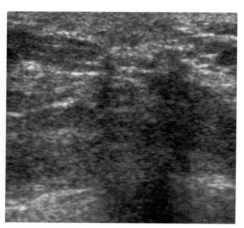

Shape	Irregular
Orientation	Parallel
Margin	Indistinct
Lesion boundary	Echogenic halo
Echo pattern	Complex
Posterior acoustic features	Shadowing
Surrounding tissue	Architectural distortion
Calcifications	None
Vascularity	Not present

a, b

Fig. 11.10 a, b Persistent postirradiation edema and fibrosis 18 months after breast-conserving surgery and postoperative radiotherapy.
a Without compression.
b With compression.

❗ Comment:
Marked sound attenuation is apparent in the noncompression scan. When compression is applied, the regenerative structures can be seen. Both scans show persistent postirradiation changes such as edematous skin thickening and increased echogenicity in the parenchyma and fat.

Table 11.3 Criteria for the evaluation of atypical scars

Shape	Irregular
Orientation	Not parallel
Margin	Indistinct
Lesion boundary	Abrupt interface
Echo pattern	Hypoechoic, not altered by compression
Posterior acoustic features	Strong shadowing, not altered by compression
Surrounding tissue	Architectural distortion (pronounced)
Calcifications	May be present
Vascularity	Not present

often an extensive structural defect that persists in all planes and is indistinguishable from carcinoma. Hypertrophic scar formation often seen after radiation therapy may involve the skin only, appearing sonographically as a circumscribed thickening of the epidermis (**Figs. 11.10 a, b, 11.11 a, b**). Rarely, keloid formation occurs, and if imaged with ultrasound using an offset pad, although unnecessary, the keloid is characteristically hypoechoic and well-defined.

It is common to find a seroma or hematoma in the initial days following breast surgery (**Figs. 11.12, 11.13**). There is no need for rash therapeutic action in these cases. Small fluid collections of only a few milliliters will usually be reabsorbed within a few weeks (**Figs. 11.12, 11.13**). If a collection is large and painfully tense on physical examination, or if there are signs of abscess formation—a rare occurrence—percutaneous aspiration may help.

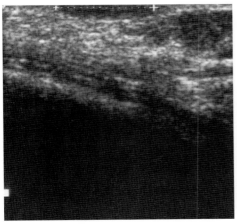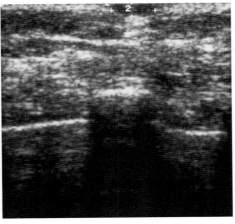

Shape	Oval
Orientation	Parallel
Margin	Circumscribed
Lesion boundary	Abrupt interface
Echo pattern	Hypoechoic
Posterior acoustic features	Enhancement
Surrounding tissue	No changes
Calcifications	None
Vascularity	Not present

a, b

Fig. 11.11 a, b Keloid formation in the skin 9 months after mastectomy. Ultrasound demonstrates the chest wall, subcutaneous fat, and thickened epidermis in the area of the scar.
a Scan along the scar.
b Scan on a perpendicular plane.

❗ Comment:
This near-focusing transducer permits superficial structures to be evaluated without a standoff pad. Because local recurrences are often manifested in the epidermis, skin evaluation is an important aspect of follow-up.

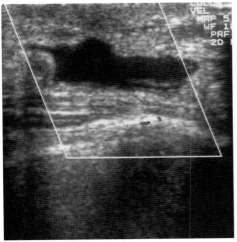

Shape	Irregular
Orientation	Parallel
Margin	Circumscribed
Lesion boundary	Abrupt interface
Echo pattern	Anechoic containing some artificial echoes
Posterior acoustic features	Enhancement
Surrounding tissue	Architectural distortion
Calcifications	None
Vascularity	Not assessed

Fig. 11.12 Seroma 10 days after breast-conserving surgery.

❗ Comment:
Following breast surgery, the wound bed often fills with fluid after the drains have been withdrawn. Generally there is no need to reopen or aspirate the wound because the small collection of fluid is usually reabsorbed without treatment and does not contraindicate postoperative radiotherapy.

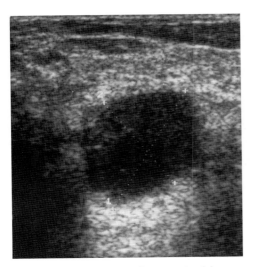

Shape	Oval
Orientation	Parallel
Margin	Microlobulated
Lesion boundary	Abrupt interface
Echo pattern	Hypoechoic
Posterior acoustic features	Enhancement
Surrounding tissue	Architectural distortion
Calcifications	None
Vascularity	Not assessed

Fig. 11.13 Small, partially organized hematoma 2 weeks after surgery for fibrocystic change.

❗ Comment:
Note the acoustic enhancement posterior to the mass. Hematomas of this size are usually reabsorbed without treatment.

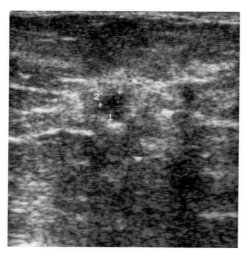

Shape	Irregular
Orientation	Parallel
Margin	Indistinct
Lesion boundary	Echogenic halo
Echo pattern	Hypoechoic
Posterior acoustic features	Shadowing
Surrounding tissue	Architectural distortion
Calcifications	None
Vascularity	Not present

Fig. 11.14 Fat necrosis 1 year after the excision of a benign lesion due to clustered microcalcifications on mammograms, identified histologically as benign breast disease, grade III. Postoperative follow-up mammograms showed increasing pleomorphic microcalcifications, and the lesion was re-excised. Histology revealed fat necrosis with foam cells, macrophages, and giant cells.

❗ Comment:
Areas of fat necrosis often show a typical mammographic features but may present as suspicious areas showing a malignant-type calcification pattern. Ultrasound can demonstrate the lesion but cannot provide reliable differentiation. Fine-needle aspiration or core biopsy is a possible alternative to excisional biopsy.

If there is surgical exploration of the axilla, which is becoming less common due to the success of sentinel node imaging as a predictor of lymph node metastases, a drain is ordinarily placed.

Hematomas often cannot be completely evacuated with an ordinary aspirating needle because of their inspissated contents, and a large-gauge venous catheter should be used. Especially for fluid collections in the axilla, the catheter poses less risk of injury than a metal needle. If the aspirate is bloody and the collection recurs within a short time, persistent postoperative bleeding should be suspected. The wound should be reopened unless the bleeding can be controlled by conservative means. Hemorrhage can be confirmed by measuring the hemoglobin concentration in the aspirate and comparing it with the hemoglobin level in current blood work.

Uncommonly, seromas and hematomas may become secondarily infected. If signs of inflammation such as leukocytosis and fever are noted clinically, the collection should be aspirated for bacteriologic analysis. A concurrent cytologic smear can furnish a more rapid diagnosis by confirming the presence of white blood cells. Severe inflammation should be managed by open treatment and drainage.

Fat necrosis and granulomas in an area of scarring can be difficult to distinguish from recurrent tumors (**Fig. 11.14**). Correlative mammograms should be sought, as they may show a characteristic appearance that can establish the correct diagnosis obviating the need for biopsy. If a recurrence is still suspected, the diagnosis should be established by percutaneous ultrasound-guided core biopsy. Because radiation therapy itself can cause cytologic atypia, fine-needle aspiration biopsy is unreliable for distinguishing treatment changes from recurrent tumor in the irradiated breast, and large needle core biopsy, with spring-activated or vacuum-assisted devices is recommended.

Differential Diagnosis

The principal dilemma in differential diagnosis is distinguishing carcinoma from scars and fat necrosis, which can have similar sonographic appearances (**Fig. 11.15**). Lesions that resemble benign tumors may develop in proximity to scars (**Fig. 11.16**). Epidermal inclusion cysts with indistinct margins can also be difficult to identify (**Fig. 11.17**). Circumscribed blood clots may form within seromas, creating a complex cystic mass in which mural nodules and septa simulate intracystic tumor (**Fig. 11.18**). If the preoperative mammograms and ultrasound examinations are reviewed, and the carcinoma a small spiculated mass or pleomorphic microcalcifications, the likelihood of recurrence as intracystic tumor is nearly zero. If doubt remains, needle biopsy can establish the diagnosis.

Diagnostic Procedures

Mammographic and sonographic findings should be correlated. Accurate interpretation sometimes depends more one modality than the other, sometimes both, and occasionally neither will be definitive. The lumpectomy site on mammograms is recognizable as a focal asymmetry, indeterminate, with regard to recurrence without reviewing previous mammograms in chronological sequence which can demonstrate scar contraction over time. Sequential ultrasound scans can depict similar decrease in size and linear elongation of the scar, and progressive resolution of radiation edema and skin thickening.

Dynamic contrast-enhanced MRI usually shows a marked increase of signal intensity in fresh and granulating scars clouding distinction between carcinoma and postoperative change. To ex-

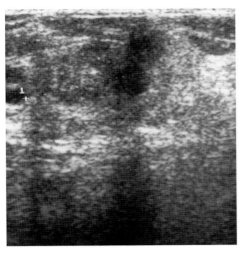

Shape	Irregular
Orientation	Not parallel
Margin	Indistinct
Lesion boundary	Echogenic halo
Echo pattern	Hypoechoic
Posterior acoustic features	Shadowing
Surrounding tissue	Architectural distortion
Calcifications	None
Vascularity	Present immediately adjacent to lesion (weak signal, only one vessel)

❗ Comment:
This case illustrates how difficult it can be to distinguish between scar tissue and cancer recurrence following breast-conserving surgery.

Fig. 11.15 Invasive breast carcinoma mimicking a scar.

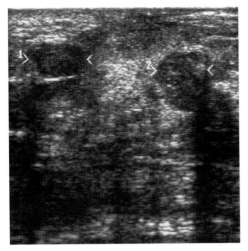

Shape	Oval
Orientation	Parallel/not parallel
Margin	Circumscribed
Lesion boundary	Abrupt interface
Echo pattern	Hypoechoic
Posterior acoustic features	No posterior acoustic features
Surrounding tissue	Architectural distortion
Calcifications	None
Vascularity	Not present

❗ Comment:
Granulomas have variable imaging features. This transverse scan shows two round lesions that resemble fibroadenomas.

Fig. 11.16 Scar granulomas 1 year after breast-conserving surgery. They were re-excised because of increasing microcalcifications.

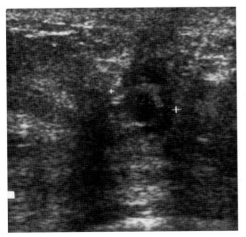

Shape	Round
Orientation	Not parallel
Margin	Circumscribed
Lesion boundary	Abrupt interface
Echo pattern	Hypoechoic
Posterior acoustic features	Enhancement
Surrounding tissue	No changes
Calcifications	None
Vascularity	Not assessed

❗ Comment:
This lesion is a cyst that formed in the area of a surgical scar. Due to sound attenuation by the scar, the cyst appears almost indistinct and is difficult to evaluate. Aspiration is useful to establish the diagnosis.

Fig. 11.17 Inclusion cyst following removal of a benign lesion.

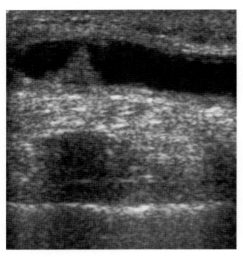

Shape	Oval
Orientation	Parallel
Margin	Circumscribed
Lesion boundary	Abrupt interface
Echo pattern	Anechoic with a hyperechoic internal structure
Posterior acoustic features	Enhancement
Surrounding tissue	No changes
Calcifications	None
Vascularity	Not present

■ Comment:
The mural hematoma resembles intracystic papilloma. When the seroma was aspirated, the structure was identified as a floating blood clot, which was partially aspirated through the needle.

Fig. 11.18 Postoperative seroma with a circumscribed hematoma.

clude recurrent tumor, MRI is useful only in the longer-term follow-up of indeterminate lesions, because it takes at least 18–24 months for the local increase in tissue blood flow to subside following surgery. In addition, the mean time to local recurrence (at or within 2 cm of the lumpectomy site) is 3 years, and if the margins of resection have been free of tumor, recurrence will be rare during the first year of follow-up. If margins have been involved, presence of tumor can be regarded as residual cancer, and recent reports suggest that the transected margin can be identified with contrast-enhanced MRI as an enhancing bulge or focal thickening within the wall of the tumor bed, itself enhancing circumferentially as granulation tissue forms. The study can be done approximately 3 weeks after surgery and may possibly contribute to focusing the re-excision.

Doppler ultrasound can show an analogous increase in signal intensity, especially after the administration of an ultrasound contrast agent. This technique, which is helpful later in distinguishing scars from recurrent tumor, is still being tested in clinical studies. The use of intravenously administered contrast agents for ultrasound is not yet FDA-approved in the United States.

Role of Ultrasound

Ultrasound ranks highly among the imaging modalities because of its capacity for dynamic investigations. Atypical scars can pose significant diagnostic problems, however. Because they usually present as circumscribed focal lesions, ultrasound-guided percu-

taneous biopsy can establish the diagnosis in doubtful cases. Fine-needle aspiration often does not yield sufficient material for cytologic analysis, because of the difficulty of aspirating cells from the fibrous tissue, and radiation-induced cellular atypia may render the cytologic interpretation indeterminate. Ultrasound-guided core biopsy is advantageous in these cases, because the hypocellular scar tissue is more easily evaluated in a histologic specimen.

Documentation

Scars should always be documented in two planes with and without compression. The spatial extent of the lesion can be appreciated in the second plane. Compression is used to determine whether echogenicity increases in response to pressure and whether the scar-related structural defect diminishes and becomes easier to interpret. In the written report, it should be explicitly noted whether the tissue is compressible and whether the lesion changes shape when pressure is applied. The written documentation should also include the precise location of a scar and its correlation with corresponding mammographic and ultrasound findings. Other important aspects include the time course of change in the lesion in relation to previous findings or results from other studies. After taking into account all other available information and the overall clinical impression, the radiologist finally makes a recommendation regarding any further diagnostic procedures that may be needed and on further follow-up intervals.

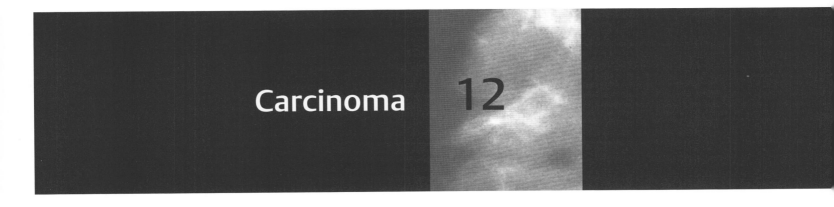

Carcinoma 12

Clinical Significance

Breast cancer is the most common malignant disease in women worldwide, with high prevalence in North America and Europe, with approximately 180 000 invasive and 62 000 in situ breast carcinomas expected to be diagnosed in the United States in 2007. The death rate has declined annually since 1990, with a 3.3% per year decrease in the death rate of women under the age of 50 years and 2.0% per year for women over 50 years. The incidence of breast cancer increases with age; the two greatest risk factors are being female and aging, with the steepest increase occurring before age 50, with increase in incidence continuing but leveling off after 50. About 25% of breast cancer patients are premenopausal, and young age should not be considered as breast cancer protection in young women, especially when imaging findings are indeterminate.

Nearly half of diagnosed carcinomas (48%) occur in the upper outer quadrant of the breast (**Table 12.1**), site of the greatest concentration of breast fibroglandular tissue, but all areas should be carefully examined because inner-quadrant tumors and peripheral lesions close to the chest wall are easily overlooked or else may not be included on poorly positioned mammograms.

Tumor size and the presence of multiple foci in one breast are of major importance in surgical planning. Several foci occurring in the same breast quadrant or separated by less than 4–5 cm are described as "multifocal," and several lesions in different breast quadrants or separated by more than 5 cm are classified as *multicentric*. If other eligibility requirements for breast conservation are met, lumpectomy may be planned for multifocal invasive or intraductal carcinoma. The incidence of multifocal carcinoma ranges from 20% to 40% in different published series. These statistics are difficult to obtain, and perhaps the growing utilization of contrast-enhanced MRI for preoperative evaluation of extent of disease in newly diagnosed breast cancer patients will shed light on an important consideration in treatment planning.

Some of the many different types of breast carcinoma are listed in **Table 12.2**. The tumors are classified by their tissue sites of origin, for the most part either ductal or lobular, and these are divided into further subtypes according to their pattern of growth. Carcinomas are also classified as invasive or noninvasive. Additionally there are several types of rare malignancy, and some lesions are metastatic from primary tumors in other organs.

The early detection of breast cancer is important in terms of providing effective treatment, and the decrease in mortality in the last 25 years, is due to earlier detection by mammography and to better treatment, which also may be enabled by more widespread

Table 12.1 Frequency distribution of the sites of occurrence of breast cancer

Site of occurrence	Frequency (%)
Upper outer quadrant	48
Upper inner quadrant	15
Lower outer quadrant	11
Lower inner quadrant	6
Central (subareolar)	17

Table 12.2 Forms and subtypes of breast cancer

Type of carcinoma	Percentage incidence
Invasive ductal carcinoma	75%
Scirrhous	
Solid	
Adenomatous	
Invasive lobular carcinoma	15%
Special forms	10%
Inflammatory	
Apocrine	
Mucinous	
Medullary	
Tubular	
Sarcoma	
Lymphoma	
Paget disease	
Squamous cell carcinoma	
Metastases from other organs	
Noninvasive carcinomas	
Ductal carcinoma in situ (DCIS)	
Comedocarcinoma	
Lobular carcinoma in situ (LCIS)	

use of mammography and perhaps to improved or new adjunctive methods of screening.

The doubling time of breast cancers is highly variable, although many grow very slowly. Ten or more years may elapse between carcinogenesis and the initial appearance of clinical manifestations. Some tumors grow much more rapidly than this, but others grow even more slowly. Besides tumor size, the lymph node status, tumor grade, and receptor status have been identified as important prognostic factors along with an increasing number of other prognostic factors, which are the subject of continuing scientific investigation.

Diagnostic Criteria

Carcinomas can have a wide variety of sonographic features. Detectability and characterization depend on technical quality of the equipment and the image produced—contrast and spatial resolution, gray scale, field of view, dynamic range—as well as recognition within the small window of the scan of subtle abnormalities such as architectural distortion that may indicate presence of tumor. As with mammography, where a white tumor is unseen against the background of white fibroglandular tissue, lack of contrast may limit perception of a mass with ultrasound. Fibro-

adenomas, hypoechoic and oval, may be difficult to impossible to identify when they are in a background of fat lobules, also hypoechoic and oval; malignant tumors, also hypoechoic, often grow within the fibroglandular layer and are conspicuous as dark (hypoechoic) masses standing out in contrast with the light gray fibroglandular tissue (**Figs. 12.1–12.3 a, b**). It is important to take these factors into account when interpreting ultrasound findings.

Typical Findings

Shape and Margins

As in mammography, a typical malignant tumor appears sonographically as a mass of variably irregular shape with margins that are not circumscribed. Within the category of masses that are not circumscribed, a lesion may exhibit any or all of the following

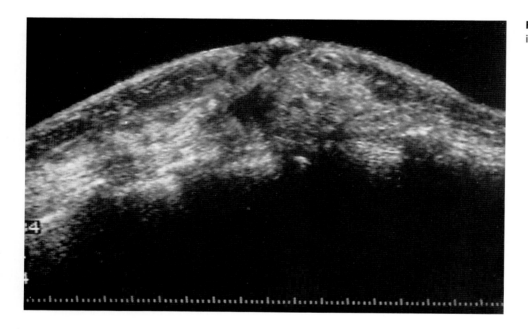

Fig. 12.1   Water-bath immersion scan of an invasive carcinoma 2 cm in diameter.

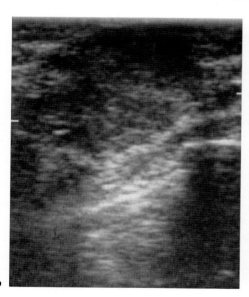 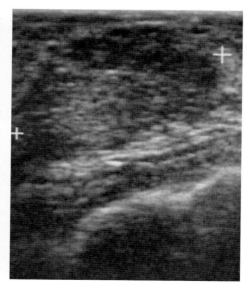

Fig. 12.2 a, b   Benign–malignant differentiation is difficult to accomplish with a simple 5-MHz linear-array transducer.
a Invasive ductal carcinoma 5 cm in diameter.
b Fibroadenoma 4.7 cm in diameter.

■ Comment:
The low resolution makes it difficult to evaluate the margins and internal structure of the lesions.

a, b

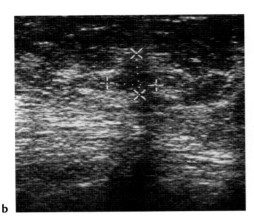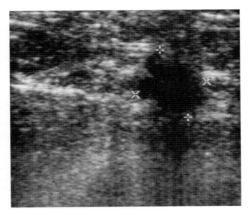

a, b

Fig. 12.3 a, b Comparison of **a** short-focused and **b** high-resolution 5-MHz transducers, shown here for an invasive ductal carcinoma 1.8 cm in diameter.

❗ Comment:
The comparison shows that, given the same frequencies, the better image processing in **b** has a significant effect on image contrast and structural resolution. The diagnostic criteria can be more accurately interpreted when a higher-resolution, appropriately focused transducer is used.

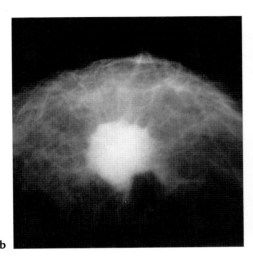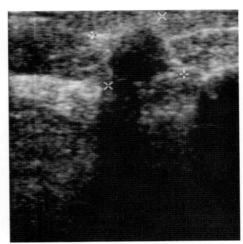

a, b

Fig. 12.4 a, b Example of an invasive ductal breast carcinoma.
a X-ray mammography.
b Ultrasound (7.5 MHz transducer).

Shape	Irregular
size	25 × 29 × 26 mm
Orientation	Not parallel
Margin	Indistinct, angular
Lesion boundary	Echogenic halo
Echo pattern	Hypoechoic
Posterior acoustic features	Shadowing
Surrounding tissue	Architectural distortion, Cooper ligament disruption
Calcifications	None
Vascularity	Present immediately adjacent to lesion

❗ Comment:
Mammography and ultrasound permit an accurate diagnosis of malignancy. The indistinct margins and acoustic shadow make it difficult to define the tumor boundaries. Often this can be accomplished by dynamic compression in a real-time examination, which can define echogenic tissue areas at the periphery of the tumor.

marginal characteristics: indistinctness, angularity, microlobulation, and spiculation (**Figs. 12.4 a, b–12.6 a, b, Table 12.3**). Variable compression of the transducer on the breast is useful technique for evaluating the tumor's shape and its margins.

Echogenicity

The echogenicity of many invasive ductal carcinomas is often heterogeneously hypoechoic and, at least in invasive ductal carcinoma, is usually hypoechoic. Malignant tumors can vary widely in their echo characteristics, however, ranging from nearly anechoic to almost entirely hyperechoic, although in real-time scanning through echogenic carcinomas, one can almost always discern at least a small hypoechoic component (**Figs. 12.4 a, b–12.7 a, b**).

Table 12.3 Criteria for evaluating typical breast carcinomas

Shape	Irregular
Orientation	Not parallel
Margin	Indistinct (angular, microlobulated, spiculated)
Lesion boundary	Echogenic halo
Echo pattern	Hypoechoic, inhomogeneous
Posterior acoustic features	Shadowing
Surrounding tissue	Architectural distortion: – Duct changes (irregularities, dilatation) – Cooper ligament changes (disruption, retraction) – Skin thickening, retraction, irregularity
Calcifications	Microcalcifications in mass
Vascularity	Present in lesion and/or immediately adjacent to lesion

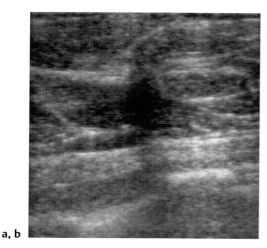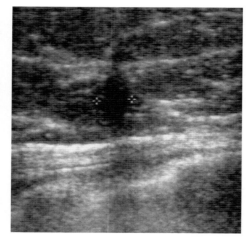

Fig. 12.5 a, b Typical appearance of invasive ductal carcinoma.
a Sagittal scan.
b Transverse scan (10 MHz transducer).

Shape	Irregular
Size	12 × 12 × 9 mm
Orientation	Not parallel
Margin	Indistinct
Lesion boundary	Abrupt interface
Echo pattern	Hypoechoic
Posterior acoustic features	Shadowing
Surrounding tissue	Architectural distortion, Cooper ligament disruption
Calcifications	None
Vascularity	Present immediately adjacent to lesion

a, b

❗ Comment:
The tumor is well delineated by its near-anechogenecity to the surrounding breast parenchyma and fat. The vertical orientation and posterior acoustic shadowing contribute to its conspicuity.

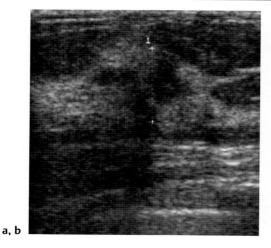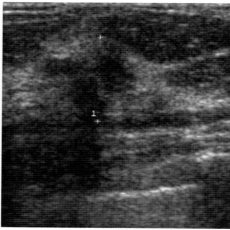

Fig. 12.6 a, b Invasive ductal carcinoma.
a Without compression.
b With compression.

Shape	Irregular
Size	11 × 14 × 14 mm
Orientation	Not parallel
Margin	Indistinct, angular
Lesion boundary	Echogenic halo
Echo pattern	Hypoechoic
Posterior acoustic features	Shadowing
Surrounding tissue	Architectural distortion, Cooper ligament disruption
Calcifications	None
Vascularity	Present in lesion

a, b

❗ Comment:
The posterior tumor margin is not defined on the uncompressed scan. When compression is applied, the firm tumor is more clearly delineated within the soft breast tissue. The tumor itself is not compressible.

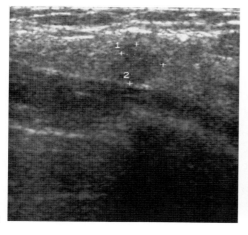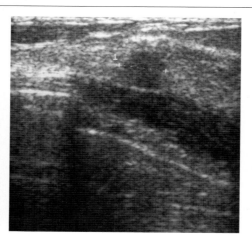

Fig. 12.7 a, b Isoechoic invasive ductal carcinoma.
a Sagittal scan.
b Transverse scan.

Shape	Oval
Size	7 × 6 × 8 mm
Orientation	Parallel
Margin	Indistinct
Lesion boundary	Echogenic halo
Echo pattern	Isoechoic
Posterior acoustic features	No posterior acoustic features
Surrounding tissue	Architectural distortion
Calcifications	None
Vascularity	Not present

a, b

❗ Comment:
This is an unusually echogenic malignancy. Only dynamic compression can clearly demarcate the tumor from the surrounding, compressible parenchyma. Both the tumor and parenchyma are hyperechoic.

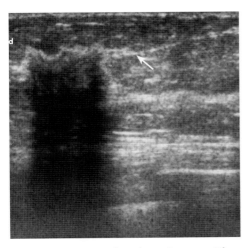

Fig. 12.8 Invasive ductal carcinoma with a strong acoustic shadow.

Shape	Irregular
Size	13 × 14 mm
Orientation	? (indeterminate because of shadowing)
Margin	Indistinct, angular
Lesion boundary	Abrupt interface
Echo pattern	Hypoechoic
Posterior acoustic features	Shadowing
Surrounding tissue	Architectural distortion, Cooper ligament disruption (arrow)
Calcifications	None
Vascularity	Present immediately adjacent to lesion

❗ Comment:
Only the horizontal extent of the tumor can be measured because of the acoustic shadow. The vertical tumor axis cannot be evaluated.

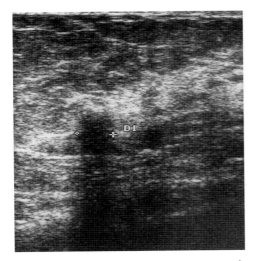

Fig. 12.9 Invasive ductal carcinoma with shadowing.

Shape	Irregular
Size	9 × 9 × 10 mm
Orientation	? (indeterminate because of shadowing)
Margin	Indistinct, angular
Lesion boundary	Echogenic halo
Echo pattern	Hypoechoic
Posterior acoustic features	Shadowing
Surrounding tissue	Architectural distortion, Cooper ligament disruption
Calcifications	None
Vascularity	Not present

❗ Comment:
This example shows that even small tumors may be associated with strong shadowing. Sound attenuation may be one of the reasons why vascularity could not be detected.

Posterior Features

Approximately 60 % of carcinomas cast acoustic shadows for several reasons. Desmoplasia, a fibrous stromal response to a tumor's presence, is strongly attenuating. Posterior acoustic shadowing may be sufficiently intense to completely obscure the breast tissue deep to the carcinoma. Marginal spicules may also be associated with this fibrous response associated with some lower-grade (1 and 2) invasive ductal carcinomas. A favorable prognosis has been associated with this sonographic pattern. Their heterogeneity also has an attenuating effect on sound through-transmission (**Figs. 12.8, 12.9**). Absence of shadowing is not a reliable criterion, however. Approximately 40 % of carcinomas are relatively cellular and either elicit no change in acoustic attenuation or enhance posteriorly (**Figs. 12.10, 12.11**). In general, these are higher grade, less

well differentiated neoplasms that have a blander ultrasound appearance related to lack of fibrotic response.

Orientation

Another criterion for malignancy is the orientation of the tumor with respect to the skin; that is, whether its long axis is parallel to the skin (synonyms: horizontal, wider-than-tall) or perpendicular (orientation not parallel to the skin, taller-than-wide). If the horizontal extent of the tumor is greater than its vertical extent and the lesion is circumscribed and no malignant features are present, the lesion is *benign* or *probably benign*. A predominantly vertical orientation is more suggestive of malignancy (**Figs. 12.12, 12.13**).

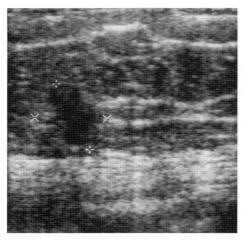

Fig. 12.10 Nonattenuating invasive ductal carcinoma.

Shape	Irregular
Size	18 × 19 × 14 mm
Orientation	Not parallel
Margin	Indistinct, angular
Lesion boundary	Abrupt interface
Echo pattern	Hypoechoic
Posterior acoustic features	No posterior acoustic features
Surrounding tissue	Architectural distortion, Cooper ligament disruption
Calcifications	None
Vascularity	Present immediately adjacent to lesion

❗ Comment:
The diagnostic criteria for this lesion are predominantly suspicious, despite the relatively well-defined margins and the absence of an acoustic shadow.

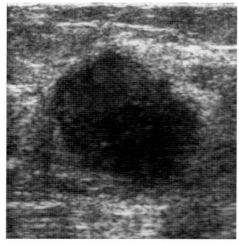

Fig. 12.11 Solid invasive ductal carcinoma with posterior enhancement.

Shape	Oval
Size	26 × 22 × 28 mm
Orientation	Parallel
Margin	Indistinct, angular
Lesion boundary	Echogenic halo
Echo pattern	Hypoechoic
Posterior acoustic features	Enhancement
Surrounding tissue	Architectural distortion
Calcifications	None
Vascularity	Present in lesion

❗ Comment:
The solid growth pattern with high cellularity of this tumor leads to posterior acoustic enhancement. These lesions often show high vascularity.

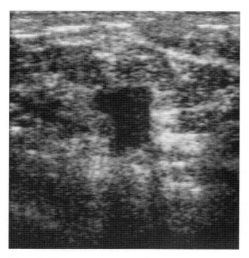

Fig. 12.12 Invasive ductal carcinoma with vertical tumor axis.

Shape	Irregular
Size	14 × 19 × 16 mm
Orientation	Not parallel
Margin	Indistinct, angular
Lesion boundary	Abrupt interface
Echo pattern	Hypoechoic
Posterior acoustic features	No posterior acoustic features
Surrounding tissue	Architectural distortion, Cooper ligament disruption
Calcifications	None
Vascularity	Present immediately adjacent to lesion

❗ Comment:
The vertical orientation of this tumor is a criterion for malignancy. This feature is very rarely seen with benign lesions, although both benign and malignant masses may have parallel (horizontal) orientation.

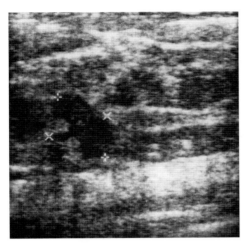

Fig. 12.13 Invasive ductal carcinoma with an oblique tumor axis.

Shape	Irregular
Size	15 × 18 × 16 mm
Orientation	Not parallel
Margin	Indistinct, micro-lobulated
Lesion boundary	Abrupt interface
Echo pattern	Hypoechoic
Posterior acoustic features	No posterior acoustic features
Surrounding tissue	Architectural distortion, Cooper ligament disruption
Calcifications	None
Vascularity	Present immediately adjacent to lesion

❗ Comment:
The major axis of this tumor is directed obliquely, but when this dimension is projected onto the vertical axis, the tumor exhibits a predominantly vertical (not parallel) orientation.

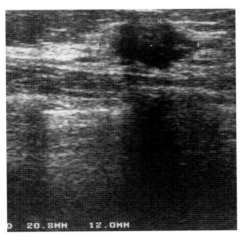

Fig. 12.14 Invasive ductal carcinoma with a horizontal tumor axis.

Shape	Irregular
Size	21 × 12 × 16 mm
Orientation	Parallel
Margin	Indistinct
Lesion boundary	Abrupt interface
Echo pattern	Hypoechoic
Posterior acoustic features	Shadowing (weak)
Surrounding tissue	Architectural distortion, Cooper ligament disruption
Calcifications	None
Vascularity	Present immediately adjacent to lesion

❗ Comment:
Most of the criteria are suggestive of carcinoma. The predominantly horizontal orientation in this case does not indicate benign etiology.

Published reports vary widely on the statistical value of this feature as a benign–malignant indicator. In our own experience, orientation is only approximately 50 % accurate in predicting benign or malignant etiology, and a vertical orientation has greater specificity and significance than a horizontal orientation, which can be associated with both benign and malignant lesions. It should be noted that the vertical extent of a tumor is difficult to measure in the presence of a posterior acoustic shadow that obscures the back wall of the lesion (**Figs. 12.8, 12.9**).

It should also be noted that a horizontal orientation is not synonymous with a benign origin, and many malignancies, including invasive lobular carcinoma, are often oriented parallel to the skin (**Fig. 12.14**). On the other hand, a vertical orientation does signify a high likelihood of malignancy if other features, such as irregular shape and ill-defined margin, are present.

 Acoustic shadows can obscure spatial orientation of a breast mass. It is essential to examine the mass in all its axes and to locate the longest axis when determining orientation. The longest axis does not always lie in the sagittal or transverse plane; it may be obliquely situated or possibly radial or antiradial (**Fig. 12.15 a, b**).

Effect on Surrounding Tissue

Because carcinomas infiltrate surrounding tissues, it is important to observe indirect signs such as architectural distortion; retraction; thickening, straightening or disruption of the Cooper ligaments, parenchyma and skin, and irregular ductal dilatation. Infiltrating tumor margins or inflammatory infiltration of surrounding tissues caused by an immune response to the neoplasm result in a more or less prominent hypoechoic zone surrounding the tumor (**Figs. 12.16, 12.17**). These are important secondary changes that are helpful in making a benign–malignant differentiation.

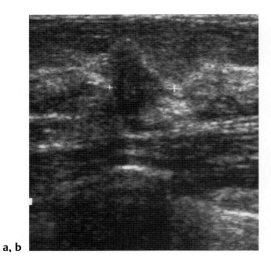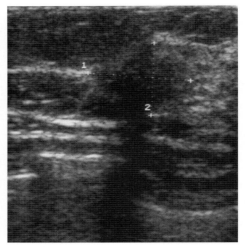

a, b

Fig. 12.15 a, b Invasive ductal carcinoma with a horizontal (parallel) tumor axis.
a Transverse scan.
b Radial scan.

Shape	Irregular
Size	17 × 12 × 11 mm
Orientation	Parallel
Margin	Indistinct, angular
Lesion boundary	Echogenic halo
Echo pattern	Hypoechoic
Posterior acoustic features	Shadowing
Surrounding tissue	Architectural distortion, Cooper ligament disruption
Calcifications	None
Vascularity	Present immediately adjacent to lesion

! Comment:
Transverse scan of the tumor (**a**) shows a vertical orientation, but the radial scan (**b**) reveals its greater horizontal extent. Note how the interpretation of different scan planes can lead to different results, accounting possibly for the differences in published reports on the statistical accuracy of this diagnostic criterion.

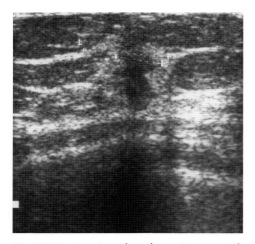

Fig. 12.16 Invasive ductal carcinoma with diffuse perifocal infiltration (hyperechoic).

Shape	Irregular
Size	14 × 17 × 12 mm
Orientation	Not parallel
Margin	Indistinct, angular
Lesion boundary	Echogenic halo
Echo pattern	Hypoechoic
Posterior acoustic features	No posterior acoustic features
Surrounding tissue	Architectural distortion, Cooper ligament disruption
Calcifications	None
Vascularity	Present immediately adjacent to lesion

! Comment:
The Cooper ligaments appear frayed and disrupted in the vicinity of the tumor. At the periphery of the tumor a hyperechoic area extends into the surrounding fat. Compression shows that this area is indurated. The carcinoma extends through the hypoechoic zone into the echogenic periphery. Tumor size is measured at the points where the surrounding structures are disrupted.

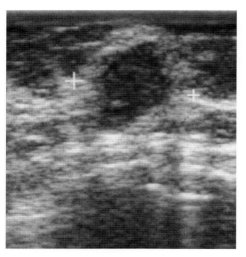

Fig. 12.17 Invasive ductal carcinoma with a hyperechoic rim.

Shape	Irregular
Size	16 × 20 × 18 mm
Orientation	Not parallel
Margin	Indistinct, angular
Lesion boundary	Echogenic halo
Echo pattern	Hypoechoic
Posterior acoustic features	No posterior acoustic features
Surrounding tissue	Architectural distortion
Calcifications	Microcalcifications in mass
Vascularity	Present immediately adjacent to lesion

! Comment:
The hypoechoic tumor is bounded peripherally by a hyperechoic zone, but the ligaments extend into this area. Histology demonstrated a lymphocytic reaction directly adjacent to the tumor.

The following variables affect the detectability of breast cancer: tumor size, echogenicity, internal echo pattern, peritumoral contrast. Optimization of both detection and characterization may depend on equipment of high quality and good examination technique. All criteria should be considered together in benign vs. malignant differentiation, because no single criterion is valid when considered in isolation. The greater the number of malignant criteria found, the higher the level of diagnostic confidence.

Less Common Findings

Hyperechogenicity

The morphologic diversity of malignant tumors leads to a variety of imaging findings, even within the group of invasive ductal carcinomas (**Figs. 12.1–12.17**). More than 90% of breast cancers are hypoechoic and are easily detected within the more echogenic parenchyma, but more diffuse lesions appear hyperechoic because of their many reflective interfaces and are difficult to identify. This applies to some invasive lobular carcinomas, which often infiltrate surrounding tissues diffusely (**Figs. 12.18, 12.19**). Careful scanning

of these hyperechoic abnormalities will commonly reveal hypoechoic components within them. It is important not to make a diagnostic judgment on the basis of one feature such as echogenicity: an echogenic circumscribed, thinly marginated mass is *benign*; an irregularly shaped, poorly defined hyperechoic area cannot be assessed as benign because of its high echogenicity alone; the marginal indistinctness places the lesion into the category *suspicious for malignancy*.

Ductal carcinoma in situ, comedo-type, spreads extensively through the ducts, and this heterogeneous pattern of involvement results in an echogenic lesion (**Fig. 12.20**). Calcifications may or may not be seen within distended, abnormally arborizing ducts.

Rarely, other histologic types of diffuse cancer, including primary breast lymphoma, may also appear hyperechoic, defined as having higher echogenicity than the reference tissue, fat, sometimes even isoechoic with fibroglandular tissue such as diffusely infiltrating ductal carcinoma and lymphoma (**Figs. 12.7 a, b, 12.21 a, b**). This echogenicity is not diagnostic, but closer scrutiny will usually reveal an architectural distortion or hypoechoic area associated with these lesions.

Although certain feature patterns can suggest a particular histology (**Table 12.4**), they do not permit an accurate histologic

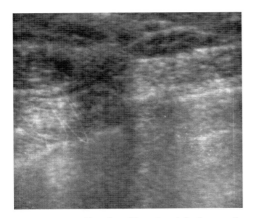

Fig. 12.18 Diffusely infiltrating lobular carcinoma.

Shape	Irregular
Size	24 × 15 × 19 mm
Orientation	Parallel
Margin	Indistinct
Lesion boundary	Difficult to define
Echo pattern	Isoechoic
Posterior acoustic features	Shadowing
Surrounding tissue	Architectural distortion, Cooper ligament retraction and disruption
Calcifications	None
Vascularity	Present immediately adjacent to lesion

■ Comment:
The echogenic tumor is poorly demarcated from the surrounding parenchyma, but there is obvious retraction of the Cooper ligaments and marked architectural distortion associated with the tumor.

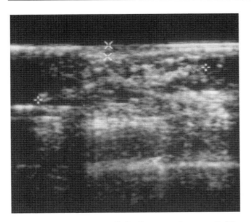

Fig. 12.19 Invasive lobular carcinoma infiltrating the skin.

Shape	Irregular
Size	42 × 11 × 24 mm
Orientation	Parallel
Margin	Indistinct
Lesion boundary	Abrupt interface
Echo pattern	Hyperechoic
Posterior acoustic features	No posterior acoustic features
Surrounding tissue	Architectural distortion—skin thickening and irregularity
Calcifications	None
Vascularity	Present in lesion

■ Comment:
Architectural alterations of breast parenchyma are not apparent, because of the superficial location of the carcinoma, but the structure of the subcutaneous tissue is distorted. The tumor is hyperechoic to fat. Histology identified the skin thickening as tumor invasion.

Table 12.4 Criteria for evaluating atypical breast carcinomas

Shape	Irregular
Orientation	Parallel
Margin	Circumscribed
Lesion boundary	Abrupt interface
Echo pattern	Hyperechoic, homogeneous
Posterior acoustic features	No posterior acoustic features or enhancement
Surrounding tissue	No changes
Calcifications	None
Vascularity	Not present

classification. Increased echogenicity is most commonly seen in lobular carcinomas, but the majority of lobular cancers, like invasive ductal carcinomas, are hypoechoic. Since these tumors tend to be multifocal, special care should be taken not to overlook echogenic tumor components (**Fig. 12.22 a, b**). Other morphologic forms or histologic subgroups such as papillary carcinoma, mixed ductal–lobular carcinoma, medullary and mucinous carcinoma, and squamous cell and tubular carcinomas can be evaluated in descriptive terms but cannot be accurately classified sonographically (**Figs. 12.23 a, b–12.28**). Based on shape, margins, and, most often, orientation, the BI-RADS assessments for these various lesions will be *suspicious for malignancy.*

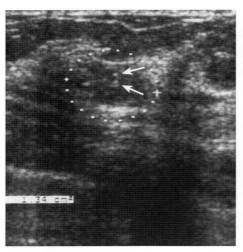 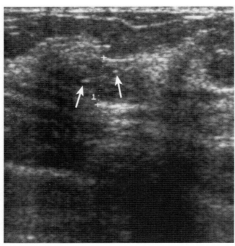

a, b

Shape	Oval
Size	14 × 8 × 10 mm
Orientation	Parallel
Margin	Indistinct
Lesion boundary	Echogenic halo
Echo pattern	Isoechoic
Posterior acoustic features	Enhancement*
Surrounding tissue	Architectural distortion
Calcifications	Microcalcifications in mass (arrows)
Vascularity	Not present

Fig. 12.20 a, b Ductal carcinoma in situ. Isoechoic comedocarcinoma in a 40-year-old woman with dense parenchyma.
a Transverse scan.
b Sagittal scan. Mammography showed clustered calcifications.

🔳 Comment:
This lesion would have been extremely difficult to detect with ultrasound alone. Mammograms usually show a typical pattern of calcifications associated with comedocarcinoma.

* The shadowing is not caused by the lesion itself but by the echogenic reactive changes adjacent to the lesion, although when calcifications are tightly grouped they may be visible on ultrasound. Individual microcalcifications occupy too little of the ultrasonic beam to cause shadowing.

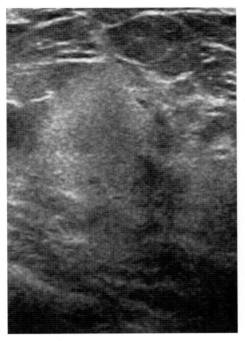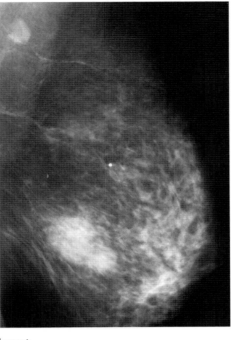

a, b

Shape	Irregular
Orientation	Nonparallel
Margin	Not circumscribed: indistinct
Lesion boundary	No abrupt interface
Echo pattern	Hyperechoic with a few hypoechoic areas
Posterior acoustic features	None
Surrounding tissue	Architectural distortion, infiltration
Calcifications	None
Vascularity	No characteristic

❗ Comment:
Small areas of hypoechogenicity within the mass are often seen in malignancies with a large echogenic component.

Fig. 12.21 a, b B-cell lymphoma, primary in the breast.
a Palpable mass in a 62-year-old woman is hyperechoic, indistinctly marginated and infiltrates the surrounding tissue. The hyperechogenicity should not suggest a benign etiology for a mass with an irregular shape, nonparallel orientation, and margins that are not circumscribed.
b Mediolateral oblique mammogram of the left breast shows a soft-tissue mass—not low density, fat-containing—in the lower breast, also with marginal characteristics that suggest malignancy, making biopsy essential.

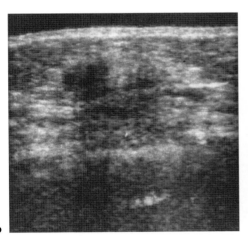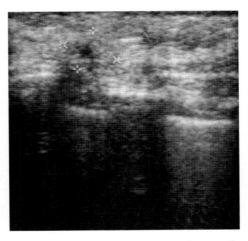

a, b

Shape	Irregular
Size	a 14 × 11 × 12 mm, b 14 × 11 × 10 mm
Orientation	Parallel
Margin	Indistinct
Lesion boundary	Echogenic halo
Echo pattern	a Hypoechoic, b complex
Posterior acoustic features	Shadowing
Surrounding tissue	Architectural distortion
Calcifications	None
Vascularity	Present immediately adjacent to lesion

Fig. 12.22 a, b Multifocal invasive lobular carcinoma. **a** Hypoechoic main tumor, **b** partially hyperechoic satellite lesion.

❗ Comment:
The complex lesion (**b**) is difficult to detect. Detection requires very close scrutiny and is essential for surgical planning.

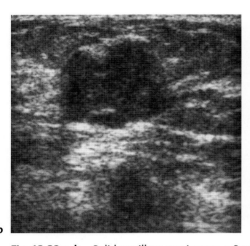 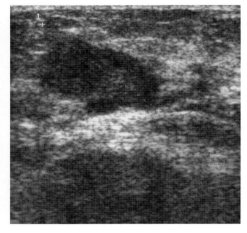

Shape	Oval
Size	20 × 17 × 22 mm
Orientation	Parallel
Margin	Circumscribed, lobulated
Lesion boundary	Abrupt interface
Echo pattern	Hypoechoic
Posterior acoustic features	Enhancement
Surrounding tissue	Architectural distortion, Cooper ligament retraction and disruption
Calcifications	Microcalcifications in mass
Vascularity	Present in lesion

a, b

Fig. 12.23 a, b Solid papillary carcinoma. **a** Sagittal scan, **b** transverse scan.

! Comment:
The posterior acoustic enhancement suggests that the lesion is a very cellular tumor. *Caution:* the pseudocircumscribed margins should not be mistaken for fibroadenoma.

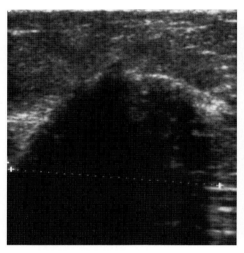 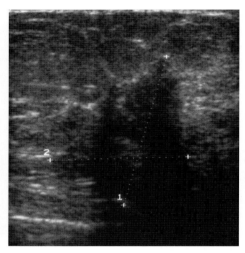

Shape	Irregular
Size	34 × 22 × 26 mm
Orientation	Parallel (difficult to assess because of strong shadowing)
Margin	Indistinct, angular
Lesion boundary	Abrupt interface
Echo pattern	Hypoechoic
Posterior acoustic features	Shadowing
Surrounding tissue	Architectural distortion, Cooper ligament retraction and disruption
Calcifications	Microcalcifications in lesion
Vascularity	Present immediately adjacent to lesion

a, b

Fig. 12.24 a, b Mixed invasive ductal and lobular invasive carcinoma. **a** Sagittal scan, **b** transverse scan.

! Comment:
This lesion is definitely suspicious for malignancy. The mixed histologic components cannot be differentiated by their sonographic features, and the pectoral muscle is obscured by shadowing and cannot be evaluated.

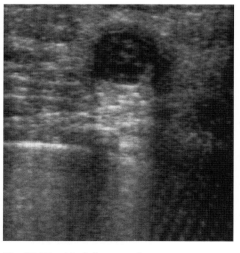

Shape	Round
Size	17 × 15 × 22 mm
Orientation	Parallel
Margin	Circumscribed
Lesion boundary	Echogenic halo
Echo pattern	Hypoechoic
Posterior acoustic features	Enhancement
Surrounding tissue	Architectural distortion
Calcifications	None
Vascularity	Present in lesion

! Comment:
Medullary carcinomas often have well-defined margins, but evaluation in multiple planes frequently shows irregularly outlined areas that are suggestive of malignancy.

Fig. 12.25 Medullary carcinoma.

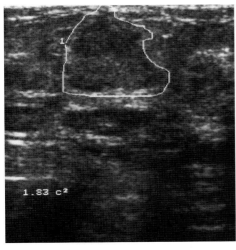

Fig. 12.26 Mucinous carcinoma.

Shape	Irregular
Size	18 × 15 × 14 mm
Orientation	Parallel
Margin	Indistinct, angular
Lesion boundary	Abrupt interface
Echo pattern	Isoechoic
Posterior acoustic features	Enhancement
Surrounding tissue	Architectural distortion
Calcifications	None
Vascularity	Present immediately adjacent to lesion

❗ Comment:
The thick mucoid material in these cancers is usually echogenic, giving the tumor a solid appearance. Because of its high echogenicity, the lesion is poorly demarcated from its surroundings. On closer scrutiny, however, a sharp tumor margin can be seen. Doubts can be resolved by core biopsy or fine-needle aspiration, which shows a typical cytologic pattern.

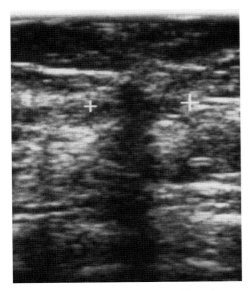

Fig. 12.27 Invasive squamous cell carcinoma of the breast.

Shape	Irregular
Size	21 × 27 × 24 mm
Orientation	Not parallel
Margin	Indistinct
Lesion boundary	Echogenic halo
Echo pattern	Hypoechoic
Posterior acoustic features	Shadowing
Surrounding tissue	Architectural distortion, Cooper ligament disruption
Calcifications	None
Vascularity	Not assessed

❗ Comment:
Because breast parenchyma has an ectodermal origin, squamous cell carcinoma may develop. This rare type of cancer does not display typical morphologic forms. An experienced cytologist can diagnose squamous cell carcinoma by fine-needle aspiration cytology, but core biopsy is more reliable for diagnosing this specific tumor type.

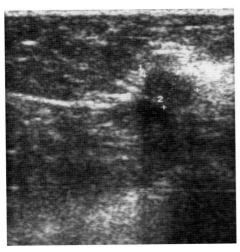

Fig. 12.28 Tubular breast carcinoma.

Shape	Oval
Size	9 × 6 × 8 mm
Orientation	Parallel
Margin	Not circumscribed: spiculated
Lesion boundary	Echogenic halo
Echo pattern	Hypoechoic
Posterior acoustic features	Shadowing
Surrounding tissue	Architectural distortion, Cooper ligament retraction and disruption
Calcifications	None
Vascularity	Present immediately adjacent to lesion

❗ Comment:
This type of malignancy has a favorable prognosis but it is less common than ductal or lobular invasive carcinomas.

Differential Diagnosis

As the examples illustrate, carcinomas are always difficult to detect when their echogenicity is increased. Differentiation is difficult if the diagnostic criteria overlap with those of other benign lesions, especially surgical scars and other types of postoperative change (**Figs. 12.29, 12.30**).

Fibrocystic breast changes cause increased sound absorption and refraction that often appear sonographically as ill-defined hypoechoic lesions. These areas can mimic carcinoma in cases where compression does not adequately improve sound penetration (**Figs. 12.31, 12.32 a, b**, see also Chapter 6, Fibrocystic Change).

As stated in Chapter 10, some carcinomas are indistinguishable with ultrasound from benign solid tumors (**Fig. 12.33**). Attention to discerning secondary signs in the tissue surrounding the mass will help differentiate a carcinoma, relatively well defined, from a fibroadenoma which will cause only compression of the surrounding tissue with no echogenic halo or architectural distortion. Using a high-frequency linear probe with center frequency between 7 and 10 MHz will help in increasing diagnostic confidence. Many physicians recommend short-interval follow-up for the probably benign lesions with a cancer likelihood of less than 2 %. If there is any doubt about a benign etiology, ultrasound-guided core biopsy should be done.

> A solid tumor should not be considered benign if any malignant features are identified, if there is any effect on the surrounding tissue such as destruction of fat planes, or until a cytologic or histologic diagnosis has been established. Abscesses can mimic malignant tumors. If multiple features suggest a benign etiology, short interval follow-up can be offered to the patient as a management option.

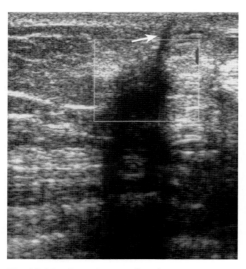

Fig. 12.29 Scar 1 year after breast-conserving surgery and postoperative radiotherapy.

Shape	Irregular
Size	12 × 14 × 10 mm
Orientation	? *
Margin	Indistinct
Lesion boundary	No echogenic halo
Echo pattern	Hypoechoic
Posterior acoustic features	Shadowing
Surrounding tissue	Architectural distortion, Cooper ligament disruption
Calcifications	None
Vascularity	Not present

* Because of strong shadowing the posterior border cannot clearly be delineated, so the orientation of the lesion cannot be recognized.

■ Comment:
This lesion is sonographically indistinguishable from carcinoma. Mammograms also frequently portray scars as spiculated densities. Differentiation is accomplished by compression, follow-up, percutaneous biopsy, or MRI (Chapter 11). As in this case, a tract from the tumor bed to the skin can often be found with US (arrow).

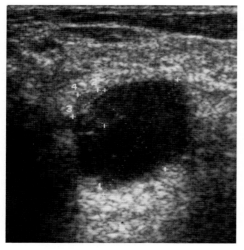

Fig. 12.30 Partially organized hematoma 4 months after tumor excision.

Shape	Oval
Size	22 × 17 × 19 mm
Orientation	Parallel
Margin	Circumscribed
Lesion boundary	Echogenic halo
Echo pattern	Hypoechoic
Posterior acoustic features	Enhancement
Surrounding tissue	Architectural distortion
Calcifications	None
Vascularity	Not present

■ Comment:
Persistent lesions resulting from the incomplete reabsorption of hematomas can create problems in postoperative management. It is important to maintain follow-up.

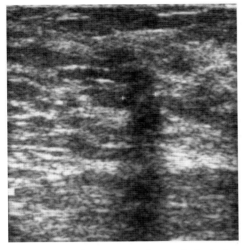

Shape	Irregular
Size	5 × 12 × 8 mm
Orientation	Not parallel
Margin	Indistinct
Lesion boundary	Abrupt interface
Echo pattern	Hypoechoic
Posterior acoustic features	Shadowing
Surrounding tissue	Architectural distortion, Cooper ligament appears disrupted
Calcifications	None
Vascularity	Not present

! Comment:
Here, when compression was applied, the lesion changed shape somewhat and the abnormality appeared to resolve. Ultimately this lesion was deemed suspicious and ultrasound-guided percutaneous biopsy established the diagnosis of stromal fibrosis and fibrocystic change.

Fig. 12.31 Indeterminate hypoechoic lesion of in a fibrocystic breast. Mammograms showed an asymmetric density. Histology revealed grade I fibrocystic change.

a, b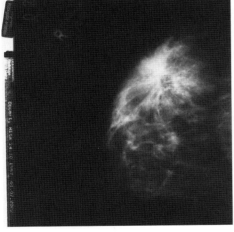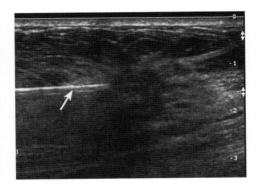

! Comment:
The lesion is indistinguishable from a carcinoma and an invasive diagnostic procedure (percutaneous core biopsy or excision) is called for.

Shape	Irregular
Size	12 × 14 mm
Orientation	Not parallel
Margin	Indistinct, angular
Lesion boundary	No echogenic halo
Echo pattern	Hypoechoic
Posterior acoustic features	Shadowing
Surrounding tissue	Architectural distortion, Cooper ligament disruption
Calcifications	None
Vascularity	Not present

Fig. 12.32 a, b Radial scar in a 46-year-old patient. Mammogram (**a**). Sonogram of core biopsy (**b**) procedure; needle (arrow).

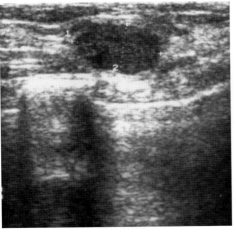

Shape	Irregular
Size	15 × 9 × 12 mm
Orientation	Parallel
Margin	Circumscribed
Lesion boundary	Abrupt interface
Echo pattern	Hypoechoic
Posterior acoustic features	Enhancement
Surrounding tissue	No changes
Calcifications	None
Vascularity	Present in lesion

! Comment:
Approximately 2–3% of carcinomas are circumscribed and resemble fibroadenomas. New palpable lesions and any solid mass that has even a single indeterminate ultrasound finding will require definitive evaluation.
Real-time scanning may allow perception of subtle findings of shape and margins that increase level of suspicion. Percutaneous fine-needle aspiration may be sufficient for a presumed benign lesion but, for a suspicious lesion, histologic confirmation by core biopsy or excision will provide the diagnosis. Increased vascularity within the lesion is highly suggestive of a malignant etiology.

Fig. 12.33 Invasive ductal carcinoma in a 27-year-old woman with physical, mammographic, and sonographic findings suggestive of fibroadenoma.

Case 1

A 42-year-old woman presented with diffuse induration of the left breast, and her gynecologist referred her for breast imaging. Mammography and ultrasound demonstrated multiple round lesions in the left breast (**Fig. 12.34 a–d**). Excisional biopsy was recommended. The referring physician did the apparently simple operation himself, without preoperative localization. When histology revealed no abnormalities, the patient was referred to the author for evaluation. As in the preoperative studies, imaging showed multiple masses with some benign features. Ultrasound-guided re-excision revealed multifocal invasive ductal carcinoma.

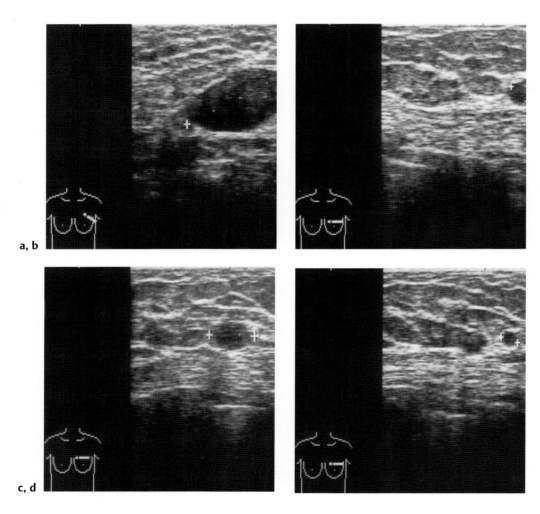

a, b

c, d

Fig. 12.34 a–d Multifocal invasive ductal carcinoma presenting as multiple fibroadenomas in a 42-year-old woman (Case 1).

Shape	Oval; round
Size	Multiple lesions, diameter 5–35 mm
Orientation	Parallel
Margin	Circumscribed
Lesion boundary	Abrupt interface
Echo pattern	Hypoechoic
Posterior acoustic features	No posterior acoustic features or enhancement (**b, c**)
Surrounding tissue	No changes
Calcifications	None
Vascularity	Present immediately adjacent to some but not all of the lesion

❗ Comment:
Palpation revealed diffuse induration. Mammography and ultrasound (**a–d**) showed multiple round lesions. Excisional biopsy was recommended, but the tumors were not found in the left upper outer quadrant. After ultrasound localization the multifocal carcinoma was removed at a second operation (Case 1).

Case 2

A 36-year-old woman in her 34th week of pregnancy felt a nodule in her right breast. Ultrasound, done elsewhere, showed a mass that was interpreted as a fibroadenoma. Mammograms showed only a slight increase in breast density compared with the opposite side. Excisional biopsy was still carried out, but diagnostic tissue was not obtained. The patient was referred to us postoperatively for further evaluation. As **Fig. 12.35** shows, the tumor was missed at excisional biopsy. The postoperative seroma indicates the boundaries of the surgical cavity. Following the induction of labor, the mass was re-excised. Frozen sections confirmed invasive cancer, and specimen histology revealed an extensive, poorly differentiated T2 carcinoma with numerous axillary lymph node metastases.

Two lessons can be learned from this unfortunate case:
1. A good preoperative evaluation is essential for treatment planning. The sonogram findings were misinterpreted in this case: the mass, which bears no resemblance to a benign fibroadenoma, has an irregular shape, angular and microlobulated margins, and a nonparallel orientation—all findings that suggest malignancy.
2. Even large tumors may be missed at surgery. Before operating, the surgeon should review the imaging findings with the radiologist to determine the spatial extent of the lesion. If the lesion is only vaguely palpable and its precise location is uncertain, it should be localized preoperatively, or tumor removal guided by intraoperative ultrasonography.

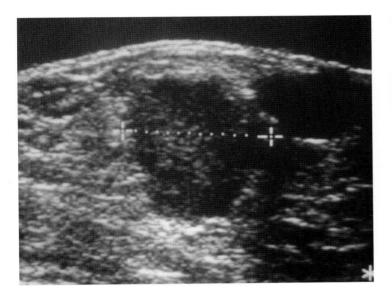

Fig. 12.35 Invasive ductal carcinoma 8 weeks after failed excisional biopsy. The tumor is at the center of the image, and the postoperative hematoma is on the right (Case 2).

Shape	Irregular
Size	33 × 30 × 28 mm
Orientation	Parallel
Margin	Circumscribed
Lesion boundary	Echogenic halo
Echo pattern	Hypoechoic
Posterior acoustic features	Enhancement
Surrounding tissue	Architectural distortion
Calcifications	None
Vascularity	Present in lesion

⚠ Comment:
A previous, inadequate excisional biopsy had been done for a presumed benign lesion. Negative histology prompted further evaluation, which showed that the biopsy had missed the tumor.

Case 3

A 42-year-old woman had screening mammograms on a regular basis. The films taken at age 40 showed symmetrical breast density. Adjunctive ultrasound revealed a small hypoechoic lesion. Because the mammograms were not suspicious, the lesion was measured but no further action was taken. One year later, interval enlargement was attributed to technical factors on the follow-up sonogram, but at 2 years significant enlargement was observed, finally prompting core biopsy and removal of the carcinoma (**Fig. 12.36 a–c**). At time of excision, the lymph nodes were negative, and the patient has remained disease free in more than 10 years of follow-up, but it would have been better to have analyzed the incidental sonographic finding at the outset enabling the diagnosis to be made at an earlier stage.

Intracystic carcinomas are relatively rare but should not be overlooked. Mammography shows only the outlines of the cyst, while ultrasound can accurately depict the walls of the cyst and its internal structure (**Fig. 12.37**). Cystic breast disease in and of itself is not associated with an increased risk of breast cancer. Breast cysts are fairly common, as are breast cancers, and they may be diagnosed at the same time adjacent to one another (**Figs. 12.38 a–d** through **12.40 a, b**). The breast imager must not fall into the tunnel vision trap of "satisfaction of search" when insonating a mammographically dense, nodular area. Don't stop looking once the cyst is seen: cysts may develop secondarily as a result of duct obstruction by tumor, or a cystic pattern may result from the necrotic degeneration of a carcinoma (**Fig. 12.41**).

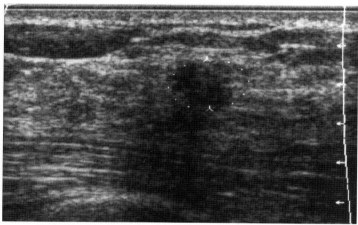

a, b

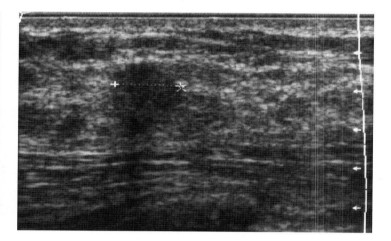

Fig. 12.36 a–c Delayed diagnosis of invasive ductal carcinoma. Follow-up sonograms over a 2-year period showed a progressive increase in tumor size.
a First examination.
b Follow-up after 6 months.
c Second follow-up after 1 year. Size increased from 6 to 21 mm.

c

Shape	Oval
Orientation	Parallel
Margin	Indistinct
Lesion boundary	Echogenic halo
Echo pattern	Hypoechoic
Posterior acoustic features	Shadowing
Surrounding tissue	Architectural distortion
Calcifications	None
Vascularity	Not assessed during the first two examinations. At the last follow-up visit, when diagnosis was confirmed, color Doppler showed vascularity immediately adjacent to lesion

! Comment:
Even at initial examination, it would have been appropriate to recommend percutaneous biopsy or close-interval follow-up. The serial images document a doubling of tumor size in 1.5 years.

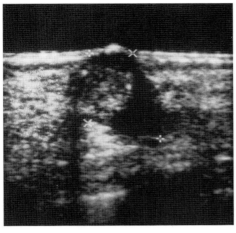

Shape	Oval
Size	28 × 21 × 22 mm
Orientation	Parallel
Margin	Circumscribed
Lesion boundary	Abrupt interface
Echo pattern	Hyperechoic
Posterior acoustic features	Enhancement
Surrounding tissue	No changes
Calcifications	Microcalcifications in mass
Vascularity	Present immediately adjacent to lesion

Fig. 12.37 Intracystic carcinoma.

❗ Comment:
Viewed in sagittal section with a skin offset, the margins of the tumor are well defined as those of an intracystic papilloma. All intracystic tumors should be excised; even negative aspiration cytology does not justify a wait-and-see approach.

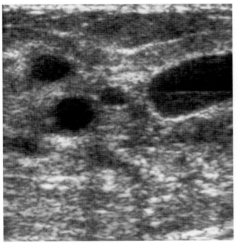
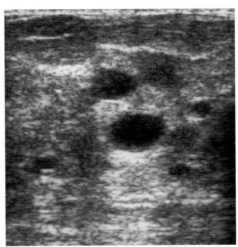

a, b

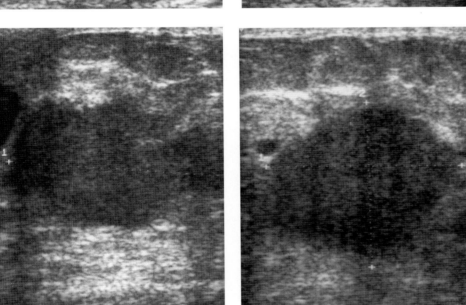

c, d

Fig. 12.38 a–d Carcinoma coexisting with cystic breast disease. **a, b** Several cysts, **c** sagittal scan of the carcinoma, **d** transverse scan.

Shape	Irregular
Size	36 × 27 × 32 mm
Orientation	Parallel
Margin	Indistinct, microlobulated
Lesion boundary	Abrupt interface
Echo pattern	Hypoechoic
Posterior acoustic features	Enhancement
Surrounding tissue	Architectural distortion
Calcifications	None
Vascularity	Present in lesion

❗ Comment:
This breast contains multiple cysts along with a large solid tumor. The patient had been followed for years for a palpable nodule in the right breast, but the large tumor had been undetected until now. Prior sonograms were unavailable for comparison.

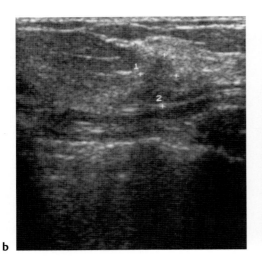

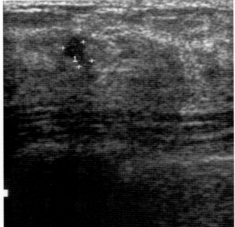

a, b

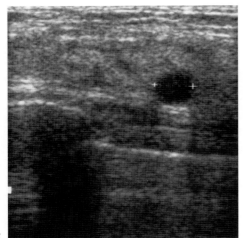

c

Fig. 12.39 a–c Multicentric invasive ductal carcinoma and cystic breast disease in a 45-year-old woman. The cystic changes had been known for several years. Current mammograms showed a new density in the lower inner quadrant of the right breast. Ultrasound showed two solid lesions (**a, b**) and cysts (**c**).

Shape	Irregular
Size	**a** 6 × 8 × 5 mm; **b** 2 × 3 × 4 mm
Orientation	Not parallel
Margin	Indistinct
Lesion boundary	Echogenic halo
Echo pattern	Hypoechoic
Posterior acoustic features	Shadowing (**a, b**)
Surrounding tissue	Architectural distortion, Cooper ligament disruption
Calcifications	None
Vascularity	Present immediately adjacent to lesion

❗ Comment:
Mammographic follow-up examinations detected the small early carcinoma. In this dense breast, however, ultrasound is invaluable for determining tumor size, detecting multicentricity, and planning surgical treatment. Alternatively, extent of disease can be studied with MRI and MR-guided biopsy.

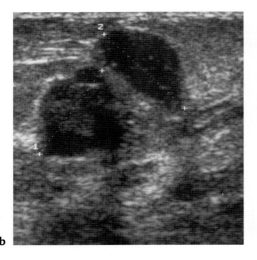

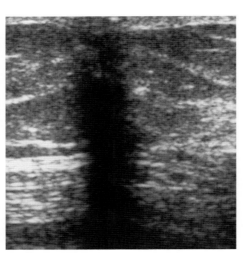

a, b

Fig. 12.40 a, b Cystic breast disease and intracystic carcinoma in a 45-year-old woman 1 year after excisional biopsy for fibrocystic change in the inner right breast.
a Transverse scan of the outer right breast shows a cyst medially and an intracystic carcinoma laterally.
b Transverse scan through the surgical scar.

	a
Shape	Irregular
Size	12 × 11 × 10 mm
Orientation	Nonparallel
Margin	Indistinct, angulated
Lesion boundary	Abrupt interface
Echo pattern	Hypoechoic
Posterior acoustic features	Enhancement (**a**); shadowing (**b**)
Surrounding tissue	No changes
Calcifications	None
Vascularity	Present in lesion

❗ Comment:
The patient was referred for ultrasound evaluation of the medial breast lesion. Scans with and without compression showed typical findings of scar tissue but in the outer right breast a large cyst with an intracystic carcinoma was found.

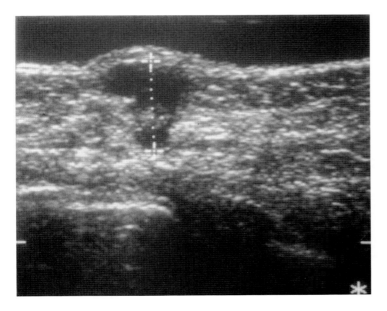

Fig. 12.41 Necrotic carcinoma in an 82-year-old woman with skin protrusion and redness and a 2 × 3-cm palpable mass. Abscess could also be considered here.

Shape	Irregular
Size	15 × 18 × 16 mm
Orientation	Not parallel
Margin	Indistinct, angular
Lesion boundary	Abrupt interface
Echo pattern	Hypoechoic and hyperechoic
Posterior acoustic features	No posterior acoustic features
Surrounding tissue	Architectural distortion, skin irregularity
Calcifications	Microcalcifications in mass
Vascularity	Present immediately adjacent to lesion

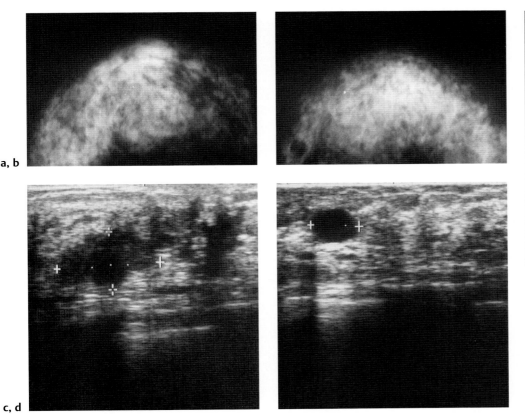

a, b

c, d

Fig. 12.42 a–d Multicentric breast cancer and cysts. Years of mammographic follow-ups showed no suspicious changes.
a, b Left and right mammograms (craniocaudal).
c, d Ultrasound now shows extensive, confluent tumor masses throughout the left breast along with cystic changes (Case 4).

❗ Comment:
Although mammography was unchanged, its sensitivity is limited by fibroglandular density, and the extensive lesion now detected by ultrasound might have been found earlier if sonography had been done.

Case 4

A 50-year-old woman with known cystic breast disease had annual screening mammograms and sonograms for 10 years. The mammograms consistently showed an extremely dense, unchanging fibroglandular parenchymal pattern in both breasts (**Fig. 12.42 a, b**). Palpation revealed bilateral coarse nodularity with no appreciable changes. The most recent follow-up examination included breast ultrasound (**Fig. 12.42 c, d**), which showed multiple confluent tumor masses 10–35 mm in diameter throughout the left breast. Histology revealed extensive invasive multicentric breast carcinoma (T2N1).

Shape	Irregular
Size	29 × 17 × 16 mm (**c, d**)
Orientation	Parallel
Margin	Indistinct
Lesion boundary	Abrupt interface
Echo pattern	Hypoechoic
Posterior acoustic features	Combined pattern
Surrounding tissue	Architectural distortion
Calcifications	None
Vascularity	Present in lesion

Further Diagnostic Procedures

All breast lesions that are indeterminate by mammography and sonography require further evaluation. If the breast tissue can be evaluated with these modalities and all focal lesions are clearly visualized, generally there is no need for further imaging studies. But a definitive diagnosis should always be established for any solid breast lesion that has an ultrasound feature uncharacteristic of a benign etiology. If fine-needle or core biopsy with ultrasound guidance yields a nonspecific or discordant result, the lesion should be re-biopsied percutaneously for histology (**Figs. 12.43, 12.44 a, b**). The advantage of core biopsy is that it provides a definitive preoperative histologic diagnosis, allowing treatment planning in advance of the surgical procedure without delay in the operating room for frozen sections diagnoses to confirm malignancy.

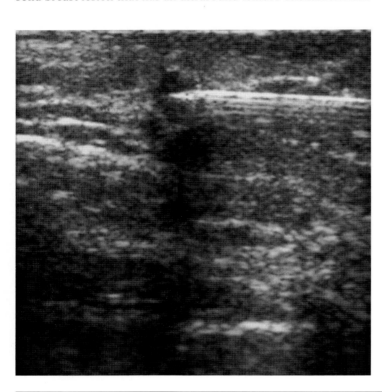

Fig. 12.43 Small carcinoma confirmed by ultrasound-guided fine-needle aspiration in an 87-year-old woman.

Shape	Irregular
Size	5 × 5 × 4 mm
Orientation	Not parallel
Margin	Indistinct, angular
Lesion boundary	Abrupt interface
Echo pattern	Hypoechoic
Posterior acoustic features	Shadowing
Surrounding tissue	Architectural distortion
Calcifications	None
Vascularity	Not present

❗ Comment:
The image shows the tumor with the aspirating needle in place. With precise needle placement, even early carcinomas can be confirmed by aspiration cytology.

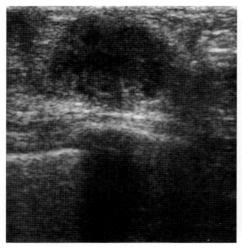
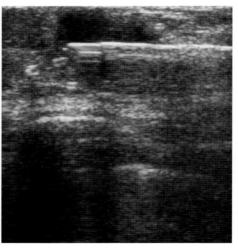

a, b

Fig. 12.44 a, b Core biopsy of invasive ductal carcinoma in an 88-year-old woman,
a Prefire image of the lesion and needle tip.
b Postfire image.

Shape	Oval
Size	19 × 15 × 17 mm
Orientation	Parallel
Margin	Indistinct
Lesion boundary	Echogeneic halo
Echo pattern	Hypoechoic
Posterior acoustic features	Enhancement
Surrounding tissue	Architectural distortion
Calcifications	None
Vascularity	Present immediately adjacent to lesion

❗ Comment:
Core biopsy under local anesthesia is rapid and well tolerated. Histologic confirmation in the 88-year-old patient allowed for prompt surgical removal of the lesion without frozen sections.

Role of Ultrasound

Ultrasound has an established role in the diagnosis of breast cancer. With modern, high-resolution ultrasound equipment, even solitary and multifocal carcinomas smaller than 1 cm can be detected and differentiated (**Figs. 12.45 a, b; 12.46 a, b**). Intraductal proliferations including DCIS and intraductal components of invasive carcinoma can frequently be detected as well. Nevertheless, ultrasound has no role yet as a primary screening modality because of its examiner and equipment dependence and the lack of equipment standards for quality assurance. But if mammograms are equivocal or of limited value due to tissue radiodensity, high-resolution ultrasound is a valuable diagnostic tool that has several important indications (**Table 12.5**). Currently, there has been increased utilization of contrast-enhanced breast MRI for evaluation of extent of disease: multifocality, multicentricity, and bilaterality. For lesions identified as indeterminate or suspicious for malignancy with MRI, percutaneous core biopsies can be done with the imaging guidance of second-look ultrasound or MRI.

With regard to tumor differentiation, all of the diagnostic criteria should be carefully evaluated using a BI-RADS feature analysis approach. No single criterion is diagnostic in itself. Malignant tumors have variable features, and only approximately 75 % display typical malignant criteria. The diagnostic criteria in breast ultrasound have changed considerably with improvements in scanner resolution. To date, however, there have been no large published series dealing with high-resolution imaging systems. **Table 12.6** presents a summary of some recently published data. It should be noted that all of the criteria were not evaluated in all studies.

Table 12.5 Indications for high-resolution ultrasound in breast cancer diagnosis

- Investigation of palpable masses
- Characterization of mammographic densities
- Cystic/solid differentiation and the detection of intracystic tumors
- Measurement of tumor size
- Detection of intraductal tumor components
- Evaluation of multifocal and multicentric lesions
- Lymph node evaluation
- Surgical planning (location, size, distance from skin and nipple)
- Preoperative localization and specimen evaluation
- Guided fine-needle aspiration, core biopsy or vacuum-assisted biopsy
- Adjunctive screening in high-risk patients

Table 12.6 Sensitivity and specificity of various ultrasound criteria in the diagnosis of breast cancer

Criterion	Sensitivity (%)	Specificity (%)
Shape	60	80
Margin	85–90	75–85
Lesion boundary	40	90
Posterior acoustic features	40	85
Orientation	45	80–90

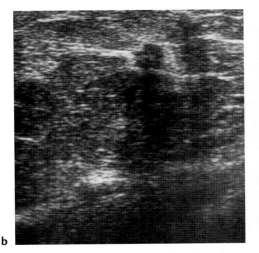 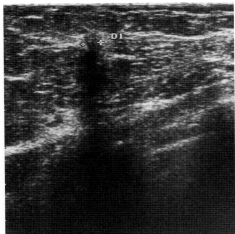

a, b

Fig. 12.45 a, b   Early invasive ductal carcinoma.
a Sagittal scan.
b Transverse scan.

Shape	Irregular
Size	5 mm diameter
Orientation	Not parallel
Margin	Indistinct, angular
Lesion boundary	Echogeneic halo
Echo pattern	Hypoechoic
Posterior acoustic features	Shadowing
Surrounding tissue	Architectural distortion, Cooper ligament disruption
Calcifications	None
Vascularity	Not present

❗ Comment:
With high-resolution technology, small lesions like this one can be seen and also differentiated. Even if no flow can be detected, the diagnostic criteria require further diagnostic workup by ultrasound guided intervention.

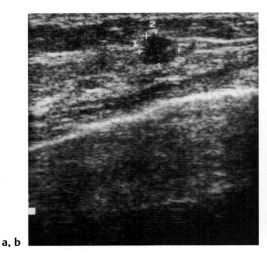 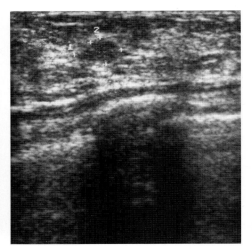

a, b

Shape	Irregular
Size	**a** 6 × 6 × 5 mm, **b** 8 × 5 × 6 mm
Orientation	**a** Nonparallel **b** Parallel
Margin	Indistinct
Lesion boundary	Abrupt interface
Echo pattern	Hypoechoic
Posterior acoustic features	No posterior acoustic features
Surrounding tissue	Architectural distortion
Calcifications	None
Vascularity	Present immediately adjacent to lesion

Fig. 12.46 a, b *Foci of multicentric invasive ductal carcinoma.*
a Lower inner quadrant of the right breast.
b Lower outer quadrant.

❗ Comment:
Ultrasound measurements direct surgical planning by indicating the diameters of both lesions and the distance of each lesion from the nipple and from each other. Presurgical or intraoperative localization of these masses will help ensure successful removal of both.

Documentation

Every tumor should be documented and measured in at least two mutually perpendicular planes, preferably in three dimensions to enable volumetric calculations to be made. Because the most common breast cancers arise from the duct system, which has a radial distribution, every suspicious tumor should also be imaged in the radial plane and its longest axis measured. This should be done for each individual lesion in breasts with multifocal (or multicentric) disease. The distances between each of the lesions and the greatest distance between the two lesions that are farthest apart should be measured and reported for treatment planning. Also to be measured are the distances from the lesion to the nipple and skin, again to assist surgical planning. Clock-face notation and distance from the nipple using the nipple as point of reference is best for documenting lesion location.

The correlation of ultrasound findings with clinical and mammographic findings should also be described, and it should be noted whether sonographic or mammographic localization is recommended or whether the mass is palpable and can be located and excised without difficulty. Axillary examination is indicated in patients with suspicious breast lesions, and abnormal-appearing lymph nodes suspected of harboring metastatic deposits should be biopsied to confirm involvement and need for going directly to axillary lymphadenectomy without the sentinel node biopsy. The internal mammary chain of nodes should be examined in patients with large or medially situated tumors.

Lymph Nodes | 13

Clinical Significance

The preoperative awareness of lymph node metastases is essential for overall treatment planning. In the past, the surgical treatment of breast cancer was far more radical than today and generally included removal of the pectoralis major muscle and the level I–III lymph nodes. Removal of parasternal internal mammary nodes was not uncommon. Current opinion favors breast conservation where possible and in general, a less radical and more selective approach to treatment to reduce surgical morbidity and other side effects. With sentinel node imaging and more frequent utilization of gadolinium-enhanced breast MRI, the risk of leaving residual viable tumor in the breast or lymph nodes of patients has lessened. There is decreased likelihood also of apparent early recurrences within a year or two of initial surgical excision. Many such "recurrences" reflect continued activity of residual carcinoma left behind after removal of the index lesion.

If sentinel node imaging is negative, in patients with no clinical evidence of level I axillary nodal involvement, many surgeons do not dissect the axilla at all. The internal mammary nodes are almost never exposed in the absence of compelling clinical concerns. This policy is questionable when we consider that the lymph nodes in the parasternal region are almost never palpable. Muscle fasciae are broadly attached to the sternum in this region, and enlarged lymph nodes deep in the intercostal spaces are virtually undetectable by physical examination. Because the fasciae create a firm boundary layer, nodal metastases in this region tend to expand inward between the ribs toward the pleura, causing indentation of the pleural cavity. As a result, these metastases remain clinically occult for a long time but can be seen with MRI or ultrasound. In principle, a tumor located anywhere in the breast can seed malignant cells to lymph nodes in this region, but it is more likely to occur with tumors located in the medial breast. It should also be remembered that the lymphatic pathways can cross behind the sternum to the opposite side to form metastases in the contralateral breast and axilla.

Although palpation of the axilla has been the traditional mainstay for clinical staging, studies have shown that preoperative detection of nodal metastases through physical examination is nonspecific. In approximately 40 % of cases, metastatic lymphadenopathy is suspected clinically in the absence of histologic metastasis. Reports vary widely on the palpability of histologically confirmed metastases, but it is reasonable to assume that only approximately 50 % of nodal metastases are palpable.

Size is an unreliable predictor of malignancy: the sizes of normal and metastatic lymph nodes are highly variable. In one large series,

an average diameter of 6.5 mm was determined for uninvolved lymph nodes and 9.7 mm for metastatic nodes, with a range from 1.8 to 40.6 mm. Thus, while larger lymph nodes tend to correlate with metastasis, even small lymph nodes a few millimeters in diameter may contain micrometastases defined as metastatic foci of diameters of 2 mm more or less.

With regard to pathways of spread, it should be noted that laterally situated tumors are drained first by the level I axillary lymph nodes, located lateral to the pectoralis minor. From there drainage proceeds medially to the level II nodes (behind the pectoralis minor muscle) and level III nodes (infraclavicular nodes medial to the pectoralis minor). If nodal metastases have developed in this region, there is a high probability of spread to the supraclavicular space and the cervical nodes. It is also very likely that tumor cells have gained access to the bloodstream, leading to hematogenous metastasis.

Diagnostic Criteria

Findings for Normal and Benign Lymph Nodes

The sonographic features of normal lymph nodes are described in Chapter 4. The cortices of normal lymph nodes are isoechoic with the axillary fat and unless the node can be identified by its more echogenic hilar fat, axillary lymph nodes may not be conspicuous with ultrasound. Nodes that are palpable and have cortices wider than 2–3 mm on ultrasound can ordinarily be found sonographically. When the cortex of a node is widened uniformly, a benign, reactive type of adenopathy is the most common explanation. The histologic interpretation of these nodes when biopsied is often "sinus histiocytosis," a reaction that can be encountered in association with breast cancers that have not metastasized. Benign reactive adenopathy also occurs in response to fibrocystic change, immune disorders, infections, and any process, such as recent biopsy, that activates the reticuloendothelial system, even if there is no clinically apparent cause.

The reactive lymph node usually displays its central echogenic hilum, which marks the entry point of the vascular pedicle. This location of these vessels should be considered in color Doppler imaging, which is occasionally used for additional support if nodal metastasis is suspected. The afferent lymph vessels pass over the convex surface of the lymph node as they approach and enter it, and the efferent vessel exits the node at the central hilum. The echogenic hilum is surrounded by a zone of low echogenicity

Table 13.1 Sonographic appearance of reactive lymph nodes

Hilum	Central, hyperechoic
Cortical zone	Hypoechoic rim of uniform width

representing the sinuses and the corticomedullary lymphatic tissues. In reactive lymph nodes, the echogenic hilum is ordinarily symmetrically positioned in the center of the node and surrounded by a cortical zone of low echogenicity (**Figs. 13.1a, b, 13.2; Table 13.1**).

Findings for Malignant Lymph Nodes

Advanced nodal metastasis is easily detected with ultrasound (**Table 13.2**). Once the hilum is invaded, the lymph node acquires a homogeneous, hypoechoic pattern (**Fig. 13.3**) although the node's hilar fat may remain, decreasing over time. Lymph node metastases may grow quite large before they penetrate the capsule, and therefore many metastatic nodes have smooth, sharp margins. The normal reniform shape of lymph nodes occasionally results in a lobulated outer contour (**Figs. 13.3, 13.4**). In some

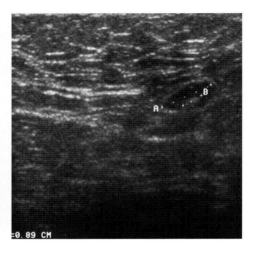

a, b

Fig. 13.1 a, b Reactive lymph node.
a Left breast, 12 o'clock (arrow).
b Level I lymph node in the left axilla.

Hilum	Hyperechoic
Cortex	Hypoechoic
Size	9 × 5 mm, hilum 4 × 2 mm

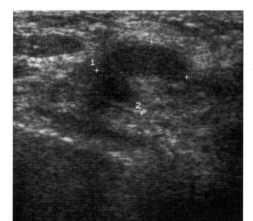

Fig. 13.2 Markedly enlarged reactive axillary lymph node.

Hilum	Hyperechoic
Cortex	Hypoechoic
Size	15 × 12 mm, hilum 7 × 5 mm

❗ Comment:
Lymph nodes of this size are often palpable and occasionally painful. The cortex is 4 mm thick. Usually no cause for the swelling can be ascertained.

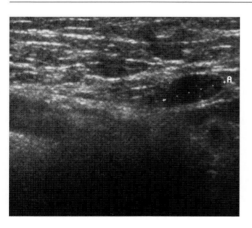

Fig. 13.3 Lymph node metastasis in the right axilla below the axillary vein. Transverse scan.

Shape	Oval
Size	11 × 5 mm
Contours	Smooth
Margins	Sharp
Internal structure	Homogeneous
Echogenicity	Hypoechoic
Sound transmission	No change posteriorly

❗ Comment:
This normal-sized metastatic lymph node was not palpable. Although it is no larger than a reactive node, no hilar fat was seen, and histology showed that it was completely permeated by tumor.

Table 13.2 Criteria for evaluating lymph node metastases

Shape	Oval
Orientation	Parallel or not parallel
Margin	Circumscribed of indistinct
Echo pattern	Hypoechoic
Posterior acoustic features	No posterior acoustic features

instances, a large metastasis may have a nodular extension that projects past the capsule (**Fig. 13.5**) in a focal bulge of echogenicity differing from that of the cortex around it.

While typical reactive and metastatic lymph nodes are easily identified, there are various intermediate patterns that result from varying degrees of metastatic involvement of the node. The hilum, which serves as an anatomic landmark, is often displaced to an asymmetric, peripheral position as metastatic involvement progresses (**Fig. 13.6**). Additional changes include asymmetric thick-

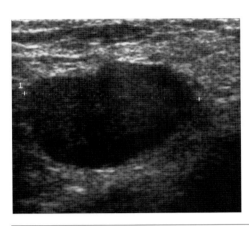

Fig. 13.4 Large metastatic lymph node in the left axilla. Sagittal scan.

Shape	Oval, lobulated
Size	21 × 18 mm
Contours	Smooth
Margins	Circumscribed
Internal structure	Homogeneously hypoechoic
Sound transmission	Enhancing

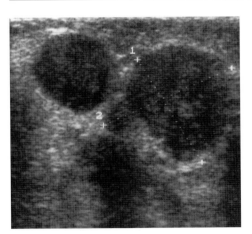

Shape	Round/oval
Size	23 × 20 mm and 15 × 13 mm
Contours	Smooth, lobulated
Margins	Circumscribed
Internal structure	Slightly heterogeneous
Echogenicity	Hypoechoic
Sound transmission	Enhanced

❗ Comment:
These lymph nodes do not display hilar structures. This finding is consistent with complete permeation of the nodes by metastatic cancer.

Fig. 13.5 Two metastatic lymph nodes in the right axilla. Transverse scan at level I.

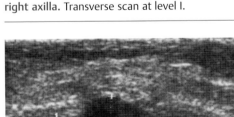

Shape	Oval
Size	18 × 15 mm
Contours	Lobulated
Margins	Circumscribed
Internal structure	Heterogeneous
Echogenicity	Hypoechoic
Sound transmission	Enhanced

❗ Comment:
A portion of the hilum, which is almost completely permeated by tumor, is visible at the left margin of the lymph node (arrow).

Fig. 13.6 Near complete metastatic permeation of a lymph node in the right axilla.

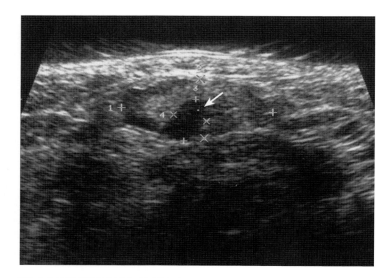

Fig. 13.7 Focal nodal metastasis involving a peripheral, circumscribed portion of the cortex.

Shape	Oval
Size	20 × 8 mm, metastasis 6 × 4 mm
Contours	Lobulated
Margins	Circumscribed
Internal structure	Hetero- and homogeneous
Echogenicity	Mixed hyperechoic and variably hypoechoic
Sound transmission	No change

❗ Comment:
The hilum displays an almost normal structure, and the cortical structure appears normal on the left and anterior aspects of the node. But the posterior cortex contains a circumscribed, markedly hypoechoic zone of metastatic involvement (arrow).

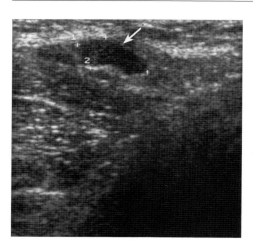

Fig. 13.8 Peripheral metastatic involvement of a lymph node.

Shape	Oval
Size	22 × 12 mm
Contours	Smooth
Margins	Circumscribed
Internal structure	Heterogeneous
Echogenicity	Mixed hyperechoic and variably hypo-echoic
Sound transmission	No change

❗ Comment:
The lymph node is markedly enlarged and roughly isoechoic to the axillary fat. However, the anterior cortex contains a distinct, hypoechoic metastasis 12 × 6 mm in size (arrow), below which is the more hyperechoic hilum.

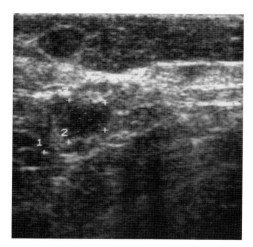

Fig. 13.9 Central lymph node metastasis in the hilar area.

Shape	Pleomorphic
Size	20 × 10 mm, metastasis 9 × 8 mm
Contours	Irregular
Margins	Ill-defined
Internal structure	Heterogeneous
Echogenicity	Mixed hyperechoic and variably hypo-echoic
Sound transmission	No change

❗ Comment:
The slightly enlarged lymph node is poorly delineated from the surrounding fibrofatty tissue. The hyperechoic hilum has been displaced outward by a central, hypoechoic metastasis.

ening of the cortical zone, where high-resolution ultrasound may demonstrate hypoechoic (or hyperechoic) structural changes within the thickened, involved nodal cortex (**Figs. 13.7, 13.8**), and ultrasound-directed fine-needle or core biopsy can be directed to these areas. It is important to note that metastases usually progress from the periphery of a lymph node toward the center, following the direction of lymphatic drainage from the capsule to the hilum. Primary hilar metastasis is a less common pattern seen in the early stage of nodal involvement (**Figs. 13.9, 13.10**).

The same morphologic changes are observed in all nodal regions. Because of their superficial location, these changes, even when still very small, are easily detected at levels II and III, in the parasternal nodes, and in the cervical nodes when normal sonographic anatomy is known (**Figs. 13.11 a, b–13.14**).

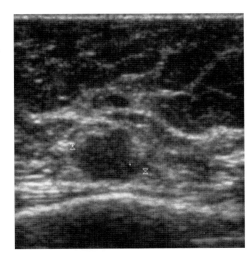

Fig. 13.10 Central metastasis in the hilum.

Shape	Oval
Size	20 × 12 mm; metastasis 13 × 10 mm
Contours	Lobulated
Margins	Microlobulated
Internal structure	Heterogeneous
Echogenicity	Mixed hypoechoic and hyperechoic
Sound transmission	No change

! Comment:
As in Fig. 13.9, this case illustrates a primary hilar nodal metastasis.

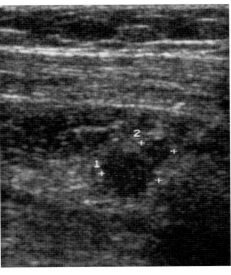
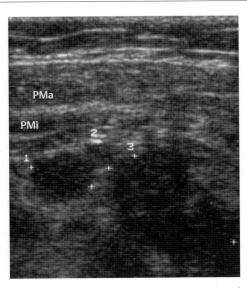

Shape	Irregular
Size	22 × 18 mm, 10 × 8 mm, and 6 × 5 mm
Contours	Irregular
Margins	Indistinct; microlobulated
Internal structure	Heterogeneous
Echogenicity	Hypoechoic
Sound transmission	No change

! Comment:
The metastatic nodes are completely permeated by tumor, and the capsule is breached, resulting in an irregular outer contour.

a, b

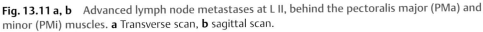

Fig. 13.11 a, b Advanced lymph node metastases at L II, behind the pectoralis major (PMa) and minor (PMi) muscles. **a** Transverse scan, **b** sagittal scan.

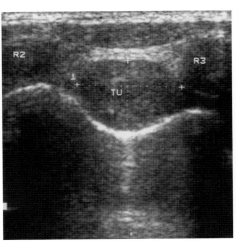
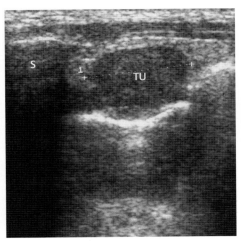

Shape	Oval
Size	17 × 12 × 18 mm
Contours	Smooth
Margins	Circumscribed
Internal structure	Homogeneous
Echogenicity	Hypoechoic
Sound transmission	Enhancing

! Comment:
Note that the anterior fascial boundary is smooth. Clinical findings were unremarkable. The metastasis has expanded downward, indenting the pleura.

a, b

Fig. 13.12 a, b Left parasternal lymph node metastasis next to the internal thoracic artery.
a Sagittal scan. The second and third ribs appear at the left and right sides of the image. Between them is the nodal metastasis.
b Left parasternal transverse scan. The sternum borders the left side of the image, and just to the right of it is the nodal metastasis.
TU = Lymph node metastasis; R2 = 2nd rib; R3 = 3rd rib; S = Sternum

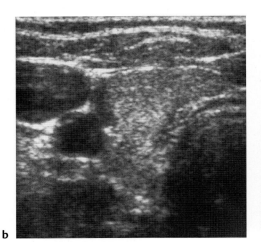
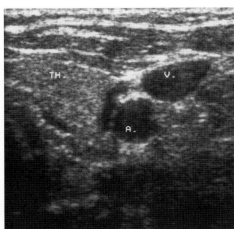

a, b

Fig. 13.13 a, b Transverse scans at the cervical level.

a Right side: The trachea is visible on the right side of the image, and lateral to it is the thyroid gland. Lateral to that are the cross sections of the carotid artery and, anteriorly, the jugular vein.

b Left side: The trachea is visible on the left side of the image. Lateral to it are the thyroid gland, carotid artery, and jugular vein.

TH = Thyroid; A = Artery; V = Vein

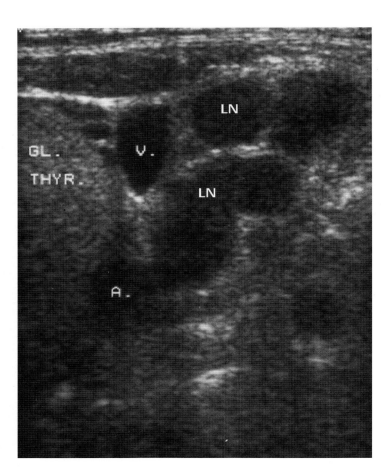

Fig. 13.14 Extensive lymph node metastasis in the left side of the neck. Several metastatic lymph nodes (LN) can be seen lateral to the thyroid gland (Gl. thyr.) and major cervical vessels (A = Artery; V = Vein).

Shape	Oval
Size	Multiple lymph nodes 5–15 mm in diameter
Contours	Smooth
Margins	Circumscribed
Internal structure	Homogeneous
Echogenicity	Hypoechoic
Sound transmission	No change

! Comment:
Metastatic lymph nodes in the neck display the same features as in other regions.

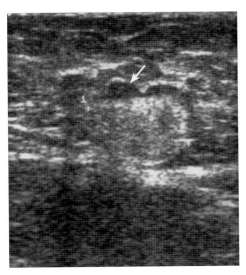

Shape	Oval
Size	18 × 15 mm
Contours	Lobulated
Margins	Circumscribed
Internal structure	Heterogeneous
Echogenicity	Predominantly hyperechoic; cortex is hypoechoic and asymmetrically thickened
Sound transmission	No change posteriorly

■ Comment:
The hilum is very hyperechoic and markedly thickened. The peripheral part of the node is hypoechoic and shows very slight, asymmetric anterior thickening. Histology confirmed a small metastatic deposit.

Fig. 13.15 Early cortical lymph node metastasis (arrow) in the right axilla (level I), transverse scan.

Differential Diagnosis

Early lymph node metastasis generally starts at the periphery of the node. Even in the absence of metastasis, it is common to find reactive nodal changes. As a result, there are lesions that cannot be positively differentiated by their sonographic features. These cases may involve a greatly enlarged reactive hilum or small, subtle cortical changes (**Fig. 13.15**). The heterogeneous permeation of a lymph node may create a generally hyperechoic or heterogeneous ultrasound appearance, making it difficult to detect the metastasis in an echogenic environment (e. g., the neck).

Further Diagnostic Procedures

Enlarged lymph nodes that do not show a symmetric reactive pattern require further evaluation. It should be noted that some normal reaction patterns can have a heterogeneous appearance. Also, there are nonmalignant changes that can mimic nodal metastases, including nonspecific granulating inflammations and tuberculosis. Lymphomas and metastases from other organs may also be detected incidentally in the axilla. This should be kept in mind even in patients with no detectable breast abnormalities. It would be unfortunate, however, if false-positive or equivocal findings were to prompt an excessive number of unnecessary interventions. Consequently, the lymph node findings should always be carefully interpreted in relation to the overall clinical presentation. If the findings remain unclear despite a careful analysis, and if malignancy is suspected, the diagnosis should be established by surgical or needle biopsy. For diagnosis of lymphomas, surgical excision of a node may be preferable even to a large-caliber needle biopsy.

If the imaging findings suggest a benign etiology, ultrasound-guided fine-needle aspiration or core biopsy can provide a reliable diagnosis at minimal cost, even if only a small portion of the lymph node is affected. A major advantage of ultrasound-guided fine-needle aspiration is that lymph nodes are considerably softer than most breast tumors. As a result, the aspirated samples are usually very cellular and are easily evaluated by an experienced cytopathologist. Level I and higher nodes, the cervical nodes, and the internal mammary nodes are all accessible to evaluation by ultrasound-guided fine-needle aspiration.

Role of Ultrasound

Mammograms occasionally demonstrate opacity of the axillary nodes. Increased nodal density is a nonspecific finding, however, and is not useful for differential diagnosis. CT scanning is too costly and time-consuming for routine applications, and results in other body regions indicate that its diagnostic accuracy is no better than that of ultrasound. Although MRI offers advantages in breast diagnosis, it generally does not provide axillary coverage. Radionuclide scanning has been used in breast imaging studies for some years, but it has been disappointing in the evaluation of nodal disease. In theory PET would provide a sensitive technique, and it may prove applicable in the future.

Recently the techniques of selective lymph node evaluation have been tested in large studies. They involve the direct injection of a radioactive tracer (technetium sulfur colloid) or vital blue dye (isosulfan blue) into a breast tumor. Several hours later, a measuring instrument is used to scan the axilla for radiotracer uptake. Lymph nodes near the tumor or axilla function as "sentinel nodes" that receive the bulk of lymphatic drainage from the injected tumor. If the removed radiolabeled sentinel nodes are free of metastases, studies have shown a high probability that axillary lymph nodes will also be negative. When sentinel node imaging is negative, axillary lymphadenectomy would not ordinarily be performed in the United States. So far this technique has not been compared with the predictive value of ultrasound. Its accuracy rate, at approximately 80%, is significantly higher than clinical examination but is still not high enough to contraindicate surgery or other testing when findings are negative. The axilla is often evaluated sonographically in new breast cancer cases, and if an abnormal axillary lymph node is found, biopsy—either fine needle or core biopsy– with ultrasound guidance can obviate need for the sentinel node procedure, going directly to surgical sampling of the axilla when the biopsied node is positive.

Documentation

The relative position of all abnormal lymph nodes should be documented so that they can be located during follow-up or surgery. Although frequently, there is no uncertainty as to which node or nodes are abnormal, if an axillary lymph node is biopsied

percutaneously with imaging guidance, a tiny marker clip can be placed in the lesion for identification in the future (for anatomic landmarks see Chapter 4, Sonographic Anatomy). Because lymph node metastases can appear as uniformly hypoechoic masses or masses with small, asymmetric fatty hilar areas and cortical bulges, the large axillary vessels or even the ribs may be mistaken for metastatic nodes when imaged in cross section. Scanning in multiple planes, application of color or power Doppler to differentiate a vessel from a solid mass (nodal or rib), and an accurate knowledge of axillary anatomy should be sufficient to avoid these errors. Suspicious lymph nodes are measured, documented in two planes, and biopsied. When reactive lymph nodes are found, at least the largest or most abnormal-appearing node should be measured and documented. If no lymph nodes are visible, an axillary scan should be recorded at the level of the axillary vein to establish that the examination was carried out.

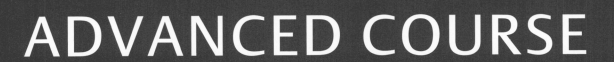

ADVANCED COURSE

14 Interventional Ultrasound 201

15 Preoperative Staging 215

16 Screening 223

17 Follow-Up and Recurrence 229

18 Three-dimensional, Extended
Field-of-View Ultrasound,
and Real-time Compound Scanning 235

19 Doppler Ultrasound 245

20 Breast Ultrasound
Review Questions 255

Interventional Ultrasound 14

Clinical Significance

It was shown in the Intermediate Course that the most common breast lesions display typical features that, in the majority of cases, allow them to be diagnosed from imaging findings. Cysts are a frequent cause of pain or palpable nodules that prompt women to seek medical attention, and can be reliably diagnosed with ultrasound. If the mammographic findings are not suspicious, there is no need for further evaluation. Nor is it necessary to further evaluate areas of breast firmness that show cyclic variations in patients who have normal sonographic and mammographic findings.

Solid circumscribed lesions present a more difficult challenge. Although many benign and malignant lesions can be distinguished by their sonographic and mammographic features, some lesions cannot be reliably differentiated. These problems were addressed in the sections on differential diagnosis in the Intermediate Course. It is important to understand that many solid masses cannot be characterized confidently on the basis of imaging findings alone. It would be inappropriate to evaluate all these lesions by surgical biopsy, as the large number of operations for benign lesions would result in an excessive financial burden as well as physical and emotional distress.

The advantage of nonsurgical interventional procedures is that they can establish the identity of an indeterminate lesion accurately with minimal effort and expense. This can be accomplished by means of various percutaneous techniques. In the past, only breast masses that were palpable were evaluated by percutaneous needle biopsy. These procedures, guided by palpation, were done as part of a "triple test" consisting of physical examination, mammography, and aspiration cytology (Hernan et al., 2003). However, manually guided aspiration was a blind technique that had a relatively high failure rate of 15–20%, because it was uncertain whether the sample came from the lesion itself or from tissue outside it.

Accuracy was improved by the introduction of stereotactic biopsy. However, this procedure can be time-consuming, requires ionizing radiation and extra mammographic views, and also requires the patient to be immobilized in a prone or seated position. Ultrasound guidance provides a rapidly performed, more comfortable, real-time alternative. As a result, ultrasound-guided percutaneous biopsies are now the procedure of choice for tissue sampling of sonographically detectable breast lesions.

Imaging-directed needle procedures are valuable not only for the histologic or cytologic sampling of indeterminate lesions but also for the aspiration of cysts and fluid collections, such as abscesses, that are painful or present as indeterminate nodules. Ultrasound can also be used for preoperative localization and to determine whether or not a nonpalpable mass has been included in the surgical specimen (**Table 14.1**). In cases where ultrasound findings are equivocal and mammograms show a suspicious lesion, usually associated with suspicious microcalcifications, the lesion should be localized preoperatively under stereotactic mammographic guidance or using an alphanumeric grid. The specimen should also be radiographed.

Research is currently being conducted into use of ultrasound to guide therapeutic procedures for breast cancer. Various means of tumor destruction—including radiofrequency, cryoablation, and high-frequency ultrasound (HIFU)—are under study, and ultrasound guidance for placement of balloon catheters for accelerated partial breast irradiation has been employed for several years (**Table 14.2**).

Needle Insertion Technique

The usage of ultrasound-guided needles for fine-needle aspiration, core biopsy, or preoperative localization should be optimized to ensure accurate needle placement and avoid complications. The reflective and refractive properties of ultrasound are an important consideration. As explained in the Basic Course, structures that are perpendicular to the ultrasound beam are optimally visualized. If the beam encounters the structure at an oblique angle, the image is poorly rendered, and a structure may not be visualized at all if it is parallel to the beam. The same geometric

Table 14.1 Indications for interventional ultrasound

> ▸ Cyst aspiration (for pain or a firm nodule)
> ▸ Investigation of indeterminate solid masses
> ▸ Preoperative histologic confirmation
> ▸ Establishing a diagnosis prior to neoadjuvant chemotherapy
> ▸ Preoperative localization of nonpalpable masses
> ▸ Localization of small lesions in the surgical specimen

Table 14.2 Interventional methods

> ▸ Fine-needle aspiration cytology or cyst aspiration
> ▸ Spring-activated core biopsy
> ▸ Vacuum-assisted large core biopsy
> ▸ Preoperative wire localization or dye injection

principle holds true for depiction of the needle: its type and gauge are less important than its angle in relation to the image plane.

In some ultrasound-guided needle procedures, the target lesion is displayed at the edge of the image to minimize the distance between skin and lesion that the needle must traverse. The needle is then inserted adjacent to the transducer and advanced toward the lesion in an anteroposterior direction (**Fig. 14.1**). Most needle guides that attach to transducers are designed for anteroposterior insertion. Although this approach may be of benefit for presurgical needle localizations and cyst aspiration, the problem with this technique for breast procedures is that the needle is visualized poorly, if at all, because of its obliquity to the image plane (**Fig. 14.2 a, b**). It should also be considered that when breast ultrasound is carried out in the supine patient, the pressure from the transducer usually results in a tissue thickness of only 2–3 cm between the transducer and chest wall. When the needle is inserted anteroposteriorly at a steep angle, there is a risk of passing through the intercostal space and entering the pleural cavity or pericardial sac. To avoid a possible life-threatening complication, automated core-biopsy devices should never be directed perpendicular to the chest wall; the angle of insertion should be shallow or parallel to the face of the transducer and to the chest wall, always under direct ultrasound visualization.

 An anteroposterior approach perpendicular to the chest wall makes it difficult to monitor the needle position and increases the risk of complications.

It is better to position the transducer so that the lesion, in view in its entirety, is 1–2 cm from the edge of the image. The convexity and compliance of the breast, along with careful positioning of the patient, usually make it possible to position the transducer roughly parallel to the chest wall while inserting the needle from the periphery in a nearly horizontal direction, directing it approximately parallel to the transducer face and chest wall (**Figs. 14.3, 14.4 a, b**). In this chest-wall parallel approach, the needle returns high specular echoes and can be monitored throughout the procedure (**Figs. 14.2 a, b; 14.5 a, b**). Even if the needle misses the lesion, there is no risk of serious injury because the needle cannot enter the pleural cavity.

If the needle is inserted at the center of the transducer and advanced at a steep angle toward the tumor, passing through the image plane, the operator sees only a punctate cross section of the needle shaft and has no idea where the needle tip is located (**Fig. 14.6**). The needle itself is not even visible until it enters the image plane. If the target is missed, it is often necessary to withdraw and reintroduce the needle. Also, the anteroposterior approach poses a risk of injury to deeper structures. As a result, beginners in particular should avoid using this technique. It should *never* be used with automated core-biopsy guns because of the risk of complications.

The best technique, illustrated in **Figures 14.2–14.4**, is to insert the needle horizontally along the image plane of the transducer. It is important to keep the needle's path straight below the center of the transducer while directing it along the image plane (**Figs. 14.4, 14.7**). Some linear transducers have a vertical seam, visible from the short end of the transducer, that joins the two halves of the probe housing. This vertical seam can be used to imagine the path

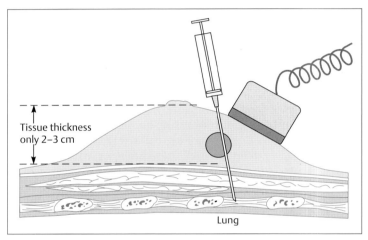

Fig. 14.1 Cave: Faulty technique of needle insertion. The needle is inserted anteroposteriorly toward the chest wall. The needle is difficult to visualize and may penetrate the intercostal space. This technique is hazardous and unreliable, and should **never** be used for core biopsy.

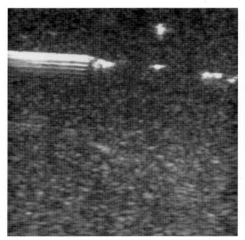
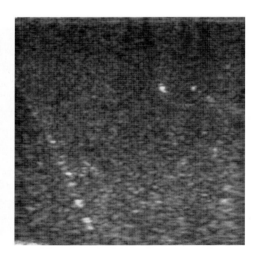

a, b

Fig. 14.2 a, b Ultrasound guidance of needle placement in a breast phantom.
a With an approach parallel to the chest wall along the scan plane, the tip of the needle is clearly visible.
b Anteroposterior insertion creates an unfavorable reflection angle, and the needle is poorly visualized.

of the ultrasound beam as it emerges in a thin sheet from the transducer. The goal would be to keep the needle within the expected path of this beam, without angling to the left or right. If the examiner inserts the needle off-center from the transducer and tries to advance it obliquely toward the lesion, the needle will pass through, rather than along, the image plane. Part of the needle will be visible on the monitor but usually not the tip, which can easily miss the target.

> The optimal direction of needle insertion is approximately horizontal and parallel to the transducer face and chest wall. With this geometry, the entire needle including its bevel will be seen, making it easier to monitor needle placement and minimize the risk of complications.

Once the appropriate path is selected and the lesion is in view, rapid completion of the biopsy will prevent the need for continual minor readjustment necessitated when the hand moves a few millimeters out of the plane of the lesion. An additional tip for successful performance of these biopsy procedures is the use of just enough gel to enable the target to be seen; the lesion has already been characterized with ultrasound, and the probe will slide away from the area to be sampled if gel is applied liberally. The probe can be stabilized further by holding it near its base, and even more so if the hand rests on sterile gauze placed around one end of the transducer. If the operator unconsciously applies ex-

cessive pressure against the breast to prevent slippage of the transducer, visualization of the needle will be diminished even if the appropriate geometry is maintained. One last suggestion is an important one: the operator's hand and body should make one smooth line as the operator moves his eyes up from the short end

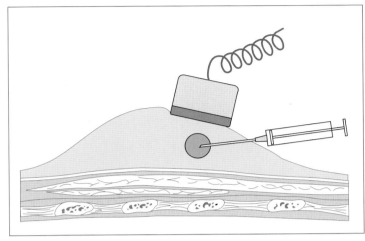

Fig. 14.3 Correct needle insertion technique. The needle is inserted from the periphery and directed approximately parallel to the transducer face and chest wall. This improves ultrasound visualization of the needle and avoids the risk of deep injury.

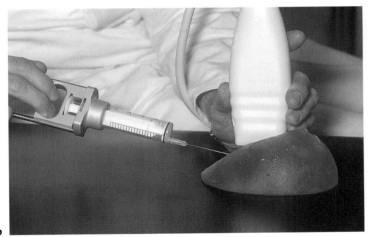

a, b

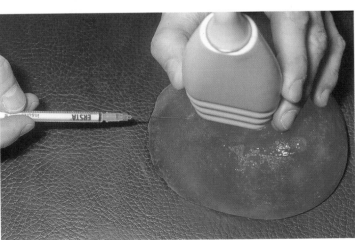

c

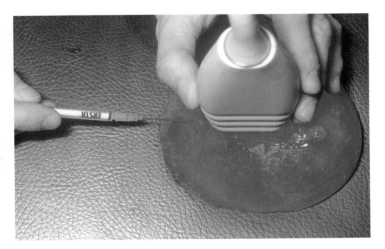

Fig. 14.4 a–c Practicing fine-needle aspiration in a breast phantom.
a The needle should be inserted from the periphery at a shallow angle.
b The needle is placed below the center of the transducer and advanced straight along the image plane.
c If inserted off-center, the needle passes through the image plane, and the position of the needle tip cannot be monitored.

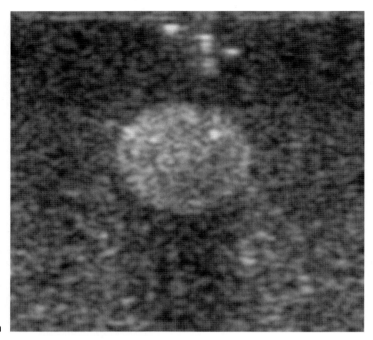
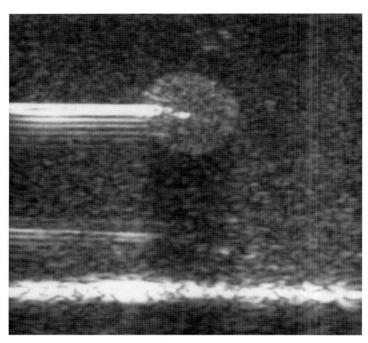

a

b

Fig. 14.5 a, b Fine-needle aspiration in a breast phantom.
a The target lesion is positioned about 1–2 cm from the edge of the image. Its depth (1 cm) can be read from a scale at the edge of the image.

b When the needle tip has entered the lesion, aspiration is started and the needle is moved in short, quick strokes at varying angles to collect cellular material.

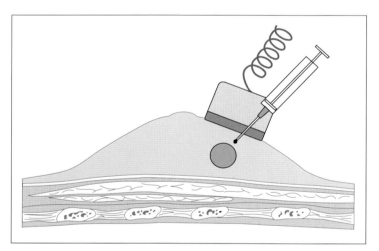

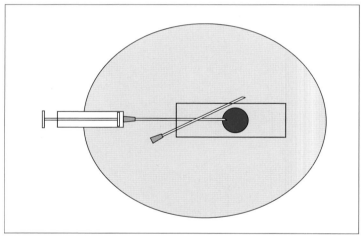

Fig. 14.6 Difficult insertion technique without constant monitoring of needle position (transducer positioned over tumor). The needle is advanced from the center of the transducer toward the tumor at a steep angle. When the needle breaks the plane of the scan, the needle shank is visible in cross section. The anteroposterior approach is hazardous (tissue beyond tumor may be aspirated as needle tip is not visualized).

Fig. 14.7 Anteroposterior view of the insertion technique. The needle should be inserted below the center of the transducer and advanced to the tumor along the image plane. An off-center needle will pass obliquely through the scan plane. In this case only a short segment of the needle can be seen and the tip is not visualized.

of the transducer on the breast to the ultrasound monitor and back again to confirm accuracy of needle passage. The success of the procedure may be compromised if the operator must twist and turn his body to look at the monitor and then again turn away from the monitor to look back at his hands and the needle.

In recording procedures, at least one set of images labeled "prefire" and "postfire" should be shown. The prefire image should capture the needle prior to firing the device, recognizing that the throw of these devices is approximately 2.0 cm. The postfire image should show the position of the needle after firing and before removal from the breast. Five passes will be accurate in 99 % of

cases, and unless pre- and postfire labeling is shown for all, after the first pass or the best one, other passes can be labeled as "pass 4," "postfire pass 4," etc.

The report of the procedure should indicate whether or not written informed consent was obtained, use of lidocaine—1 % is used most commonly—in what amount, what device was used, gauge of the needle (ordinarily 12 to 16G for spring-activated devices), placement of a marker clip and radiographic confirmation, complications if any, and, later, when the histopathology interpretation is received, an addendum containing the pathology diagnosis, who was notified and when (usually the referring physician and the patient), and the names suggested for surgical consultation or the imaging and clinical follow-up.

In the United States, written informed consent is expected for all image-guided procedures. Only experienced examiners should attempt needle procedures in danger areas such as the axilla, intercostal spaces, and neck region, and biopsying areas close to an implant shell may cause some hearts to race, although when a spring-activated device with needle passage horizontal to the chest wall is fired, the needle will recoil a millimeter or so upwards, not down toward the prosthesis.

When these procedures are done by trainees, a reasonable number should be supervised at the outset, and it is advisable to practice on biopsy phantoms before doing the first procedures on patients. Several breast biopsy phantoms are available. They are fairly expensive and can be used only a limited number of times, as every pass leaves a permanent needle track. However, the cost is justified by the fact that the structural characteristics of the phantom mimic the acoustic properties of breast tissue. Once the technique has been mastered in a phantom, it can easily be applied to patients. Available products include the BB-1 breast biopsy phantom manufactured by ATS (ATS Labs, Bridgeport, CT, USA), the rmi 429 US biopsy phantom (Gammex rmi, Middleton, WI, USA, and Giessen, Germany), and the CIRS phantom (CIRS, Norfolk, VA, USA).

Fine-Needle Aspiration Cytology

Solid Lesions

In fine-needle aspiration cytology (FNAC), a thin-gauge needle is used to aspirate cellular material from breast lesions for cytologic analysis (**Fig. 14.8**). If the diameter of the needle is too large, there is a greater likelihood of aspirating blood, which is undesirable in fine-needle aspirations. The thin needles used for manually guided aspirations are relatively short; we prefer a 20G needle (0.9 mm diameter) 70 mm long, used with a 20-mL syringe to achieve sufficient negative pressure. Needles of 23G and 25G are also suitable. To coordinate movements of the needle and transducer, the examiner should hold the transducer in one hand and the needle in the other. We use a pistol-grip syringe holder (e. g., Cameco [Precision Dynamics Corp., Burbank, CA, USA], or Inrad [Inrad, Inc., Kentwood, MI, USA], the latter used with a 10-mL syringe) to facilitate the aspiration.

The needle is inserted into the lesion without suction. When the needle tip has entered the lesion, suction is applied while short needle excursions are performed in a fan-shaped pattern. This technique samples material from all areas of the mass and avoids filling the needle with extraneous parenchyma or fat. Aspiration should be done only while the needle is inside the mass. With an adequate aspiration, fluid will usually be seen rising through the transparent hub, indicating that the needle has filled with material. It is difficult to aspirate cells from fibrous lesions. Usually in these cases the needle must be moved back and forth 10–20 times at varying angles while suction is applied. Fewer excursions are needed for soft lesions and for most malignancies. Lymph nodes can be sampled with very little needle movement, because they are soft and yield a very cellular aspirate.

When sufficient material has been aspirated, the needle is withdrawn from the breast without suction, and the material is expressed from the needle onto a glass slide. A second slide is used to smear the aspirated material, similar to the technique used in preparing a blood smear. If it appears that insufficient material has been sampled, the aspiration can be repeated. A single aspiration is sufficient in most cases. At some sites, a cytopathologist or cytotechnologist can be present in the breast imaging suite at the time of the procedure to confirm adequacy of the aspirate for interpretation.

For fixing and staining, most cytopathologists prefer the May–Grünwald–Giemsa stain for breast cytology, in which case

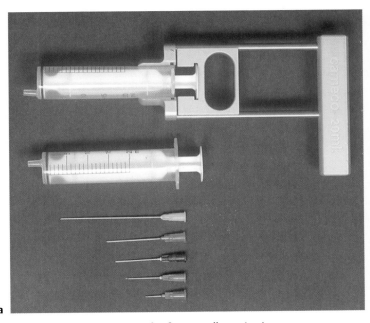
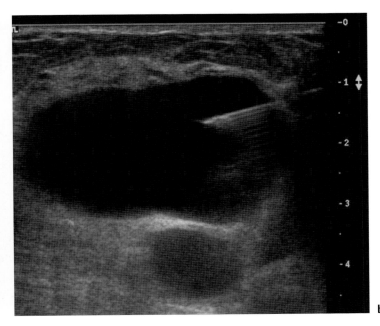

a

b

Fig. 14.8 a, b Instruments for fine-needle aspiration.
a 20-mL syringe, Cameco pistol-grip syringe holder, and assorted aspirating needles. We prefer a 7-cm 20 G needle.
b Aspirating needle placed in a large cyst for aspiration.

the smear is fixed by air drying. Papanicolaou stain, which is standard for cervical smears, is less commonly used for breast cytology; it requires alcohol fixation. At the outset, the radiologist should consult the cytopathologist to determine specimen preparation and the preferred stain for breast cytology. Choice of a particular stain will also determine the fixation method. A sample that is improperly fixed and stained cannot be interpreted.

The breast imager should have a basic knowledge of cytodiagnosis to compare the cytologic findings with the sonographic findings and interpret them accordingly. This is particularly important if the cytology report is inconclusive, as is frequently the case if typical tumor cells cannot be identified. The aspiration of fibromas and lipomas generally yields connective tissue cells, fat cells, and perhaps a few ductal epithelial cells. These are normal constituents of breast tissue, and so a specific tumor diagnosis cannot be made from the cytologic findings. An experienced examiner who knows the ultrasound findings, has formed a tentative diagnosis, and knows what cellular constituents are likely to be found in the cytologic sample, will be able to interpret the "equivocal" result accordingly. In the United States, except for facilities with outstanding cytopathology, most image-guided biopsies are large-needle core or vacuum-assisted sampling procedures which enable specific and more definitive histopathologic diagnoses to be made.

Fibroadenomas are typical lesions that can be evaluated by fine-needle aspiration biopsy (**Fig. 14.9 a, b**). They show a uniform cytologic pattern with coherent clusters of ductal cells. In the absence of proliferative changes, surgical biopsy is not required. Problems may arise in the diagnosis of a hamartoma or adenofibrolipoma, whose echogenicity varies with the amount of connective tissue present in the lesion. On dynamic examination, however, the sharply circumscribed mass is found to be soft and compressible. Cytology usually shows only clusters of adipose and connective tissue cells (**Fig. 14.9 c, d**), and the cytologist, unaware of the radiologic findings, will often return an inconclusive report. This aspirate does, however, suggest a diagnosis when interpreted

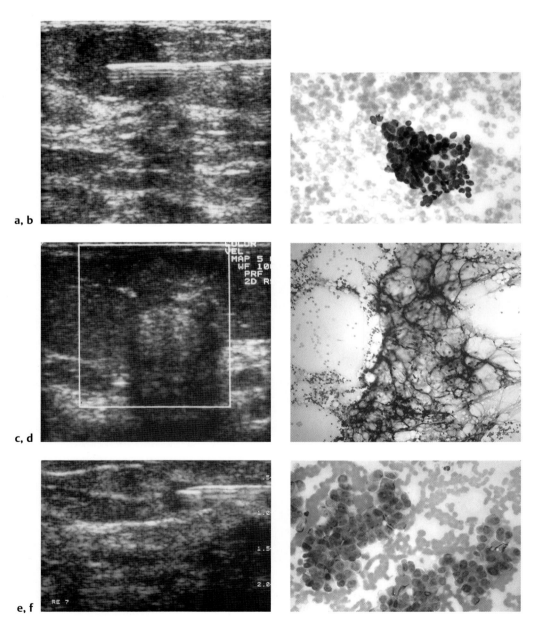

Fig. 14.9 a–f Examples of typical cytologic findings.
a Ultrasound appearance of a fibroadenoma during fine-needle aspiration.
b Cytologic appearance of a fibroadenoma.
c Ultrasound appearance of a fibrolipoma during aspiration.
d Cytologic appearance of a fibrolipoma.
e Ultrasound-guided fine-needle aspiration of a carcinoma.
f Cytologic appearance of the carcinoma.

a, b

c, d

e, f

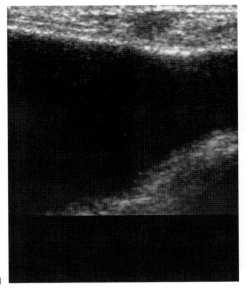
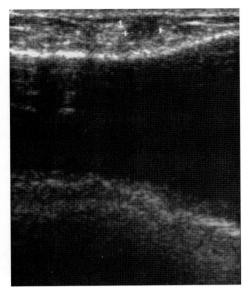

Fig. 14.9 g–l
g Ultrasound appearance of a silicone breast implant following mastectomy and reconstruction. The two indeterminate lesions anterior to the implant were aspirated.
h Smear prepared from the tumor recurrence.
i Apocrine metaplasia.
j Foam cells.
k Aspiration of an inspissated cyst.
l Inspissated cyst aspirate on a glass slide.

g

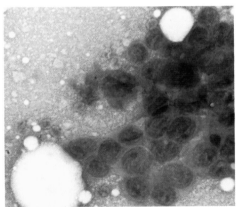
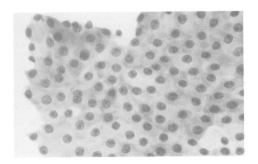

h, i

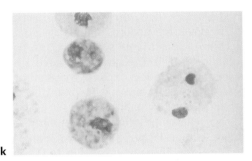
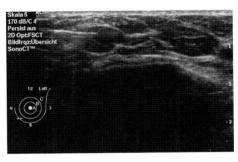

j, k

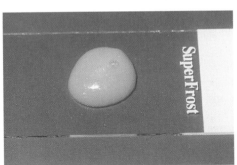

l

in conjunction with the sonographic findings. Mammography can obviate the need for any diagnostic procedure by depicting the thin capsule enclosing the heterogeneous, fat-containing material within. On physical examination, these lesions are palpable but soft, and if the typical mammographic findings are demonstrated, the mass is assessed as a BI-RADS category 2 lesion, a benign finding for which routine follow-up is appropriate.

Aspiration is rarely indicated for malignant tumors. Whenever possible, in cases with suspicious mammographic or sonographic findings (categories 4c and 5) the diagnosis should be confirmed preoperatively by core biopsy. In some cases, however, aspiration cytology can confirm the tentative diagnosis of an indeterminate lesion by demonstrating nuclear pleomorphism (**Fig. 14.9 e, f**).

Ultrasound-guided aspiration can sample diagnostic material from difficult areas, such as a suspected recurrent tumor over a breast implant (**Fig. 14.9 g, h**). Histologic confirmation by core biopsy or malignant cells on FNA is particularly useful for surgical planning in breasts that contain multiple lesions.

In the United States, percutaneous cytologic or histopathologic sampling is preferred to more costly, invasive open surgical procedures for diagnosis. For lesions highly likely to be carcinoma based on imaging criteria, ultrasound-directed, stereotactically guided, or MRI-guided biopsies of solitary or multiple lesions can provide reliable histopathologic diagnoses. This is of value particularly when lesion distribution would indicate multicentricity, should malignancy be confirmed. In addition, the use of sentinel node imaging, where indicated, is an important part of surgical treatment planning that is made possible by having a histologic diagnosis of invasive tumor prior to the excision.

Fluid-filled Lesions

The fluid from most cysts aspirated with ultrasound direction or guided by palpation can be discarded. Exceptions are bloody fluid obtained from a nontraumatic aspiration procedure or purulent material, sent for Gram stain, culture, and antibiotic sensitivity as well as cytologic analysis. After a cyst has been aspirated, the cyst fluid can be sent directly to the laboratory if it can be processed within 24 hours. More prolonged storage or transport may cause the cellular components of the cyst fluid to break down. The safest method is to centrifuge the fluid (10 minutes at 2000 rpm), discard the supernatant, and prepare a cytologic smear from the sediment.

Aspirated cyst fluid is usually acellular and contains precipitated material. It is common, however, to find cells of apocrine metaplasia and foam cells (**Fig. 14.9 i, j**). These are normal degenerative or transformed cellular constituents of cysts and fibrocystic lesions and do not require further evaluation, provided the pathologist finds no evidence of proliferative changes.

Inspissated cysts can be difficult to aspirate (**Fig. 14.9 k, l**). These lesions frequently appear solid at ultrasound, and obtaining this paste-like material can be challenging. However, the real-time image will show that the needle is freely mobile within the mass and no flow will be observed within the mass when color or power Doppler is used. Injection of saline or some lidocaine may help to liquefy the contents of the cyst, and use of a 16G or 18G needle may increase the chance of a successful aspiration. Often the radiologist must be patient and work for some time before finally aspirating the viscous fluid through the needle.

Large Needle Biopsy: Core, Vacuum-assisted, and Other Technologies

Many breast imagers prefer core biopsy over fine-needle aspiration in the belief that histologic specimens furnish a more accurate diagnosis. With the reported inadequacy of samples obtained by FNAC ranging from 0 to 37%, this preference may be justified at facilities where the inadequacy rate is at the high end. Where FNAC works well, the preferences of the breast imager and the

pathologist together should be honored. Even core biopsy can yield a false-negative result, however, for many different reasons: faulty needle placement, collection of necrotic tissue, sampling beyond the lesion (miscalculation of size of lesion, length of throw, and site of device activation as causes), or incomplete processing of the tissue block omitting the lesion itself from the prepared slides. With both FNAC and core biopsy, the acceptance of the pathology interpretation relies on careful correlation with the imaging assessment. If there is discordance, the procedure and all of its steps should be reviewed to determine the cause, the need for re-evaluation of the specimen, and the indications for re-biopsy.

False-negative results were common in the days of manually guided Tru-Cut needle biopsies The activation of tight, strong springs in current automated core biopsy systems can result in collection of a tissue sample at high speed, providing a significantly better tissue core than was possible previously (**Fig. 14.10**). In addition to establishing a histologic diagnosis preoperatively, eliminating the need for intraoperative frozen sections if a patient goes directly to surgical excision, receptor status and other prognostic factors can be determined from tissue cores, and large, extensive, or inflammatory carcinomas can be diagnosed as a prelude to instituting preoperative neoadjuvant or primary adjuvant chemotherapy.

In the United States, where the advantages of sampling techniques that can provide a histologic rather than a cytologic diagnosis are accepted, acceptance of core biopsy has become pervasive. The teaching of interventional procedures has become an essential part of the curriculum for radiology residents and for breast imaging fellows, who should become very experienced during the intensive post-residency breast imaging fellowship year.

The use of vacuum-assisted devices is associated with higher equipment costs, acknowledged by higher third-party reimbursements for vacuum-assisted biopsies than for core biopsies using spring-activated devices. The powerful vacuums in these systems, which enable rapid collection of intact large specimens, can be used with ultrasound guidance as well. The spring-activated automated core biopsy devices are much less expensive and allow fanning through various areas of a mass, and may be preferred to sample large masses with ultrasound guidance.

The vacuum-assisted devices that collect multiple large samples can also be used to remove benign lesions such as papillomas causing nipple discharge or painful fibroadenomas (**Fig. 14.11**). In addition to the very efficient vacuum-assisted devices requiring only one insertion to collect multiple samples by rotation of the instrument (**Fig. 14.12**), there are simpler, cordless, battery-operated devices utilizing syringes within the device to create the negative pressure that optimizes the cutting mechanism, resulting in increased tissue yield per core. These devices have to be removed from the breast and reinserted to obtain each specimen (**Fig. 14.13**). These devices, as with the more elaborate vacuum-assisted devices with electronic cords, can be used with or without a throw of approximately 2 cm.

Relatively recently, devices have been developed that use freezing to cause tissue to adhere to a metallic biopsy instrument. Following nondestructive tissue adherence achieved with CO_2, a cutting device sheaths the needle-like spike, and the device is then removed from the breast for collection of the specimen. This equipment (Cassi, Siemens Medical Inc., Pleasanton, CA, USA) does

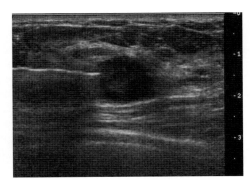

Fig. 14.10 a–d Core biopsy.
a Biopsy device with needle inserted.
b Prefire ultrasound view of needle placement.
c Postfire view.
d Histologic tumor specimen.

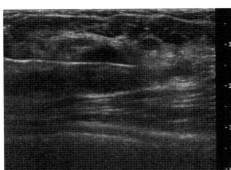
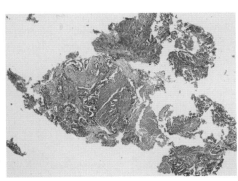
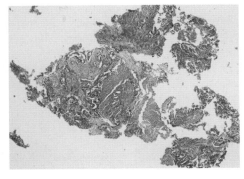

a, b

c, d

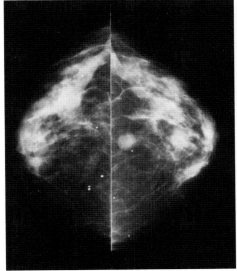
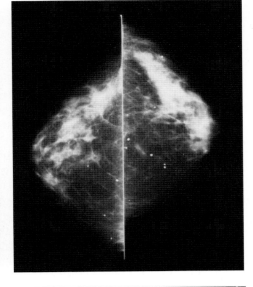

a, b

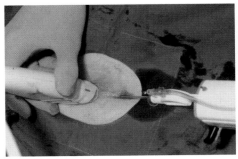
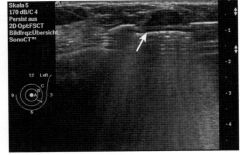

c, d

Fig. 14.11 a–d Complete resection of a fibroadenoma with the Mammotome (Ethicon Endo-Surgery, Cincinnati, OH, USA).
a Mammography (CC projection) of both breasts.
b Mammography 6 months after tumor resection with the Mammotome demonstrates complete removal without visible scar formation.
c After local anesthesia and skin incision the vacuum biopsy needle is inserted and tumor resection starts under ultrasound guidance.
d Ultrasound image with the open vacuum biopsy needle placed behind the tumor (arrow). Ideally the procedure starts at the posterior margin of the tumor, which permits observation of tissue resection until the lesion is completely removed.

Case 1

Patient had a high anamnestic risk for breast cancer. Screening mammography had detected a new rounded density. US showed a circumscribed hypoechoic lesion. Because of high familial risk factors core biopsy was recommended to confirm the benign lesion. The patient agreed with histopathologic confirmation but wanted the tumor removed at the same time without open surgery. This is an ideal indication to perform vacuum-assisted core biopsy as a benign lesion can be confirmed and at the same time be completely removed.

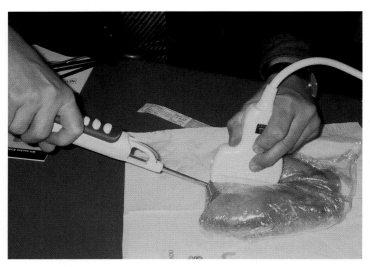

Fig. 14.12 Practicing hand-held vacuum biopsy in a breast biopsy phantom (turkey breast filled with targets). (Mammotome, Ethicon Endo-Surgery, Cincinnati, OH, USA).

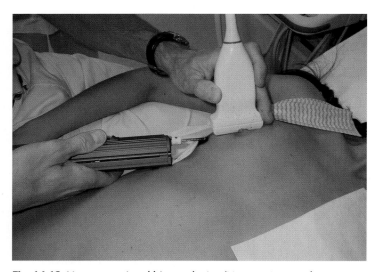

Fig. 14.13 Vacuum assisted biopsy device (Vacora, C.R. Bard, Inc., Murray Hill, NJ, USA) used for minimally invasive resection of a fibroadenoma.

not have a throw, and the specimen is collected at the location where the device is placed. The needle-like entry into tissue is 19G and the collecting cannula that cuts the specimen is 10G. Because it remains where it is placed with ultrasound guidance, rather than advancing with activation, we have used it to provide excellent samples of the cortex of axillary lymph nodes thought to harbor metastases. One or two samples will suffice, and with continuous ultrasound visualization of the cortical target, we have incurred no complications to date. The effectiveness of a device (Visica, Sanarus, Inc., Pleasanton, CA, USA) causing tissue alternately to freeze to a spike, form an ice ball, and then thaw for several cycles until the tissue is deemed to be destroyed, is being tested for effectiveness in ablating cancers in a multicenter research protocol.

The needle–transducer geometry described above pertains to the technique for all of these procedures, which can be carried out safely when the needle enters the breast as parallel as possible to the face of the transducer as well as the chest wall and perpendicular to the ultrasound beam.

Automated core and vacuum-assisted biopsy specimens are placed in formalin as they are collected, with a separate jar used for each site sampled, and submitted for histopathologic interpretation. Both for large lesions, for which downsizing may be attempted with neoadjuvant chemotherapy, and for small lesions that may be difficult to recognize following large-needle biopsies, marker clips of different shapes should be placed within each lesion at the conclusion of the biopsy procedures. The small markers are generally preloaded into needles and can be inserted with US guidance into the biopsied lesions. Craniocaudal and 90° lateral mammographic images to show location of the marker clips will complete the procedure.

Ultrasound-Guided Localization

Either needle–hookwire assemblies (**Fig. 14.14**) or the injection of methylene blue dye (**Fig. 14.15**, **Fig. 14.16**) can be used for ultrasound-guided preoperative localization. The use of activated charcoal as a marking material is not FDA-approved in the United States. The advantage of wires is that they can be placed long before the operation. One disadvantage is the need to dissect along the wire at surgery, although other surgical approaches are also successful, and the lesion-plus-wire can be delivered through an incision distant from the entry point of the wire into the breast. If the wire is cut it is difficult to find the distal end, although many types of wire have been adapted to make transection less likely either by braiding or by using alloys that are difficult to cut, such as nickel–titanium. When ultrasound is used as the imaging guide, the needle–hookwire assembly can be placed using the shortest and most direct path to the lesion, a route shorter than that for mammography using an alphanumeric grid with the needle required to be parallel to the chest wall.

Although many surgeons prefer the injection of methylene blue dye, it is used less and less commonly in the United States. The dye may be injected into the center of the lesion or at its periphery. The advantage of dye localization is that it provides the surgeon with a visible guide for dissecting to the lesion and widely encompassing it (**Fig. 14.16**). One disadvantage is that surgery must be started within 30 minutes of the injection because of the diffusion of the water-based dye. Frequently the dye has been cleared from the tumor within 2–3 hours of the injection, and the lesion can no longer be located. When dye localization is used, the direction of needle insertion should be indicated on a line drawing, because usually there is retrograde staining of the needle track. The surgeon should know this, so that he will not inadvertently resect the dye along the needle track and leave the tumor behind.

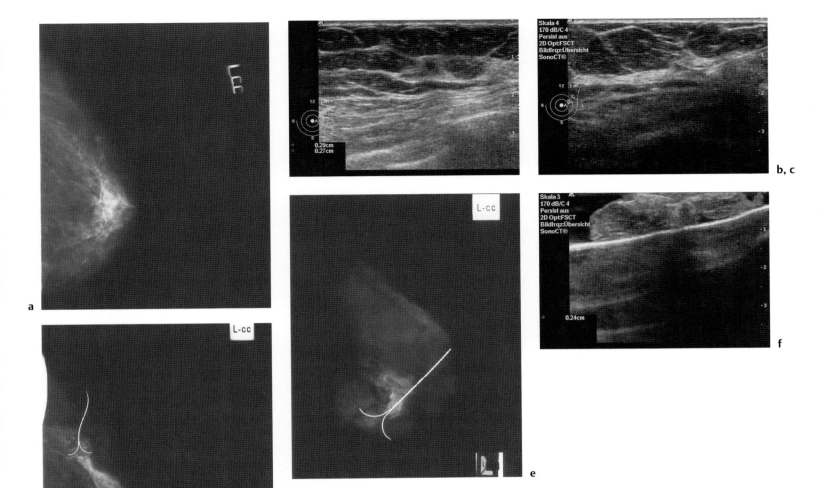

Fig. 14.14 a–f Ultrasound-guided preoperative hook wire localization of an early invasive ductal carcinoma, diameter 4 mm.
a Mammography of the left breast. CC projection showing a 4-mm irregular density.
b Displaying the lesion by ultrasound.
c Placement of the hook wire into the lesion under ultrasound guidance.
d Radiologic control of the correct placement of the hook wire.
e Radiography of the excised specimen.
f Specimen ultrasound of the excised tissue.

❗ Comment:
Nonpalpable lesions require preoperative localization. If the lesion is visible on ultrasound and mammography, the sonographic approach is easier and more accurate to perform. However, in small lesions it is essential to reassure that the same lesion is represented by both imaging methods. In this case the localization was simply performed under ultrasound guidance and an ensuing mammogram was taken to correlate with the mammographically suspicious lesion.

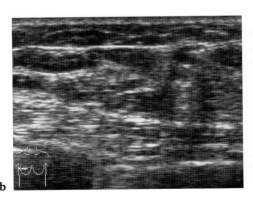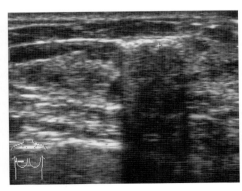

Fig. 14.15 a, b Ultrasound-guided dye localization.
a Needle placement in the lesion.
b After injection of the dye.

❗ Comment:
In the dye injection technique, it is common to inject some air from the needle into the tumor. This creates a bright echo with an acoustic shadow. Usually the air is absorbed within a few minutes.

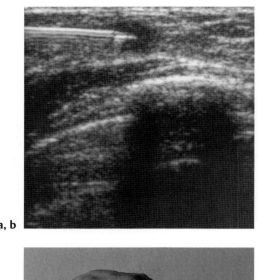
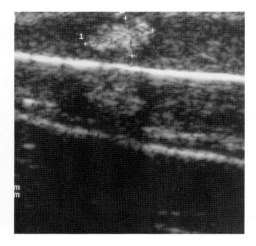

a, b

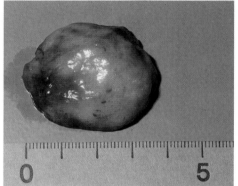
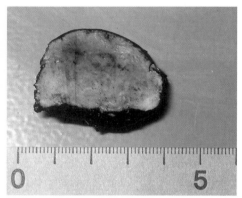

c, d

Fig. 14.16 a–d Ultrasound-guided dye localization.
a Needle placement in the lesion.
b Lesion following injection of the dye.
c, d Surgical specimen (fibroadenoma).

⚠ Comment:
Tiny air bubbles scattered throughout the tumor cause it to appear hyperechoic on the postinjection scan.

Specimen Ultrasonography

Specimen imaging is required for all lesions, benign and malignant, excised following needle localization. When there is uncertainty regarding successful excision of palpable masses, specimen radiography and/or ultrasound can confirm removal of the lesion (**Fig. 14.17**). The technique should be considered for nonpalpable but sonographically visible lesions in cases where complete removal cannot be verified by other means.

In the older water-bath scanners, the entire surgical specimen was placed in a thin plastic vessel or wrapped in film for examination. When a real-time scanner is used, the entire specimen is placed into a shallow dish and covered with film to avoid soiling the transducer (**Fig. 14.17**). After ultrasound gel is applied, the tissue can be examined by contact scanning. The lesions in the surgical specimen have the same ultrasound appearance as they did within the breast (see **Fig. 14.14**). If findings are equivocal, compression can be applied to distinguish areas of fatty infiltration from firm tumors . Just as in vivo, the tumors in the excised specimen should be scanned and measured in multiple planes. The size of the tumors can be compared with preoperative images to confirm that the lesions coincide (**Fig. 14.18**) and the localizing wires, if still engaged in tissue, can be traced to the lesion. If the lesions are small, the pathologist may find it difficult to cut at the right place when processing the material. Particularly in the case of

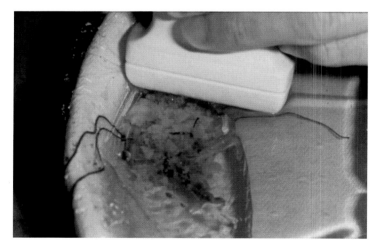

Fig. 14.17 Placement of the transducer on to the surgical specimen immersed in water and covered with a plastic sheet.

small multifocal tumors, it can be difficult to find each focus within the specimen. Ultrasound can help in these cases by directing the insertion of needles or wires into the tumor foci. Once in place, the localizing needles can guide the pathologist in processing the specimen (**Fig. 14.18**).

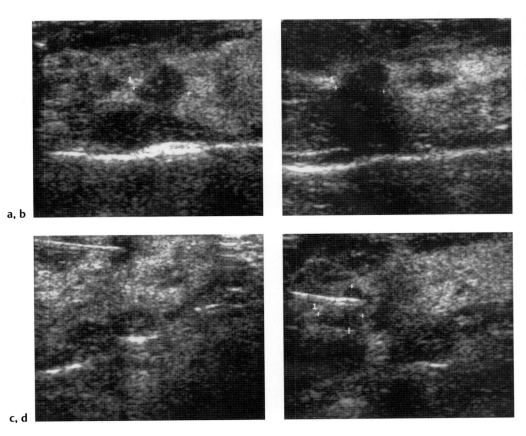

a, b

c, d

Fig. 14.18 a–d Specimen ultrasonography of multifocal carcinoma. Needle localization of the tumor foci is performed under sonographic guidance.

ℹ Comment:
In the pathologic workup of the specimen, it is not sufficient to find the main tumor; it is also important to establish multifocality or multicentricity. If the disseminated tumors are small and nonpalpable, presurgical localization may aid the pathologist in identifying additional foci.

Summary

Ultrasound-guided fine-needle aspiration allows a higher confidence level in the evaluation of indeterminate breast lesions, and core or vacuum-assisted biopsy can provide a diagnosis. These procedures are simple, rapidly accomplished, and safe when done by an experienced examiner. Ultrasound guidance is also advantageous for the preoperative localization of tumors. Specimen ultrasonography helps to eliminate uncertainties in the excision of nonpalpable lesions (Hernan et al., 2003).

Preoperative Staging | 15

Clinical Significance

In a dramatic departure from modified radical mastectomy, in the last two decades breast-conserving surgery has become the most frequently selected surgical therapy for breast cancer. Today it accounts for 60% or more of breast cancer operations. Where removal of the breast or large segmental excisions are required, various options are available for reconstruction including silicone or saline prostheses, transverse rectus abdominis myocutaneous flaps, and, for subtotal excisions, latissimus dorsi flaps.

Once malignancy has been confirmed, the determination of surgical management relies upon defining the extent of the disease process. Before the era of survey ultrasound and bilateral MRI, the incidence of multifocal and multicentric tumors was still largely unknown. In typical cases the main tumor was detected clinically or through mammographic screening, surgically removed, and histologically evaluated. If clear margins were confirmed, further surgery was withheld and postoperative radiotherapy was instituted. Numerous studies have shown that 20–40% of breast cancer patients have multifocal or multicentric tumors. Most of these lesions are clinically occult. Because premenopausal women are commonly affected, the small multifocal lesions are often undetected by mammography, hidden within the dense fibroglandular tissue. There is evidence from therapeutic studies, however, that the incomplete removal of multifocal carcinomas increases the likelihood of tumor recurrence even when radiotherapy is provided. Consequently, the goal of surgical treatment must be to remove all macroscopic tumor components. Multifocality is not a contraindication to breast-conserving therapy if the foci are in the same quadrant as the index lesion or separated by no more than 4–5 cm, but if no effort is made to locate them, they may remain in the breast, because most breast surgeons keep their excisions as small as possible to achieve good cosmetic results.

In recent years the additional information regarding extent of disease has prompted many centers to include MRI (or survey ultrasound) in the preoperative work-up of new or suspected breast cancer patients, because of its high sensitivity in the detection of mammographically occult breast tumors.

Because high-resolution ultrasound is also capable of detecting subclinical tumors, tumor extension, and early carcinoma, H. Madjar conducted a prospective study to assess the accuracy of ultrasound in preoperative staging. The results of the study were very positive, and we have therefore adopted preoperative ultrasound staging as a routine clinical procedure.

Tumor Size

Tumor size is one of the most important prognostic indicators. In a fatty breast it can be determined with reasonable precision by mammography. In a dense breast, however, superimposed glandular tissue prevents accurate tumor delineation. MRI is also reliable in establishing tumor size, as is a tomographic technique where contrast between background parenchyma and hypoechoic tumor remains. Ultrasound can also define tumor boundaries accurately when a standardized measuring technique is used (Table 15.1).

Three orthogonal planes measured from two perpendicular views can be used to compute tumor volume, which may be useful in assessing response to neoadjuvant chemotherapy. The longest axis of a mass should be sought and measured; a measurement

Table 15.1 Standard measurements of suspected malignant tumors

Scan plane	Direction of measurement
Sagittal	Horizontal and vertical
Transverse	Horizontal
Radial	Horizontal

Also: measure in plane of maximum diameter (unless already measured in other standard planes)

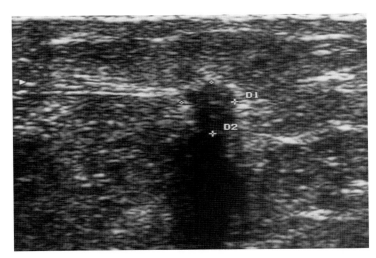

Fig. 15.1 Invasive ductal carcinoma with irregular contours, 5 × 5 mm. Although there is an echogenic rim, the sharp delineation of the tumor from healthy tissues permits a very accurate determination of tumor size.

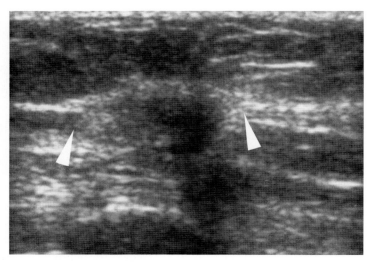

Fig. 15.2 Invasive ductal carcinoma with an irregular shape and ill-defined margins, making it difficult to measure actual tumor size. It can be estimated by including the area of architectural distortion (arrowheads) around the hypoechoic tumor. Tumor size 15 × 8 mm.

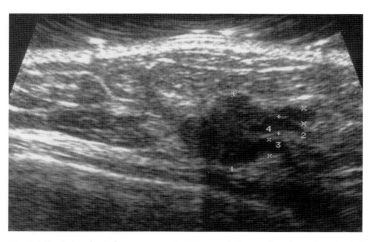

Fig. 15.3 Intraductal component at the periphery of an invasive ductal carcinoma. Radial scan in the upper outer quadrant of the right breast. Intraductal extensions should be included in the measurement of lesion extent.

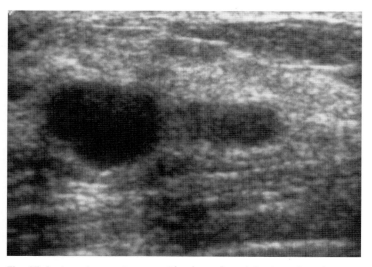

Fig. 15.4 Invasive carcinoma with a lateral, nodular intraductal extension. Radial scan in the lower outer quadrant of the left breast.

perpendicular to this provides the second measurement, and the third measurement can be obtained from the orthogonal view. The measurements should be reported. Also, at the time of excision, particularly if the tumor has been localized before surgery, the radiologist should communicate the orientation of the tumor on the localization images to the surgeon to ensure correlation with the surgical specimen, so that the pathologist can examine representative sections with knowledge of the locations of the various margins. Specimen radiographs and sonograms should be made available to the pathologist for reference in conjunction with preparation of the sections.

The vertical dimension can be difficult to measure in cases where an acoustic shadow obscures the posterior boundary of the tumor. In most cases, dynamic examination with compression, transducer angulation, or increasing the gain setting will help to define the posterior tumor margin. In malignant tumors with irregular contours, the maximum tumor diameter can be easily measured as long as the boundary between the tumor and surrounding tissue is sharply defined (**Fig. 15.1**). Frequently, however, malignant tumors have ill-defined margins or a hyperechoic rim, in some cases causing a marked discrepancy between the sonographic measurement of the hypoechoic center and the histologically determined tumor size (**Fig. 15.2**). In those cases, the report might include the dimensions of the hypoechoic portion of the tumor as well as the echogenic part.

Intraductal Carcinomas and Intraductal Components

In the measurement of overall tumor extent, it is important to include any intraductal component that may be present. When the area around an invasive ductal carcinoma is looked at closely, it is common to find microcalcifications or other signs of intraductal extension that directly adjoin the main tumor and permeate the surgical specimen to a variable extent. In these cases it is difficult for the surgeon to decide on an adequate safety margin for tumor excision. When a high-resolution scanner is used for a careful preoperative examination, it is often possible to locate these intraductal extensions at the periphery of the invasive tumor, especially on radial scans, and to ascertain their extent (**Figs. 15.3, 15.4**).

It should be added, however, that intraductal proliferation in fibrocystic change or enlarged ducts with inspissated secretions can have a similar sonographic appearance (**Fig. 15.5**) (see also Chapter 6). Another problem is multifocality, as it can be difficult to locate small in-situ foci that are not directly adjacent to the main tumor but are distant from it (**Figs. 15.6 a, b, 15.7 a, b**). MRI can also be helpful in tumor mapping, but here again, benign proliferative changes can show enhancement following administration of gadolinium contrast agents. For proof of cancer extension, image-guided percutaneous core biopsy may be necessary.

Carcinomas in situ may also occur in isolation. Their early detection is the domain of mammography, which in many cases can depict the typical pattern of microcalcifications that suggest intraductal carcinoma. Calcifications in the echogenic parenchyma are very difficult to locate with ultrasound unless the examiner knows precisely where to look, based on the mammographic findings. Ultrasound is advantageous, however, in its superior soft-tissue delineation and its direct, anatomic visualization of the mammary

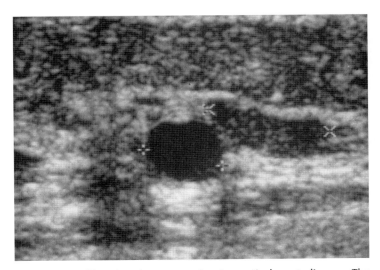

Fig. 15.5 Proliferative duct expansion in cystic breast disease. The expanded duct, which contains internal echoes, is indistinguishable from the intraductal extension of carcinoma in **Figure 15.4**.

ducts. Because most intraductal cancers are associated with cellular proliferation in the ducts, these lesions are often manifested by areas of irregular ductal dilatation. It is difficult, however, to interpret these changes and distinguish them from benign intraductal proliferations (**Fig. 15.8**). Small intraductal foci in a fibrotic breast (see also Chapter 6) are also inconspicuous. Another limitation of ultrasound, and other imaging modalities, is the detection of lobular carcinoma in situ, ordinarily an incidental histologic finding in surgical or percutaneous specimens directed to removal of suspicious microcalcifications seen on mammogram. With ultrasound, one may see a dense breast with extensive fibrocystic changes and areas of irregular ductal dilatation (**Fig. 15.9 a–d**). Although this pattern cannot be classified as normal, it is equivocal for differentiating carcinoma from severe forms of fibrocystic change. These borderline cases are an indication for image-guided fine-needle aspiration cytology or core biopsy, and at the very least, close interval follow-up. Not all forms of ductal carcinoma in situ (DCIS) are detectable by imaging procedures. Tumor cells that grow in thin sheets, as in Paget carcinoma, may not cause appreciable duct expansion (**Fig. 15.10**). But other ductal

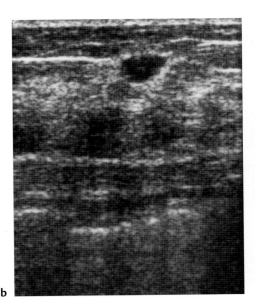
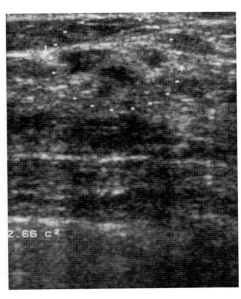

a, b

Fig. 15.6 a, b Invasive ductal carcinoma (**a**) with an extensive intraductal lesion distant from the primary tumor (**b**). The distance between the invasive and intraductal lesions should be reported, to help in presurgical planning. Each focus is biopsied percutaneously, a marker clip of different shape placed in each, and the procedure concluded with craniocaudal and lateral mammograms which enable the distances to be measured accurately.

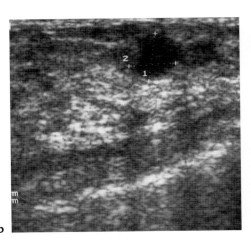
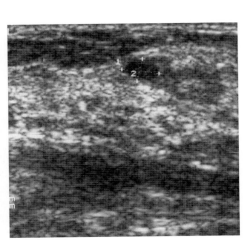

a, b

Fig. 15.7 a, b Invasive ductal carcinoma (**a**) with a small peripheral intraductal component and (**b**) a small intraductal focus distant from the primary tumor.

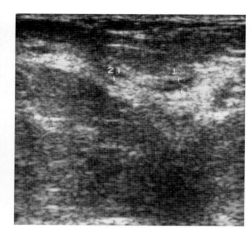

Fig. 15.8 a, b Intraductal carcinoma in two subareolar duct segments. Radial scan of the left breast at the 3 o'clock position.

a, b

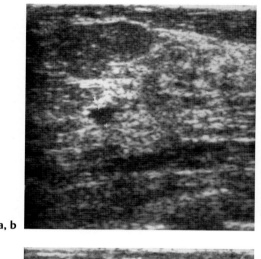
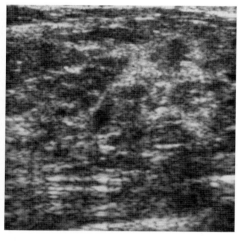

Fig. 15.9 a–d Extensive lobular carcinoma in situ (LCIS). The focal lesions resemble pronounced fibrocystic change. The four image sections show multiple small irregularly-shaped masses in the right breast of a 50-year-old woman with mammographically dense parenchyma. Clinically there were no visible or palpable abnormalities.

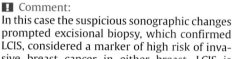 Comment:
In this case the suspicious sonographic changes prompted excisional biopsy, which confirmed LCIS, considered a marker of high risk of invasive breast cancer in either breast. LCIS is thought to be an incidental finding in specimens of biopsies most often done for calcifications.

a, b

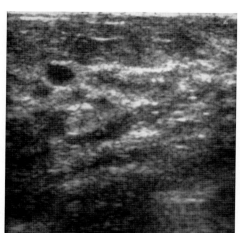
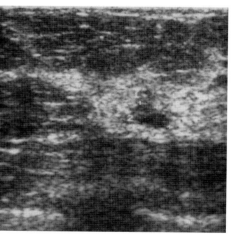

c, d

cancers such as high-grade DCIS (comedocarcinoma) can produce complex intraductal growths, giving rise to an echo pattern that is difficult to interpret (**Fig. 15.11**). Mammography can show intraductal cancers in cases where characteristic microcalcifications are present, but not in every case. Uncommonly, DCIS presents as a mass, either small or quite large, up to or larger than 5 cm, as seen in some noninvasive intracystic papillary carcinomas found in men as well as women. It is therefore important to integrate interpretations of the sonographic and mammographic findings.

Multifocality and Multicentricity

The detection of multiple tumor foci in one breast is important for treatment planning. In cases where multifocal lesions are closely spaced or the intraductal component is nearby, it is reasonable to consider a breast-conserving resection with a margin of healthy tissue. But if there are multicentric lesions in two or more quadrants, breast-conserving surgery is no longer an option.

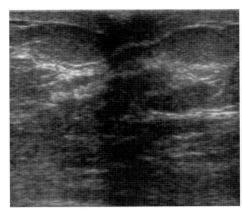

Fig. 15.10 Paget disease. Histology showed clusters of pagetoid cells in the thickened nipple, pictured here, and in the underlying breast tissue. In typical cases, ultrasound does not reveal gross morphologic changes. Mammography may show microcalcifications in ducts near the nipple, and occasionally in a large duct in the nipple itself.

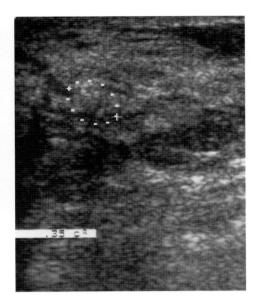

Fig. 15.11 Small, hyperechoic focus of comedocarcinoma 5 mm in diameter.

! Comment:
Mammography in this case showed clustered microcalcifications. The only correlative ultrasound finding is a hyperechoic, noncompressible tissue area.

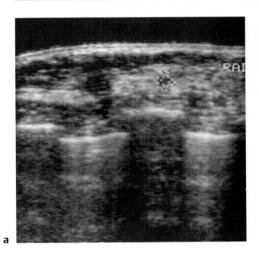

a

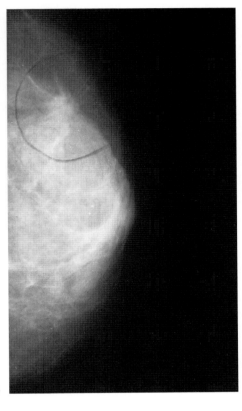

b

Fig. 15.12 a, b Multifocal carcinoma with a primary tumor 6 × 7 mm in size.
a Ultrasound reveals a second 3 × 3-mm lesion (calipers) below the primary tumor.
b Mammography shows a typical malignant-type spiculated density with no evidence of multifocal disease.

! Comment:
If surgical planning had been based on mammograms alone, the smaller tumor mass would have been missed. Adjunctive techniques such as survey ultrasound or contrast-enhanced breast MRI are important aids in preoperative assessment.

In a prospective comparative study of mammography and ultrasound by Madjar (1993), 39 of 100 breast cancer patients were found to have multifocal disease. The multifocality was detected in 4 patients by palpation and in 13 patients by mammography. When breast ultrasound was used, multifocality was detected in 34 cases. The study was carried out 15 years ago using a 5-MHz transducer. The results affirmed the value of preoperative sonographic staging, and since then ultrasound has often been used in the planning of breast operations. The subsequent improvements in image processing and higher scanning frequencies have reinforced expectations of the benefits of preoperative scanning, particularly in women with dense breasts in whom mammography successfully detected the primary tumor but not the occult foci (**Fig. 15.12 a, b**). Multifocal or multicentric tumors are being found with increasing frequency when the high-resolution transducers are used, not just in preoperative studies but also in the extended screening of high-risk patients (**Figs. 15.13 a–d** through **15.15 a–i**).

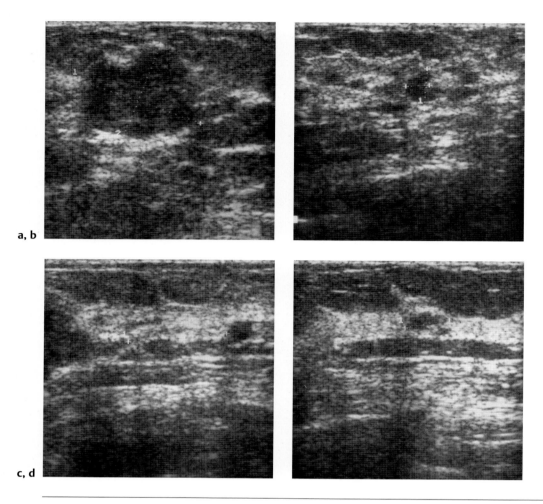

a, b

c, d

Fig. 15.13 a–d High-resolution ultrasound of multicentric invasive ductal carcinoma with multiple invasive and in situ lesions throughout the breast. The scans show the main tumor, measuring 21 × 17 mm (**a**), and numerous small tumors 5–7 mm in diameter in other quadrants of the breast (**b–d**).

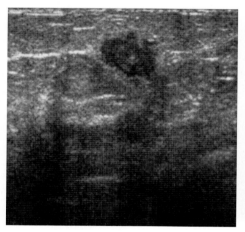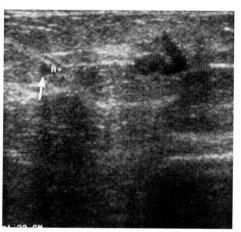

a, b

Fig. 15.14 a, b High-resolution ultrasound of multifocal invasive ductal carcinoma.
a The sagittal scan shows small extensions at the tumor periphery.
b On the radial scan, an isolated 2 × 2-mm focus (arrow) is seen 1.2 cm lateral to the main tumor.

Surgical Planning

A key question to be answered is whether the lesion in question is malignant or most likely benign. If the diagnostic criteria are inconclusive, the diagnosis should be established by fine-needle aspiration or core biopsy. Often this will obviate the need for surgery when benignancy is confirmed. In positive cases, it will facilitate preoperative consultation and the preparations for surgery. Accurate information is needed on tumor location, size, ex-

tent, and relation to neighboring structures to plan the incision and ensure a technically sound operation (**Table 15.2**).

All appropriate imaging modalities should be utilized to characterize the breast abnormalities and to determine extent of the pathology and most suitable surgical therapy. Presurgical localization procedures can be planned. For example, if mammograms show clustered pleomorphic microcalcifications in a dense parenchymal background, ultrasound examination can ascertain whether or not an underlying mass or ductal abnormality is present. If the calcifications are present in the mass, the vacuum-

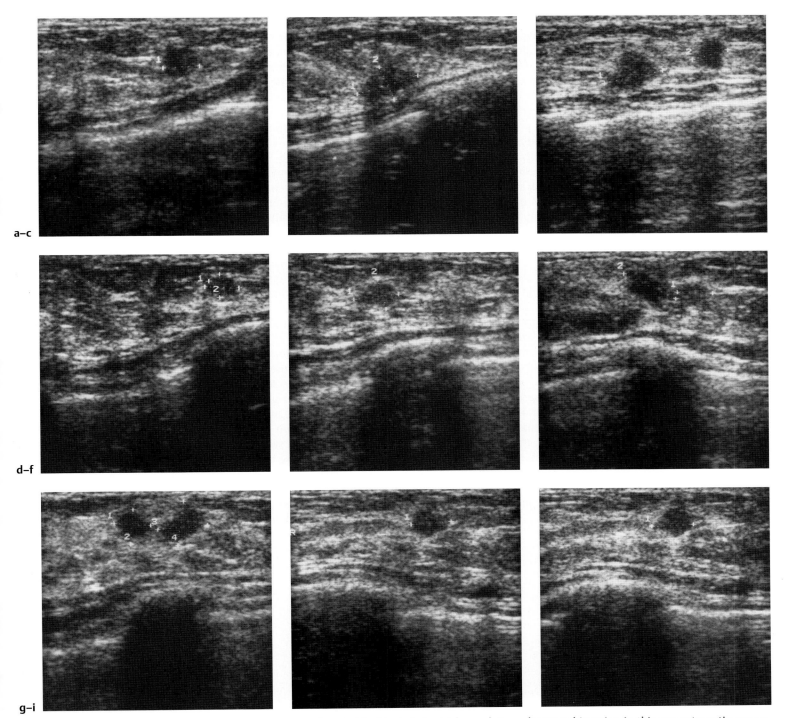

Fig. 15.15 a–i Extensive multicentric carcinoma was detected incidentally by high-resolution ultrasound imaging in this asymptomatic premenopausal patient. Bilateral mammography is indicated, as would be ultrasound of the contralateral breast if not already done, or bilateral MRI.

assisted or automated core needle biopsy can be done under ultrasound guidance, the specimens radiographed, and a marker clip placed in the area of biopsy. If enhancing foci or segmental regions of enhancement are seen on MRI, it should not be assumed that these additional areas are malignant: biopsy following second-look ultrasound or MRI-guided biopsy is required to confirm that the additional areas are part of the malignant process. Following the evaluation for extent of disease, presurgical localizations can be planned. Where DCIS is confirmed adjacent to the index invasive lesion, the involved area can be demarcated by two or

Table 15.2 Diagnostic data used in surgical planning

> ▸ Tumor size
> ▸ Tumor margins
> ▸ Tumor location
> ▸ Distance from skin
> ▸ Distance from nipple
> ▸ Multifocal or multicentric lesions
> ▸ In-situ components (location and total extent)
> ▸ Invasion of the skin or chest wall
> ▸ Lymph node status

more hookwires inserted with mammographic guidance. These bracketed localizations help to ensure removal of the entire area of tumor with the goal of obtaining free margins. If the lesions are masses, they can be bracketed with ultrasound guidance.

Among the imaging guides that can be used for presurgical localization, ultrasound is the most direct and rapidly accomplished method, preferred for masses and other lesions identified sonographically. Following the localization procedure, craniocaudal and lateral mammograms should be taken to confirm that the localization conforms to the area where microcalcifications were detected. If the localizations have been done in the breast imaging suite, labeled radiographs and the sonogram should be sent to the operating room, either electronically or as hard copy. A written description of the procedure should accompany the images—the type of needle–hookwire assembly, placed from what approach—lateral, medial, cranial or caudal, distance from the skin to the wire's hook or lesion.

On sonograms, tumor location is most accurately designated using clock-face notation and the distance of the lesion from the nipple. It should also be noted whether the tumor location is superficial, central, or prepectoral, and distance from the skin to the center of the lesion can be given. Tumor size is a determinant of the feasibility of breast conservation. Although T1 (up to 2 cm) and T2 (up to 5 cm) tumors are eligible for lumpectomy, mastectomy is needed if the tumor is too large in relation to breast size or if it is in a location where its removal would cause a deformity. Lesion margins are also important, because extent of the tumor is more difficult to map with poorly defined carcinomas than with sharply marginated tumors, and larger resections may be necessary to achieve margins free of tumor involvement. Multicentric disease largely precludes breast-conserving surgery. For multifocal lesions, the precise location and distribution of the foci must be known so that they can be found and removed at operation.

If there is suspicion of an intraductal component directly adjacent to the tumor, the resection margins should be broadened. The skin-to-lesion distance is important, for in the case of peripheral tumors even mastectomy can pose a high risk of recurrence if the breast is outlined with a transverse elliptical incision from which breast parenchyma is dissected out of the subcutaneous tissue. If the tumor is superficially placed and extends into the subcutaneous fat, even a mastectomy may leave some tumor cells in the tissue. This should be considered for each individual lesion in cases of multifocal disease. Breast-conserving surgery usually involves making a skin incision directly over the tumor. If the tumor is near the skin, it is easy to include an elliptical skin area in the surgical specimen. If the tumor is far from the skin, an elliptical skin excision may be omitted or the incision site may be modified somewhat for cosmetic reasons.

The distance of the tumor from the nipple should also be considered in deciding between breast conservation and mastectomy and in planning the operation. Especially in cases where mastectomy with primary reconstruction is proposed, it is important to decide whether the nipple–areola can be conserved or whether the whole breast should be excised through an elliptical incision.

Surgical planning is also influenced by chest wall invasion, as this may necessitate a change in preparations. With regard to lymph node status, the surgeon should have detailed information on the presence and location of enlarged lymph nodes and any matted nodes, especially at levels II and III or in the parasternal region, so that these nodes can be selectively approached. Abnormal-appearing lymph nodes that are confirmed by FNAB or core biopsy as metastatic will obviate the need for sentinel node imaging at time of surgery. Color Doppler imaging is particularly useful in the axillary region to assess the relation of involved nodes to major blood vessels and the thoracodorsal neurovascular bundle. If any anatomic difficulties are detected preoperatively, the surgical team can prepare for them in advance.

Clinical Significance

Screening involves examining asymptomatic individuals to detect an epidemiologically significant disease. A successful screening program requires a disease of high prevalence where early detection can affect the course of the disease, standardized technique of examination and interpretation, patient compliance, effective treatment, accessibility to the population at risk, and a low-risk cost-effective approach, not to mention the need for suitable equipment and trained personnel. In the United States and western Europe, breast cancer is without question an epidemiologically significant disease.

In the United States in the last several years, the number of newly diagnosed female breast cancer patients has ranged from 180 000 to over 200 000 annually. In randomized controlled trials of X-ray mammographic screening over several decades the mortality reduction attributable to mammographic screening is over 20 %, and has been reported in László Tabár's long-term Swedish studies to be as high as 60 %. Tabar includes 40–50-year-old women. Postmenopausal women and women over the age of 50 years screened with mammography have also shown mortality reduction, the measure of success in breast cancer screening as opposed to survival, which can be affected by biases such as when detection occurred in the temporal course of the disease. In spite of published data, discussions about the value of screening in premenopausal women continue. Although the incidence of breast cancer rises with increasing age, breast malignancies occur in significant numbers of women under the age of 50 and measurably in women younger than 40 years. Younger women tend to have denser breasts, where mammography is less sensitive than in the fatty breasts of older women. This is only a generalization, however, and many postmenopausal women have dense breast tissue related to fibrous tissue, and some premenopausal women, particularly multiparous women, have fatty breasts that are easy to evaluate mammographically.

Although the incidence of breast cancer is lower in women aged 40–50 than in those over 50 years of age, mammography-related mortality reduction in women under 50 supports screening, and the American Cancer Society recommendations in the United States call for annual screening mammography in asymptomatic women from the age of 40 years (**Fig. 16.1 a–c**). There is no agreed-upon age at which screening should be stopped.

The benefits of mammographic screening and the recommendations for its use are based on statistical evaluation of the prevalence of breast cancer in a population at average risk. For women whose risk of developing breast cancer is extremely high—women with a young, first-degree relative (mother, sister, daughter) with premenopausal breast cancer, particularly if bilateral—the advice is for mammography is to commence 5–10 years earlier than the age at which the affected relative was diagnosed.

Target Group for Extended Screening

In discussing screening issues, we must consider that many premenopausal women have clinical symptoms or see their doctor because of cancer fears. In particular, women who are at risk for breast cancer because of a positive family history or previous surgery for atypical proliferative fibrocystic change cannot be placed in the same category as other screening patients. They should be offered a screening program in which negative results will afford these women a reasonable degree of assurance that they do not have breast cancer detectable at the time of the examination. Everyday clinical experience and the results of screening studies teach us that mammography alone cannot accomplish this goal in young women with radiographically dense breasts (**Fig. 16.2 a, b**). This had led to uncertainty among many women and physicians about the need for screening mammography at all, and adoption for screening of other imaging modalities unproven through randomized controlled trials to reduce breast cancer mortality. Unfortunately, recognition of the limitations of mammography may have tended to reduce patient compliance for this medically necessary screening examination. What is under study, however, are the benefits of *supplemental* screening with other imaging modalities for women at high risk of breast cancer with mammographically dense breasts. Currently, the two imaging modalities most likely to be used in addition to mammography are ultrasound and MRI.

Prerequisites for Extended Screening

As shown in the preceding chapters, modern high-resolution handheld ultrasound techniques can detect early breast cancer (**Fig. 16.3**). It is unreasonable to expect, however, that this kind of service can be provided on a mass scale. So far there are no guidelines for the use of suitable ultrasound equipment in screening for breast cancer, just as ultrasound screening itself is not listed

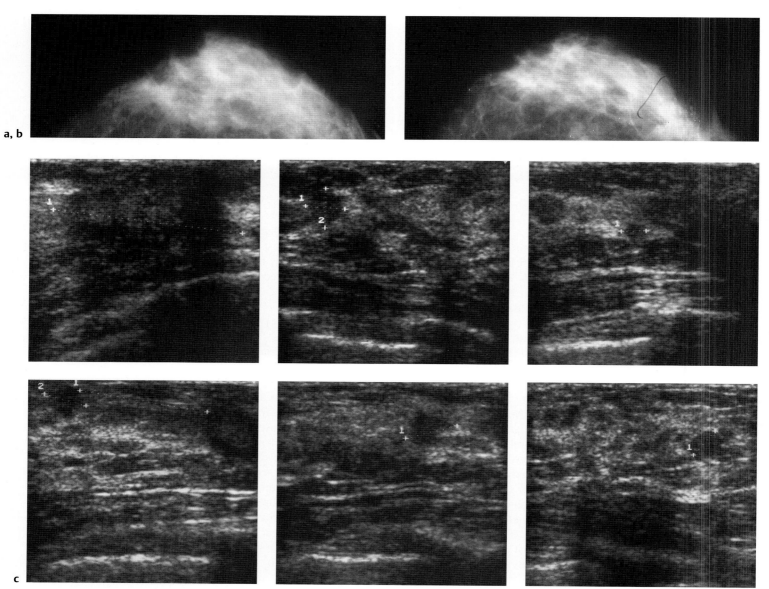

Fig. 16.1 a–c Multicentric breast cancer in a 47-year-old woman.

a Screening mammogram taken 1 year before. Craniocaudal projection of the left breast shows dense parenchyma that is difficult to evaluate but does not show suspicious focal abnormalities.

b Current mammogram. There is no change in overall breast density, but there is an ill-defined density (thin, black, linear marker) not observed in prior films.

c High-resolution ultrasound of the palpable mass shows a hypoechoic lesion with irregular shape, ill-defined margins 32 × 20 × 36 mm in size. Many small tumor masses are also visible on multiple scan planes. Histology confirmed multicentric carcinoma (pT2N1).

▌ Comment:
Given the extensive lesions and the minimal change in mammographic findings, one may question presence of the carcinoma 1 year earlier and its detectability with high-resolution ultrasound.

among the indications for breast ultrasound in the American College of Radiology's Practice Guideline for the Performance of the Breast Ultrasound Examination. Although supplemental survey breast ultrasound is being used at individual sites, public discussions are replete with confusion and misconceptions regarding the true capabilities and limitations of ultrasound, particularly among those who are inexperienced in its use.

A second problem is the examination technique, also not standardized. The optimal utilization of modern equipment for early detection is possible only if the breast can be completely and systematically surveyed. To ensure this, it is necessary to improve training and quality control guidelines. Nevertheless, it is not feasible to implement a screening program utilizing handheld equipment on a mass scale because of the time requirements, the cost, and the examiner-dependence of the diagnostic procedure. It would, however, be desirable to be able to offer additional screening to preselected high-risk patients.

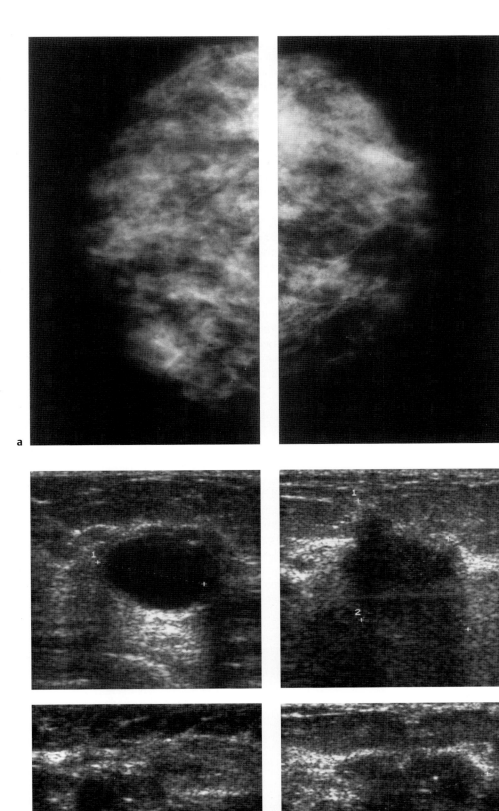

a

b

Fig. 16.2 a, b Multifocal breast cancer in a 50-year-old woman who had been followed for several years for cystic breast disease.

a Current bilateral craniocaudal mammograms show typical dense fibrocystic breasts. These findings are unchanged relative to prior mammograms.

b Ultrasound scan of the round lesion demonstrates an anechoic simple cyst (upper left). The other images represent multiple scans of a breast carcinoma. The main tumor, measuring 28 × 29 × 27 mm, is located in the upper outer quadrant.

! Comment:
The breast cyst and other fibrocystic changes in the generally dense parenchyma may have caused the carcinoma to be missed on earlier screening mammograms.

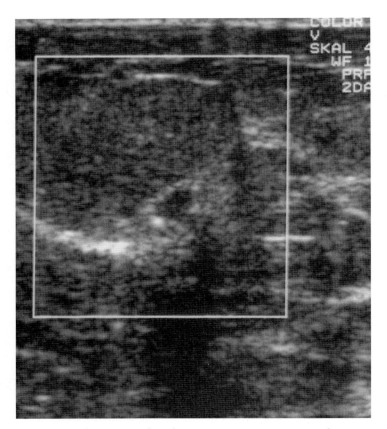

Fig. 16.3 Early invasive ductal carcinoma, 5×5×4 mm, in the involuted breast of a 55-year-old woman. The lesion was discovered on screening mammograms and confirmed by ultrasound.

⚠ Comment:
Even small carcinomas can be detected with ultrasound. This is possible even in advanced fatty involution, although mammography is also accurate and indicated in this setting. With tiny masses, success with ultrasound relies on good equipment and a systematic examination technique.

Studies on Ultrasound Screening

No hard data have been published on sonographic screening, because the large Japanese studies employed ultrasound exclusively, without the benefit of mammograms for comparison of sensitivities and specificities of the two modalities. In addition, there are no data on mortality reduction, and it is questionable at this time, for reasons of both cost and ethics, whether a randomized controlled trial with an end point of mortality reduction can be performed either for ultrasound or for MRI breast cancer screening. Studies in large populations have clearly shown, however, that asymptomatic cancers can be detected by ultrasound and MRI in addition to mammography.

Clinical series in the United States indicate that when ultrasound is used concurrently with mammograms, depending on breast density and risk of breast cancer, 2–6/1000 clinically and mammographically occult lesions can be detected. A multicenter study at 21 sites in North America and one in Argentina is under way. The goal of the project, under the auspices of the American College of Radiology Imaging Network (ACRIN) and the National Cancer Institute (NCI), is to assay the independent contribution of

ultrasound in the detection of cancers that are unsuspected clinically and mammographically. Mammography and ultrasound scanning are carried out and interpreted independently by two different physicians in 2809 women, and findings from the two studies are brought together and patient management determined. Preliminary results suggest that ultrasound can increase the yield of cancers detected by mammography. Participants are women with 25 % or greater lifetime risk of breast carcinoma and whose breast tissue on mammograms is heterogeneously or extremely dense. The sonograms are done by experienced breast imaging physicians after a training course to standardize the survey protocol.

One criticism of ultrasound as a screening modality has been its dependence on the experience of the examiner and the difficulty of determining how much experience an examiner needs—a question addressed in the protocol of the ACRIN study as well as at our site, where we conducted a study of similar design. A pilot study was conducted at our center within the framework of a doctoral thesis. A doctoral candidate received training and instruction in breast ultrasound for a period of 3 months. Over the next 3 months, she performed a systematic breast ultrasound examination on all women who were seen as outpatients or inpatients for non-breast-related problems at our gynecologic clinic.

Results of the Freiburg Screening Study

In total, 1016 women were examined. Fibroadenomas were found in 19 women, circumscribed or diffuse fibrocystic changes were found in 231, and breast cancer was detected in 4. The results of the prospective, blinded ultrasound examinations were compared with subsequent mammographic findings. If either modality revealed a lesion requiring further evaluation, percutaneous or open biopsy was used to establish a diagnosis. Thirty-five benign lesions and four malignant lesions were diagnosed cytologically or histologically. The results are summarized in **Tables 16.1 and 16.2**.

Both ultrasound and mammography yielded suspicious findings for two of the breast cancers. One of these involved multifocal

Table 16.1 Examination results for 4 malignant tumors in 1016 women

	Mammography		
	Suspicious	Benign	Total
Ultrasound			
Suspicious	2	1	3
Benign	–	1	1
Total	2	2	4

Table 16.2 Examination results for 35 benign lesions in 1016 women

	Mammography		
	Suspicious	Benign	Total
Ultrasound			
Benign	15	16	31
Suspicious	1	3	4
Total	16	19	35

disease, which was detected only by ultrasound. Another 7-mm cancer was detected only sonographically. Despite the large number of ultrasound examinations, only seven yielded suspicious findings, and cancer was confirmed in four cases. Histology identified the remaining three cases as fibrocystic change. Sixteen of the mammographic examinations were suspicious, and two of these were histologically confirmed as cancer. One case involved papillomatosis and nine involved fibrocystic changes that were manifested by clustered microcalcifications. Five cases of grade I–II fibrocystic change presented mammographically with suspicious densities or microcalcifications. Two of these were associated with a coexisting fibroadenoma and one with a solitary breast cyst. Two other cases with suspicious densities represented proliferative grade III fibrocystic change. Ten mammograms were classified as indeterminate, and one of these involved fibrocystic change. Of the 17 cases that had microcalcifications, eight were classified as benign and nine as suspicious on the basis of mammographic criteria. Malignancy was confirmed in two of the suspicious cases, and the remaining seven had only fibrocystic changes.

Conclusions of the Freiburg Screening Study

While our study was small and cannot be considered to be a fully fledged screening study, it was conducted in an asymptomatic population. And while it cannot be compared with randomized mammographic studies, the results show that ultrasound screening is feasible in principle and that the experience acquired by sonographers can be transferred to other physicians.

It is interesting to note that the incidence of 4 carcinomas in approximately 1000 patients conforms to the expected prevalence of breast cancer in the corresponding population. It should also be considered that this study was done more than a decade ago using standard equipment for that time: an Acuson 128 unit with a 5-MHz transducer (Siemens Medical Systems, Mountain View, CA, USA). The results attainable with modern, state-of-the-art equipment are at least as good. We cannot evaluate the sensitivity and specificity of the routine examinations now being carried out at our center, because this can be done only within the limited framework of a blinded, prospective protocol. However, ultrasound is used routinely as a complementary study to investigate mammographically indeterminate findings (**Figs. 16.1 a–c, 16.2 a, b**). Additionally, our experience to date has led us to utilize high-resolution ultrasound for the extended screening of high-risk patients (**Fig. 16.4 a–d**). As the incidence of breast cancer is significantly higher in these patients than in the general population, the extra cost is justified. Our day-to-day experience with high-risk patients continues to support the benefits of ultrasound screening in this selected group, as it is common to detect occult carcinomas that, without ultrasound, would presumably have been detected clinically or mammographically at a later time.

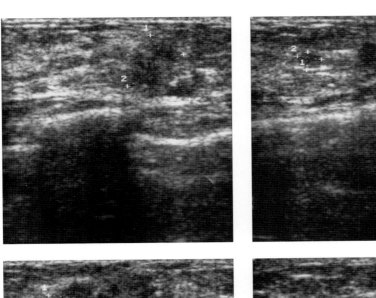
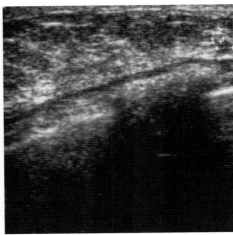

a, b

c, d

Fig. 16.4 a–d Multicentric carcinoma in a 41-year-old woman. This patient was enrolled in an extended ultrasound screening program because of her positive family history. She had no clinical manifestations of breast disease. No abnormalities were observed in the other breast. The patient underwent mastectomy of the affected breast, indicated because of multicentricity.

Follow-Up and Recurrence 17

Clinical Significance

The large number of breast cancers diagnosed per year—approximately 200 000 in the United States—and the concomitantly large number of diagnostic and therapeutic interventions carried out each year underscore the important role of follow-up. A local recurrence diagnosed at the average time of 3 years after lumpectomy at or near a lumpectomy site, which is then treated with mastectomy, does not alter the survival outlook of a patient, bleaker when an early chest wall recurrence is found following mastectomy.

In addition to follow-up for recurrence, another very important role for clinical and imaging follow-up is to reassure patients that they remain cancer-free. The response to therapy—particularly radiation—will change the appearance of the breast drastically, and post-treatment changes of edema, skin thickening, and a spiculated scar can resemble carcinoma. Monitoring the slow resolution of these breast alterations is very important not only in detection of recurrence but also to allay the nearly constant anxiety and the potentially significant change in life circumstances: psycho-oncology has come to play a major role in the care of breast cancer patients.

Because the diagnosis of tumor recurrence initiates a chain of events, one should question whether the detection of certain changes has real therapeutic implications or will merely exacerbate the patient's fears. Until a few years ago, it was common to conduct intensive pretreatment staging or follow-up programs that included X-rays, radionuclide scans, CT, MRI, ultrasound, and costly laboratory tests to detect metastases to the bone, lung, liver, and CNS. More recent studies have shown, however, that in most cases, particularly when the carcinoma is likely to be Stage 1, the detection of distant metastases and subsequent treatment measures will not improve the prognosis and will at best offer a chance for palliation. Clinical examination remains important in the detection of metastases and can direct the initiation of appropriate palliative treatment. Research continues, however, in identifying successful treatments for advanced cancer patients and there has been recent increased utilization of PET and PET-CT when metastatic activity is suspected or highly likely.

In the case of local and locoregional recurrences of breast cancer following conservation therapy, however, early detection is meaningful, for it enables the lesion to be treated before it disseminates. Consequently, the use of high-quality imaging equipment is essential in diagnosing this type of recurrence.

Detection of Locoregional Recurrences

Recurrent tumors may develop in the chest wall following mastectomy, or within the breast itself following a breast-conserving excision. The contralateral breast may be involved by a second carcinoma or by a metastatic spread from a recurrent tumor. It is equally important to examine the axillary lymph nodes, the supra-clavicular and infraclavicular nodes, the internal mammary nodes, and the neck (**Table 17.1**). A variety of diagnostic methods are available for this (**Table 17.2**).

The selection of diagnostic methods depends on prior treatment and the clinical situation. Mammography is ineffective in evaluating the chest wall following mastectomy, and mammography is unnecessary on the side of mastectomy except for using a spot compression view to alleviate anxiety in a patient who questions a mass or thickening in redundant tissue in the mid-axillary line. The contralateral breast should be screened annually with mammography. Prepectoral recurrences in the subcutaneous tissue or epidermis are diagnosed clinically. Recurrences within or deep to the pectoralis muscle are difficult to detect clinically, however, and ultrasound is the method of choice in these cases. CT or MRI can be helpful as well.

Table 17.1 Locoregional recurrences of breast cancer

▸ Local
▸ Intramammary
▸ Chest wall
▸ Contralateral breast
▸ Lymph nodes
▸ Axilla
▸ Internal thoracic artery
▸ Supra- and infraclavicular
▸ Neck

Table 17.2 Methods for diagnosis of locoregional recurrence

▸ Inspection and palpation
▸ Ultrasound
▸ Mammography
▸ MRI
▸ CT
▸ Radionuclide imaging and PET
▸ Fine-needle aspiration or core biopsy

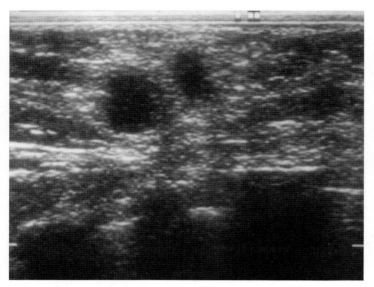

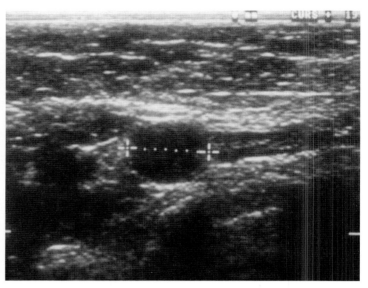

Fig. 17.1 Chest wall recurrence in a patient who underwent right-sided mastectomy. Ultrasound shows several prepectoral hypoechoic masses with irregular, ill-defined margins in the subcutaneous fat. The masses do not cast acoustic shadows but do exhibit an echogenic halo.

Fig. 17.2 Sagittal scan of a lymph node metastasis in the right axilla of the patient in Fig. 17.1.

❗ Comment:
The lymph node resembles a vessel imaged in cross section, but scanning in two planes identifies it as a discrete mass. Color Doppler can confirm it as nonvascular, if doubt remains.

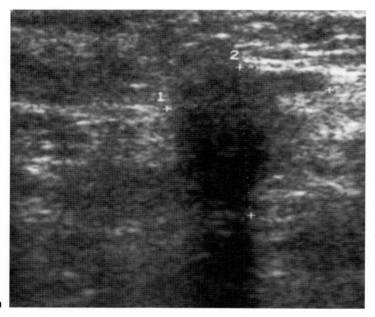

a

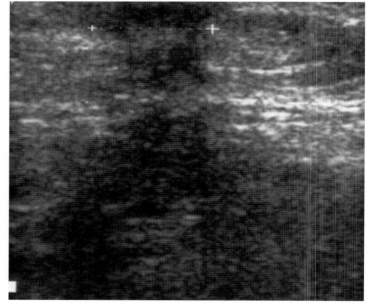

b

Fig. 17.3 a, b Recurrence in the left chest wall and axilla of an 85-year-old woman. The patient underwent mastectomy and axillary lymphadenectomy 9 years earlier for a pT1pN0 tumor (ER and PR positive).
a Sagittal scan of the left chest wall shows a heterogeneous, hypoechoic, shadowing mass with irregular margins invading the chest wall.
b Sagittal scan of the left axilla shows a heterogeneous, hypoechoic, shadowing mass with indistinct margins infiltrating the skin.

For the axilla, ultrasound is excellent in sorting out where induration due to postoperative scarring, usually extending to the skin, can make it difficult to palpate recurrent disease (**Figs. 17.1–17.3 a, b**). Axillary ultrasound can also be used to define the relationship of recurrent lesions to the major vessels, which may influence treatment planning (**Fig. 17.4 a–d**). Because local recurrences can give rise to extensive local metastases that are clinically occult, the whole region spanning the chest wall, axilla, supra-clavicular region, and neck should be examined with ultrasound. In some cases, a local or axillary recurrence is detected clinically, and subsequent ultrasound will show additional tumors in regions that are inaccessible to definitive surgery. These tumor masses may serve to contraindicate excision of a local recurrence where the surgery would merely remove the tip of the iceberg. A better option in these cases is radiotherapy or chemotherapy (**Fig. 17.5 a–c**).

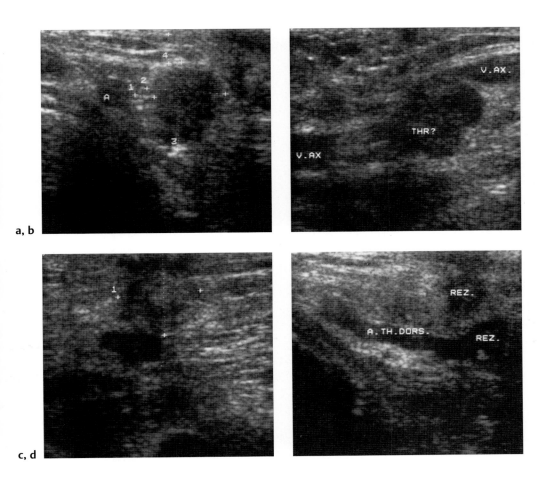

a, b

c, d

Fig. 17.4 a–d Extensive left axillary metastases with thrombosis of the axillary vein, involvement of the thoracodorsal artery, and invasion of the skin. The 44-year-old woman underwent breast-conserving surgery with axillary lymphadenectomy 3.5 years previously, followed by radiation to the left breast for a pT1N1 tumor. She underwent six cycles of CMF chemotherapy. The first recurrence appeared in the axilla 15 months after surgery. Cicatricial changes were palpable at follow-up, but a discrete mass was not detected clinically. The images show several scans of the left axilla.

a Sagittal scan. At the left is the axillary artery, and to the right of it is a larger, hypoechoic mass with irregular margins. The axillary vein is not visible.

b Transverse scan below the axillary artery, showing a segment of the axillary vein. A thrombus is visible at the center of the image.

c Transverse scan through the mid-axilla shows a hypoechoic mass with irregular margins, 14 × 14 mm, infiltrating the skin.

d Sagittal scan over the mass shows how the tumor is related intimately to the thoracodorsal vessel. (REZ = Recurrence; A.TH.DORS = Thoracodorsal artery)

❗ Comment:
Defining the anatomic complexity of the tumor and its surroundings with ultrasound allows for appropriate preoperative preparations, including consultation with a vascular surgeon.

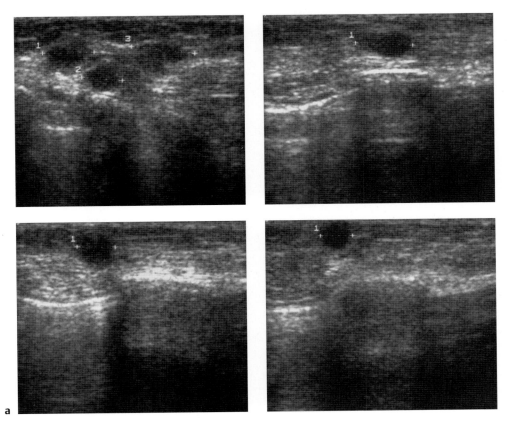

a

Fig. 17.5 a–c Case report: The 63-year-old patient underwent left mastectomy with axillary lymphadenectomy 1 year earlier for a pT4N2M1 tumor (grade III, ER positive, PR positive). Postoperatively she underwent six cycles of CMF chemotherapy. She now presented at follow-up with lymphedema of the left arm. Clinical examination of the left axilla revealed a deeply situated, firm, immobile nodule 2 × 3 cm in size. Ultrasound shows multiple tumor masses involving the left chest wall, the left axilla, and the lymph nodes on both sides of the neck.

a Scans of the left chest wall show multiple metastases in the pectoralis major muscle.

Fig. 17.5 b, c ▷

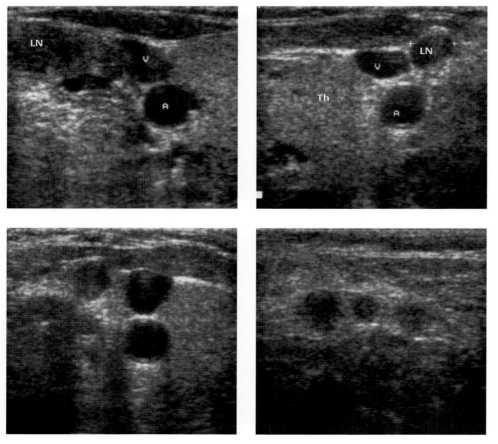

Fig. 17.5

b Several scans of the left axilla show metastases of varying size. The image at lower right shows a metastasis in the deltoid muscle.

Fig. 17.5

c These scans depict the right side of the neck (upper and lower left), the left side of the neck (upper right), and the left nuchal region (lower right). Several lymph node metastases can be seen lateral to the carotid artery and jugular vein. Medial to the vessels is the thyroid gland. Nuchal metastases are also visualized. A = Artery; V = Vein; Th = Thyroid gland; LN = Lymph node

Ultrasound is not useful for the primary diagnosis of chest wall, pulmonary or pleural metastases, which are best detected by physical examination, chest radiographs, and/or CT scans. If pleural effusion has been detected, ultrasound is useful for estimating the fluid volume and determining a safe route for percutaneous aspiration and drainage. On occasion, an asymptomatic pleural effusion may be detected incidentally during a routine follow-up examination of the chest wall in which scanning covers the more deeply situated areas behind the pectoralis muscle (**Fig. 17.6 a, b**).

Ultrasound is an important part of follow-up in patients who have had breast-conserving surgery and postoperative irradiation. As described in Chapter 11, postoperative changes can be difficult to evaluate mammographically. Particularly after radiotherapy, the density of the breast is substantially increased, and radiation changes may limit mammograms for up to the first 2 years follow-

ing radiotherapy (see **Fig. 11.2**). Nevertheless, the early detection of a recurrence is as important as primary early detection in preventing distant metastases. This can be accomplished by supplementing mammography with careful examination of the breast with high-resolution ultrasound (**Fig. 17.7 a, b**). Scars are compressible in most cases, and this property distinguishes them from true recurrences. Occasionally, however, scars can be extremely difficult to differentiate, especially in first-time patients who have no prior images for comparison (**Fig. 17.8 a, b**). If a recurrence cannot be excluded by imaging alone, there is always the option of ultrasound-guided fine-needle aspiration or core biopsy, which are generally successful in averting unnecessary surgery.

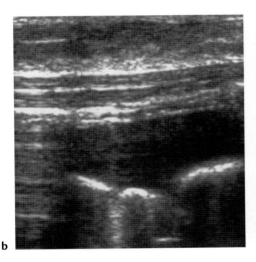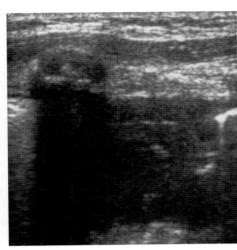

a, b

Fig. 17.6 a, b Case report: The 41-year-old woman underwent mastectomy with axillary lymphadenectomy 5 years earlier for a pT4N1 tumor. Postoperatively, she underwent chemotherapy. She was now asymptomatic. The chest wall was smooth at follow-up, but ultrasound revealed a fluid collection deep to the chest wall within the pleural cavity, consistent with a pleural effusion.
a Transverse scan in the intercostal space.
b Sagittal scan.

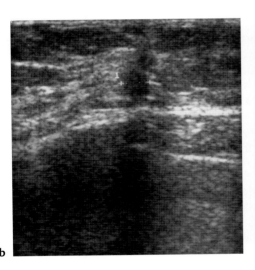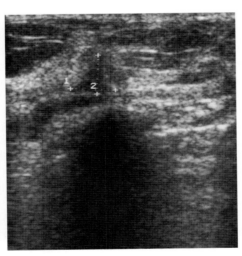

a, b

Fig. 17.7 a, b Case report: The 47-year-old woman underwent breast-conserving surgery in the upper outer quadrant of the left breast, axillary lymphadenectomy, and postoperative radiotherapy 6 years earlier. Six weeks earlier a recurrence was excised from the upper outer quadrant of the left breast, because a marked change had been detected clinically and mammographically. The rest of the breast appeared clinically and mammographically normal. The patient now presented for further treatment planning. An ultrasound examination was done as a routine measure and revealed a mass, 5 × 7 × 6 mm, in the lower outer quadrant of the left breast, distant from the surgical site.
a Transverse scan.
b Sagittal scan.

⚠ Comment:
The differential diagnosis included a scar granuloma because of the previous operations. But because the mass was located outside the surgical cavity, it was evaluated by fine-needle aspiration biopsy. This study raised suspicion of malignancy, which was confirmed histologically. The nodule was locally excised, and the patient has been disease-free for 2 years.

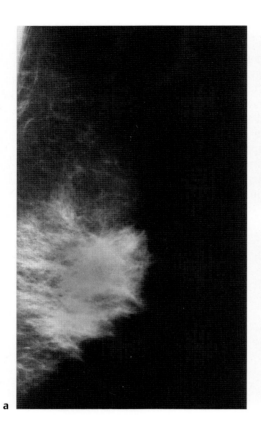

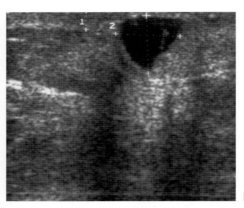

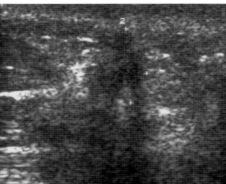

Fig. 17.8 a–c Case report: The 49-year-old woman underwent breast-conserving surgery in the lower inner quadrant of the left breast, axillary lymphadenectomy, and postoperative radiotherapy 1 year earlier for a pT1N0 tumor. At mammographic follow-up 6 months after primary treatment, the irradiated breast was very dense. Current follow-up showed a decrease in radiodensity, but ill-defined densities in the area of the tumor bed raised suspicion of a recurrence.

a Mediolateral mammogram, **b, c** ultrasound scans.

b Sagittal scan in the lower inner quadrant of the left breast shows a seroma measuring 11 × 9 × 13 mm. The skin in this area is 3 mm thick.

c Medial to the seroma is a poorly marginated, hypoechoic mass with an acoustic shadow and marked structural defect. Since ultrasound cannot positively identify the lesion as a recurrence or a scar, ultrasound-guided core biopsy was done and showed no evidence of a recurrence.

Role of Ultrasound Compared with Other Modalities

Ultrasound has a unique and important role in the diagnosis of locoregional recurrence. It can be used without difficulty in patients who have undergone mastectomy. When the areas most likely to harbor recurrences are scanned thoroughly, subclinical metastases can be detected with a high degree of confidence, and equivocal clinical findings can be accurately evaluated. PET-CT or MRI can be used if ultrasound findings are negative and there is high clinical suspicion of locoregional failure.

Mammography is also an established part of breast cancer follow-up after breast-conserving therapy as well as after mastectomy. Following unilateral mastectomy, the contralateral breast should be screened annually for the early detection of metastasis or a second tumor. It is unnecessary to do mammography routinely on the side of mastectomy, whether or not there has been reconstruction,

Although the value of mammography is often limited by posttreatment changes during the initial months after breast-conserving surgery and radiotherapy, the first follow-up mammograms should be obtained at 6 months postoperatively to establish a baseline for future follow-ups.

The great advantage of mammography is that the entire breast is imaged in standard planes, providing a relatively simple means for conducting serial observations. Postirradiation changes subside slowly over time, allowing for an accurate mammographic evaluation by 18–30 months after lumpectomy (see **Fig. 11.2**). Because scars often appear as spiculated densities, the appearance of the scar as it contracts should be documented over time to permit the early detection of any pattern changes that may signify local recurrence. Although there is no universally accepted protocol for mammography after breast-conserving therapy, following the 6-month baseline mammograms of the treated breast, continued follow-up at 6-month intervals for 2 years will provide a sequence of studies done frequently enough to confirm resolution of changing features such as edema, skin thickening, and scar contraction, and confident exclusion of local recurrence at or near the tumor bed. Annual mammography of the contralateral breast should not be forgotten.

If there is ambiguity about mammographic signs of recurrence near a mature lumpectomy site, and ultrasound has not shown a new mass, dynamic contrast-enhanced MRI may be helpful in confirming suspicion and in directing biopsy. To date, there have been no studies comparing MRI with ultrasound in follow-up after breast conservation although women participating in ACRIN 6666, an ultrasound breast cancer screening study, are offered MRI as well as ultrasound and mammography during the third and final follow-up round. Many of these women are breast cancer patients, most of them treated with lumpectomy and radiation therapy, and the addition of MRI should be useful in estimating the relative sensitivities of the three imaging modalities—mammography, ultrasound, and MRI. Just as the success of ultrasound depends on an experienced examiner and good, high resolution equipment, MRI is also operator dependent to some degree in its performance and without doubt in its interpretation, where there is a steep learning curve. Mammography combined with ultrasound is adequate for routine follow-ups, provided the physicians and sonographers have sufficient experience with breast ultrasound. MRI is a more costly and complex procedure that can be used selectively for the noninvasive investigation of equivocal findings.

Three-dimensional, Extended Field-of-View Ultrasound, and Real-time Compound Scanning

Clinical Significance

3D ultrasound imaging has attained a high level of quality, but its dependence on the examiner continues to be a problem. The ability to visualize structures in three dimensions plays a major role in this regard. The ability to form a three-dimensional mental picture varies greatly among different examiners, and it can be learned only to a degree. Examiners who are poor visualizers will have great difficulties in conducting examinations and interpreting the findings. This leads to yet another problem: documentation and reporting the findings to another physician. Even if the sonographer has acquired a good three-dimensional impression of the disease process, it is still difficult to share that impression with another physician. This problem is particularly acute in cases where the recipient of the ultrasound report will also carry out the breast surgery. As a rule, the ultrasound documentation consists of two-dimensional images that show a lesion in cross section but do not convey a spatial impression of the lesion or its location in the tissue. This also makes it difficult to compare ultrasound findings with the results of other studies such as mammography or MRI. A common makeshift solution is to make line drawings of the lesion and describe its location as accurately as possible. But because malignant tumors are not simple geometric figures, it is very difficult to document and describe their shape and extent, especially if the lesions are multifocal. Given the complexity of breast anatomy, then, a reasonable approach is to represent the lesion and the surrounding organ in three dimensions. This can be accomplished by acquiring and storing three-dimensional image data and rendering the images in an extended or three-dimensional format. This also permits other examiners to repeat the breast examination and review suspicious findings even when the patient herself is no longer available.

Extended Field-of-View Ultrasound

Another problem of ultrasound is that the small field of view under the transducer demonstrates only a small section of the whole breast. A sectional image of the lesion without the surrounding tissue makes planning for surgery and also comparison with mammography and MRI difficult. A panoramic scan enables the investigator to produce a two-dimensional cross-sectional image of the whole breast. In comparison with the small field of view under the real-time transducer, this allows much better recognition of the whole breast anatomy and the localization of a lesion within the breast.

Real-time Compound Scanning

In conventional ultrasound sound is always transmitted in one direction only, producing a simple scan image. One of the important physical limitations of ultrasound is that good reflection of sound is only given if the ultrasonic beam hits structures in a perpendicular angle. If the angle of sound inclination is oblique, refraction occurs and the structure cannot be displayed. Breast anatomy is rather complex with many reflectors in variable directions. Therefore conventional ultrasound is limited with regard to demonstrating all breast structures. Compared with simple scanning, a compound image is created by image reconstruction from multiple scan directions. This improves the display of architectural details considerably.

Technical Principles – 3D

The principle of three-dimensional ultrasound is based on the acquisition and storage of numerous two-dimensional images in contiguous or closely spaced planes of section. Generally this requires a direct mechanical linkage and an automated method of moving the transducer through the various image planes so that the planes can be accurately localized. Systems have been designed for accomplishing this electronically, but this requires a very smooth, steady movement of the transducer combined with a time-triggered relay that stores the sectional planes at equally spaced intervals. The stored image data can be processed and displayed in various ways. Perhaps the most realistic display mode would be a transparent image in which the tumor could be viewed in three dimensions through the normal breast anatomy. In fetal examinations, for example, such a transparent display is excellent owing to the high contrast between the tissue (fetus) and the surrounding amniotic fluid, but because of the large number of similar gray levels that coexist within the breast it poses serious technical difficulties at present. High contrast is also desirable for constructing three-dimensional surface-rendered images. But this degree of contrast is unusual within the breast, and so for the time being other means are needed for representing structures in three dimensions. The simplest method is to image a representative sectional plane and then reconstruct the two planes that are perpendicular to the original plane to create an orthogonal multiplanar display (**Figs. 18.1–18.6**). If these planes were reconstructed along fixed, predefined spatial axes, they could not depict the complex geometry that is typical of malignant tumors. However,

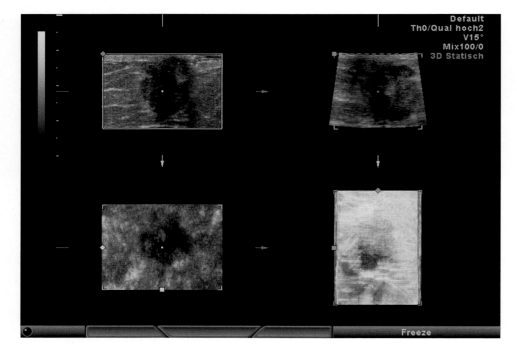

Fig. 18.1 Invasive ductal carcinoma, size 12 × 17 × 14 mm. Sectional planes reconstructed from the volume acquisition: sagittal (upper left), transverse (upper right), horizontal (C scan, lower left), and transparent display (lower right). The slice thickness for the transparent mode has been selected to large. Therefore the tumor is partly covered from the surrounding breast tissue. The C scanning plane clearly shows the typical retraction pattern of carcinomas.

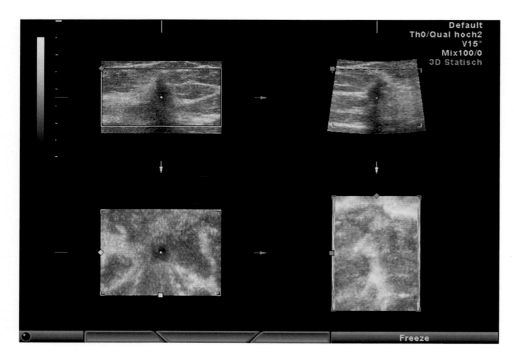

Fig. 18.2 Early invasive ductal carcinoma, size 5 × 6 × 5 mm. The horizontal C plane at lower left clearly shows the retraction sign. The lower right image displays the transparent mode. As in Fig. 18.1 the slice thickness has been selected to large and therefore the tumor is completely hidden through the surrounding fibroglandular tissue.

complex growth patterns can be appreciated if the image planes can be freely rotated in space. At present, three-dimensional structures in breast ultrasound are most clearly represented by a volume block in which a sectional slice from the tumor can be interactively displayed in arbitrary spatial planes (**Figs. 18.1–18.7**).

Extended Field-of-View-Ultrasound

Another method of image reconstruction involves extending the image plane itself. A basic limitation of ultrasound is the small field of view, especially with high-resolution transducers, which usually have an image field width of 4 cm or less. The old water-bath immersion scanners had a great advantage in this regard, as they could provide two-dimensional survey images of the entire breast. Today, real-time scanners are used almost exclusively because of their better spatial resolution, but the small field of view taxes the examiner's ability to visualize the breast anatomy (see also Chapter 2, Examination Technique). The manufacturers of high-end ultrasound equipment used for breast sonography all offer the possibility of achieving extended fields of view with high-resolution transducers. One such imaging process recently developed by Siemens (Siemens Medical Systems, Mountain View, CA), called SieScape, combines the advantages of high-resolution real-time ultrasound with a dramatically extended field of view. In SieScape imaging, the transducer can be moved freehand along the image

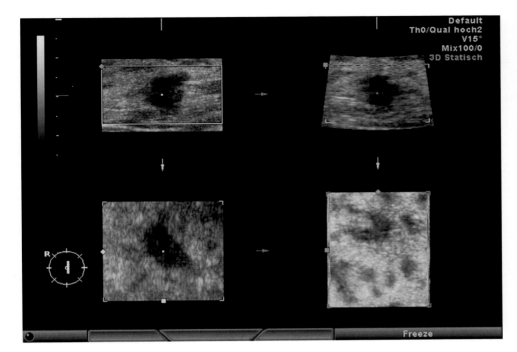

Fig. 18.3 Multifocal invasive ductal carcinoma, size 13×16×14mm, imaged on orthogonal planes which show the very irregular shape of this mass to advantage. The C scan (lower left) shows a moderate retraction sign. Volume rendering (lower right) demonstrates several small tumor foci surrounding the index lesion.

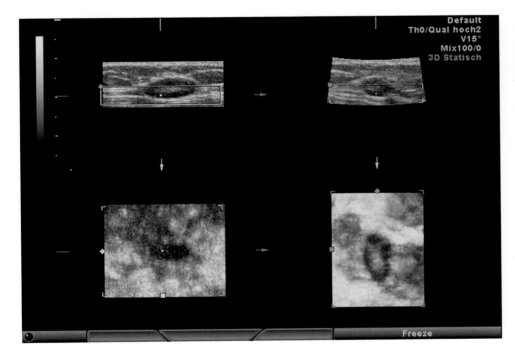

Fig. 18.4 Three-dimensional image of a normal reactive lymph node which became clinically apparent as an indeterminate lump in the periphery of the glandular breast cone. The three orthogonal sections define the spatial extent. The C plane shows an indeterminate pattern. Volume rendering highlights the typical lymph node structure.

plane without a position sensor. The fast electronic image processing correlates the successive planes of section and assembles them seamlessly into a two-dimensional panoramic view of breast anatomy. These SieScape views are static images that closely resemble the older whole breast water bath scanning technique of the 1980s. Their advantage is that they can document an entire cross section of the breast, and therefore both the breast anatomy and the relationship of abnormalities to anatomic structures can be documented in one image. At the time of writing, many other manufacturers of ultrasound equipment are developing 3-D and 4-D capability suitable for breast imaging. They include Philips, General Electric, Toshiba, U-Systems, and others.

Real-time Compound Scanning

This technique is a relatively new image-forming technology which is available in some instruments in the upper price class. The principle is described in detail in Chapter 2, and for better understanding of real-time compounding it is recommended to study this chapter and the corresponding images. In simple scanning images are formed by sound reflections from one scan direction. In real-time compounding the crystal groups of the electronic multi-array transducer are not only fired in different sequences for focusing each single beam (see Chapter 1); sequences are also created to form different scanning directions (see **Fig. 18.13 a, b**).

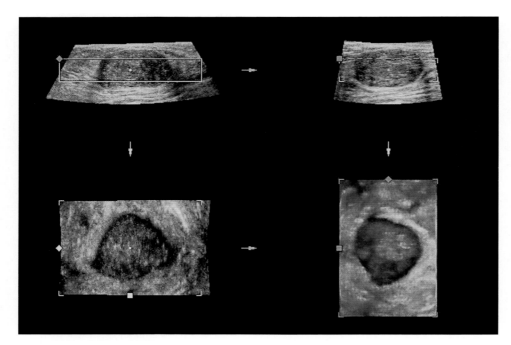

Fig. 18.5 Three-dimensional display of a fibroadenoma, size 28 × 12 × 20 mm. The C plane shows a compression sign, typical for benign tumors. The C plane and the three-dimensional volume rendering outline the circumscribed margin of the lesion.

! Comment:
The homogeneous internal structure, circumscribed margins and abrupt interface, visible on all the sections, are in contrast to the appearance of carcinomas.

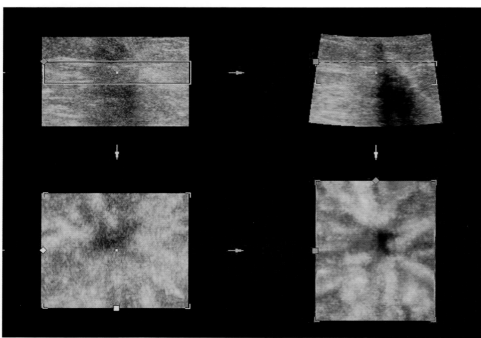

Fig. 18.6 Orthogonal multiplanar display of an invasive ductal carcinoma, size 10 × 8 × 12 mm. The C plane shows the typical retraction sign. With optimized selection of slice thicknes, volume rendering highlights this phenomenon.

This greatly improves image quality, which depends on sound inclination angles. It improves the display of anatomical details and reduces artifacts.

Sample Applications of Three-dimensional Ultrasound

The reconstruction of arbitrary spatial planes from the stored image volume offers advantages in terms of image documentation and interpretation. The outer margins of a tumor are the most important criterion for differential diagnosis. Tumor margins can be clearly appreciated by viewing multiple orthogonal planes in one image, as opposed to two-dimensional imaging where the examiner must scan the tumor in all spatial planes and document the images individually (**Figs. 18.1–18.7**).

The volume of a lesion cannot be accurately determined using two-dimensional ultrasound. It can be approximated by measuring the lesion along three spatial axes, but this method becomes less precise as the shape of the lesion becomes more complex. In these cases three-dimensional reconstruction offers a much more accurate method of determining surface area and volume, and this can be advantageous in tumor diagnosis and measuring response to neoadjuvant chemotherapy for which, traditionally, lesion diameter has been the only criterion used in monitoring response. But volumetry would detect changes in tumor size with much greater precision.

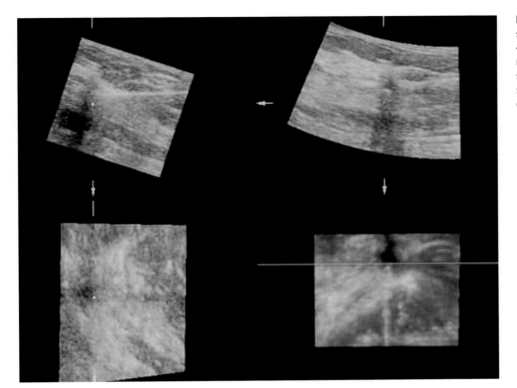

Fig. 18.7 Three-dimensional targeting of a small invasive ductal carcinoma, size 4×4×5 mm. The position of the core biopsy needle is precisely displayed in all three dimensions. In particular, the volume rendering mode shows exactly the position of the needle in the center of the lesion.

Sample Applications of Extended Field-of-View Imaging

As mentioned earlier, panoramic view provides broad images using real-time equipment. The real-time ultrasound survey examination starts in standard fashion with a complete survey of the breast. A plane is then selected for panoramic scanning, panoramic view is switched on, and the transducer is moved smoothly and without stopping along the plane over the desired region (**Fig. 18.8**). This yields an extended field-of-view image that clearly depicts the relative position of the lesion, or even multifocal lesions within range (**Fig. 18.9**). This technique allows for the visualization of masses that exceed the transducer's field of view (**Fig. 18.10**). Even with benign masses, it is important for surgical planning to determine the precise extent and location of the lesions, especially if they are nonpalpable.

Figure 18.11 illustrates an intraductal papilloma located at the nipple margin. With the panoramic scan, the radiologist can demonstrate the location of the lesion within the long axis of the duct and indicate to the surgeon exactly where the incision should be placed for accurately excising the small mass.

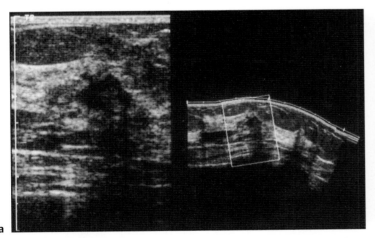
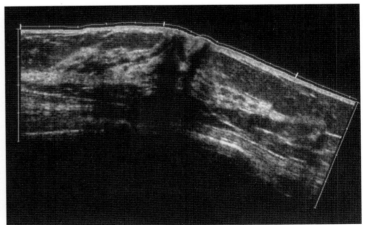

a

b

Fig. 18.8 a, b Panorama scans of invasive ductal carcinoma with an intraductal extension to the nipple region of the left breast (upper outer quadrant).
a Sagittal scan. The panoramic view appears on the right. On the left, in the same image, is a close-up view of the tumor itself.
b Radial panoramic view of the intraductal extension into the nipple region.

! Comment:
This case illustrates how the panoramic view can be combined with a close-up view to document in one image both the location of the tumor in the sagittal plane and its high resolution, detailed features.

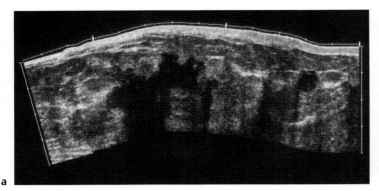

a

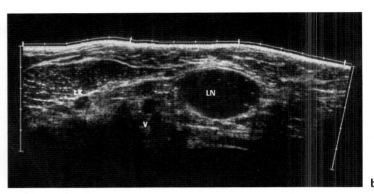

b

Fig. 18.9 a, b Multifocal invasive ductal carcinoma with level I and II axillary metastases.

a Sagittal scan of the outer left breast. The index lesion is visible in the left (cranial) half of the image. In the right half of the image, a second, small tumor mass is visible in the lower part of the breast.

b Oblique scan through the upper axilla. A small lymph node metastasis is visible below the pectoralis major muscle. A much larger nodal metastasis can be seen farther to the right, below the axillary vein.

⊞ Comment:
The complex spatial geometry and anatomic relationships of the tumor and metastases can be clearly appreciated in the panoramic scan. This can be very helpful in reporting the findings to the surgeon and planning the operation.

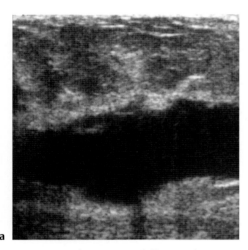

a

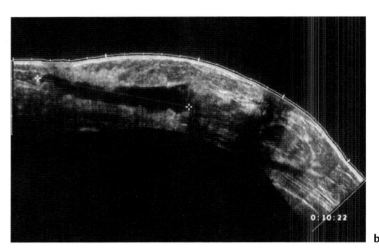

b

Fig. 18.10 a, b Seroma following breast-conserving surgery in the upper outer quadrant of the right breast.

a Ordinary sagittal scan, **b** panoramic sagittal image.

⊞ Comment:
The seroma is demonstrated on standard sagittal scans, but its extent and relative location are best appreciated on the panoramic image.

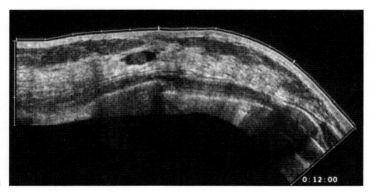

a

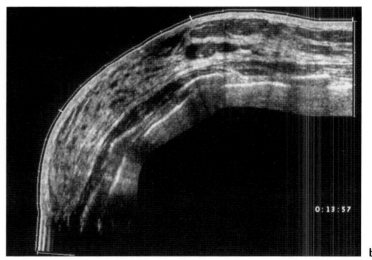

b

Fig. 18.11 a, b Appearance of intraductal papilloma on panoramic scans.

a Parasagittal panorama scan of the right breast, medial to the nipple.
b Radial panoramic view of the right breast.

⊞ Comment:
Both panoramic scans show the abnormal duct along with segments of normal ducts. The radial scan demonstrates the very close proximity of the papilloma to the nipple.

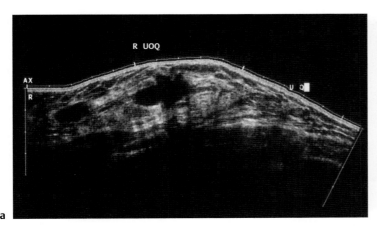

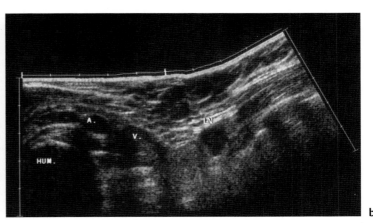

a

b

Fig. 18.12 a, b Solitary invasive ductal carcinoma with level I axillary nodal metastases.

a Oblique panoramic scan extending from the upper outer quadrant (UOQ) to the lower inner quadrant of the right breast. The scan starts in the anterior axilla (AX), where a nodal metastasis is visible on the axillary tail of the breast parenchyma. The poorly marginated, hypoechoic mass is visible at approximately the center of the image.

b Oblique scan through the axilla at level I. The humerus (HUM) is seen on the left side of the image, and next to it are the axillary artery and vein. Below them, at mid-level I, is a small lymph node (LN) metastasis.

■ Comment:
The panoramic image clearly demonstrates the solitary nature of the carcinoma and also defines the location of the nodal metastases.

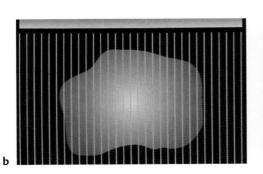
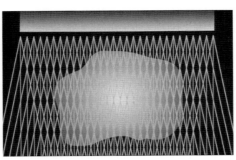

a, b

Fig. 18.13 a, b Comparison of an electronic linear array transducer in simple and compound scanning mode.

a Standard real-time technique with multiple parallel scanning lines in one direction (simple scan).

b Real-time compound scan: The image is acquired by multiple repetitions of different pulse sequences in different scan directions. This results in a compound image, which reduces sound artifacts such as speckle and improves display of anatomical details by optimizing sound inclination angles.

Wide field-of-view imaging can also be advantageous in the axillary region, where anatomic orientation is particularly difficult for inexperienced examiners. The panoramic view of normal anatomic structures such as the pectoralis major and minor muscles and large blood vessels, combined with the visualization of abnormal lymph nodes, provides a vivid representation of the axillary anatomy and pathologic changes (**Fig. 18.12**).

Sample Applications of Compound Scanning

Improvement of recognition of anatomical details can easily be appreciated by comparing images in simple and compound technique (**Figs. 18.13–18.17**). Compounding evidently improves detection of distinct anatomical disorders and small lesions. This technique has been rapidly and widely accepted over the past few years because of the improved image quality, but studies have not yet been performed to evaluate whether this technology has an influence on early tumor detection.

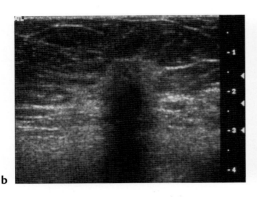 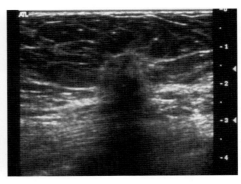

Fig. 18.14 a, b Invasive ductal carcinoma, size 15 × 18 × 16 mm.

a Simple scan (conventional real-time scanning technique): the typical carcinoma with indistinct margins and posterior shadowing is clearly visualized.

b Compound scan: speckle reduction in the subcutaneous tissue and breast parenchyma is clearly visible. Display of the lesion boundary shows much more detail. Shadowing as one typical sign for malignancy can still be recognized, but it is less pronounced compared with the simple scan.

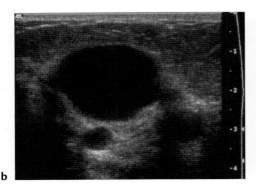 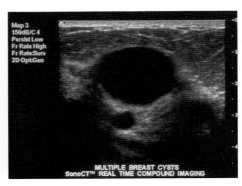

Fig. 18.15 a, b Fibrocystic disease.

a Simple scan with a slightly noisy image (speckle artifacts) and lateral boundaries are not well defined.

b The compound scan shows speckle reduction and improved display of all margins and boundaries.

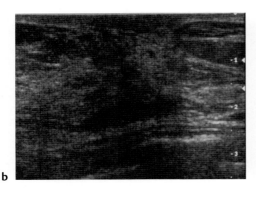 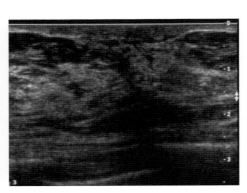

Fig. 18.16 a, b Retroareolar region in simple and compound scan. The central glandular breast cone is often difficult to visualize because of unfavorable sound inclination angles.

a Simple scan with poor sound penetration.

b Compound scan showing improved sound penetration and better display of the retroareolar structures.

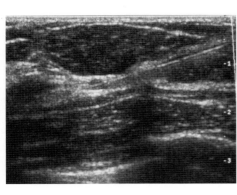 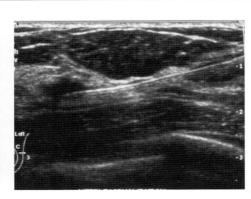

Fig. 18.17 a, b Fine-needle aspiration of a lesion. Because of the deep location of the tumor the needle approach is in an unfavorable angle, with poor sound reflection at the needle.

a Simple scan: because of sound refraction the needle is not clearly visible.

b Compound scan: optimization of sound inclination angles improves display of lesion boundaries and the needle.

Discussion and Outlook

Examination technique and spatial interpretation in standard real-time ultrasound are not a problem for experienced examiners who are skilled at visualizing structures in three dimensions. Nevertheless, a major ongoing problem in routine diagnostic situations is the reporting of ultrasound findings to physicians who are not trained in ultrasonography. Despite its high information content, ultrasound is frequently omitted in radiologic consultations in favor of other modalities, because of a lack of display options. Three-dimensional image reconstruction and two-dimensional panoramic views provide a means of presenting complex findings in formats that can be clearly understood even by those unfamiliar with ultrasound. With their realistic portrayal of anatomic relationships, these techniques are also excellent for reporting findings to surgeons and planning breast operations.

Three-dimensional image reconstruction at high enough resolution to be useful in breast imaging is probably at the threshold of its development. Until recently, the storage and rendering of an image volume was a process that took many minutes to complete. Today it can be accomplished in a few seconds, in actual fact in real time. There have also been rapid advances in the image quality of three-dimensional reconstructions. Image quality is limited chiefly by the resolution of the transducer and the number and spacing of the image planes that are stored in the volume image. Both are constantly being improved (**Fig. 18.8 a, b**). Extended field-of-view ultrasound is an elegant method of making ultrasound images easier to understand and interpret. Although the images created are not three-dimensional, the panoramic views still represent a significant advance. They address the problem of a small, real-time field of view unable to encompass structures that project beyond the image field boundaries. This provides a rationale for research and development of high-resolution ultrasound systems that can depict the entire breast in thin, tomographic sections and more than one plane, and that are semi- or completely automated and could be used for screening as well as treatment planning.

Real-time compounding is one of the most significant technological advances of the past few years. Besides many other techniques for improvement of image quality, it does not only reduce artifacts but also enhances the display of anatomical details. It facilitates image interpretation and has the potential to further improve early tumor detection.

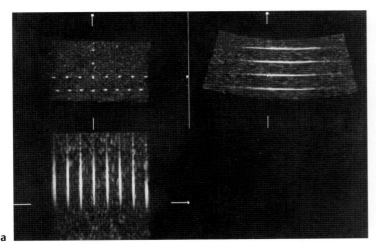 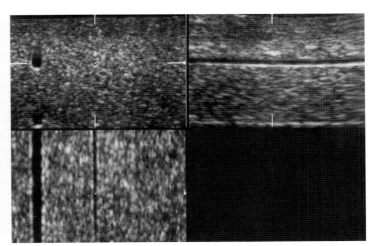

Fig. 18.18 a, b Appearance of the target structures in the test phantom in three-dimensional reconstruction. The test demonstrates uniformly high resolution in all three spatial planes.
a Line targets (nylon threads 0.05 mm in diameter).
b Anechoic cylinders for cyst simulation (1 mm in diameter).

Clinical Principles

The vascularization of malignant tumors is a phenomenon well known from pathologic, biochemical, and angiographic studies, and we know that the degree of neovascularization correlates with the biologic behavior of the tumor. Thermography, once widely used as an adjunct to clinical examination, can detect the change in surface temperature associated with the focal increase in blood flow to a breast malignancy. However, it has been discredited as a screening method for breast cancer because of its low sensitivity, poor specificity (inflammatory processes as well as cancer are associated with local heat), and lack of precise anatomic localization (Williams et al., 1990). Contrast-enhanced MRI is also based on angiogenesis in malignant tumors as well as other factors such as membrane permeability. For many cancers, but certainly not all, there is an intense rapid rise followed by signal washout after the administration of a paramagnetic contrast agent, most commonly a gadolinium chelate such as gadopentate dimeglumine.

The measurement of tumor blood flow is more applicable to lesion characterization than to screening. But there are anatomic situations that hamper evaluation of the breast tissue, and there are tumors that do not display typical diagnostic features, and the measurement of tissue blood flow can be helpful in evaluating problem cases of this kind. It should be understood, however, that the measurement of tumor blood flow is a nonspecific assessment that cannot differentiate lesions with absolute confidence. The degree of blood flow correlates with tissue metabolism. Thus, while fast-growing malignancies generally have a copious blood supply, blood flow is also increased in proliferative benign tumors, in pregnancy and lactation, and in inflammatory conditions.

Historical Development

Doppler ultrasound has been used for more than 20 years to analyze blood flow in breast tumors. Initially only continuous-wave (CW) Doppler systems were available. These devices are very sensitive, but they require an experienced user and it is difficult to examine nonpalpable lesions.

Pulsed Doppler systems became popular in the early 1980s, as they allow for selective flow sampling in vessels that are located by ultrasound imaging. Tumor vessels are very small, however, and usually cannot be visualized in the B-mode image. It is tedious to move the Doppler sample volume through the image while searching the tumor and its surroundings for blood vessels. Also,

most of the older duplex scanners used a low frequency and were relatively insensitive in detecting tumor vessels. As a result, duplex scanning did not find significant applications in tumor diagnosis.

Color flow imaging paved the way for the use of Doppler ultrasound in tumor diagnosis. The first instruments had poor sensitivity. By the 1990s, however, color Doppler technology had advanced sufficiently to permit the effective localization of tumor vessels (**Fig. 19.1**). This was achieved through the use of higher Doppler frequencies and improved signal processing. The recording of Doppler spectra was also improved and provides additional information on tumor blood flow (**Fig. 19.2**). Nevertheless, color Doppler demonstrates only a portion of the vessels. This is due to the limited sensitivity of Doppler in detecting microscopically small vessels and the dependence of the Doppler principle on the beam–vessel angle. Vessels that are perpendicular to the beam direction are poorly detected. Blood flowing in the direction

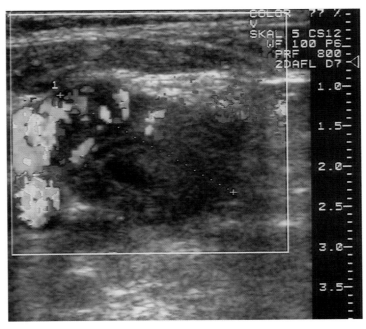

Fig. 19.1   Color Doppler image of invasive ductal carcinoma. The greatest vascular density is found at the periphery of the tumor. Note the predominantly radial pattern of vessels converging on the tumor.

▶ The high sensitivity setting, with a PRF of 800 Hz, often leads to aliasing in the vessels due to the high flow velocities. This must be tolerated, since increasing the PRF would decrease Doppler sensitivity and reduce the number of detectable vessels.

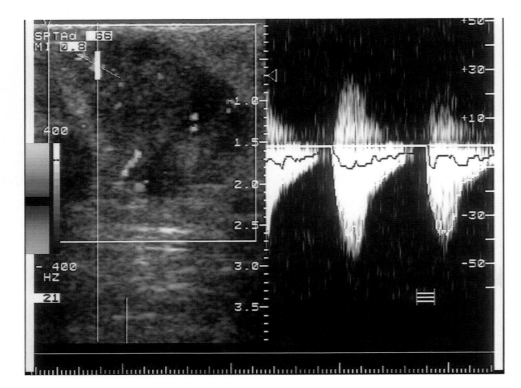

Fig. 19.2 Color Doppler and duplex sonography for the measurement of blood flow. Again, most vessels are found at the tumor periphery. The Doppler spectrum shows a high systolic blood flow velocity (37.9 cm/s) and an absence of flow in diastole (RI = 1.0). This high resistance pattern is typical of breast carcinoma.

▶ Breast carcinomas often have a firm consistency, exerting a pressure that collapses the blood vessels within the tumor. As a result, only peripheral vessels can be seen in most cases and the flow resistance is high.

of the beam results in a higher frequency shift and a better recorded signal.

To improve the visualization of small vessels and avoid the problem of insonation angle, a different method of signal processing was developed. This technique, called power Doppler, does not register the angle-dependent frequency shift but the intensity (amplitude) of the reflected signals, which depends on volume flow. As a result, the course of tumor vessels is more clearly visualized (**Fig. 19.3 a, b**). This technique is susceptible to artifacts, however, and much experience is needed to interpret the images correctly. Another disadvantage is that, for the present, power Doppler imaging yields nonquantitative information. The image is interpreted subjectively, and there are no objective parameters that can be used for tumor differentiation. For these reasons, color Doppler is still preferred. It is easily combined with duplex technology for concomitant flow imaging and flowmetry. However, this requires a sensitive instrument with optimum settings. Given the range of variation among different instruments, standardization is difficult to achieve.

Examination Technique

In our previous studies at the University of Freiburg, we used the ATL UM9 HDI (Philips Medical Systems, Bothell, WA) color flow imager with a 10–5-MHz linear-array transducer. We used a 50–100 Hz filter and a pulse repetition frequency (PRF) of 800–1000 Hz. The power and gain were set as high as possible, that is, just below the noise level.

Doppler ultrasound is used to investigate focal abnormalities rather than to scan the entire breast. Given the variability of tumor blood flow, all vessels should be sampled for the quantitation of flow. Because vessels often are not visualized within malignant tumors, particular attention should be given to feeding vessels that enter the periphery of the mass.

With just enough pressure to maintain contact, the transducer should be placed lightly on the breast to avoid vascular compression. Before any vessels are sampled, various insonation angles should be tested to obtain an optimum Doppler signal. First a slow scan through the tumor is done in the color Doppler mode so that all the vessels can be located and counted. Then the examination is completed by analyzing flow signals in the duplex mode. Usually the course of the vessels can be seen, and so the probe angle can be adjusted to ensure an accurate measurement of flow velocity.

Duplex analysis should include the determination of maximum systolic velocity *(S)* and end-diastolic velocity *(D)*. This provides information on total blood flow and makes it possible to calculate indices from the Doppler spectra. The most important index to be determined is usually the resistance index (RI) or the AB ratio:

RI = $(S - D)/S$

AB ratio = S/D

The pulsatility index (PI) is less frequently determined because it requires fitting an envelope curve to the Doppler spectrum. This is time-consuming and fraught with potential errors. Our comparative measurements have shown, moreover, that this index correlates closely with the RI and the AB ratio.

Flow velocity analysis provides a basis for various calculations. For example, the vessel with the highest-velocity flow can be used for tumor differentiation. It is also possible to calculate the mean value for all the flow velocities measured in a particular tumor. Because carcinomas are supplied by many small, low-flow vessels in addition to a few large vessels, the mean velocity may be low despite a high total blood flow. A better way to assess total blood flow is to add together all the flow velocities measured in the tumor. It would be simpler and more accurate to use a computer to extract the total blood flow from the color Doppler data.

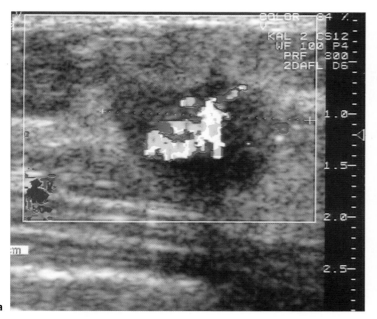
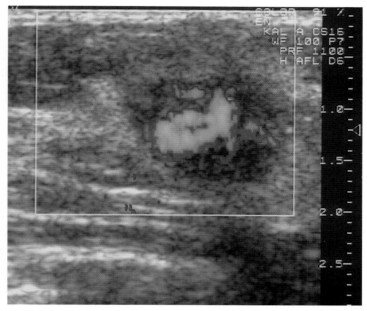

a

b

Fig. 19.3 a, b Color Doppler and power Doppler images of a solid cellular carcinoma. The relatively soft consistency of this tumor accounts for the central vascular density.

a Branching vessels can be identified in the color Doppler image.

b The course of the vessel is seen somewhat more clearly in the power Doppler image, but individual vascular branches are not defined.

Interpretive Criteria

Malignant tumors are associated with an increased number of blood vessels (**Fig. 19.1, Table 19.1**), which converge on the tumor and enter it in a radial pattern. Often, however, only vessels at the tumor periphery are visualized while vessels inside the tumor are collapsed as a result of the very firm consistency of most carcinomas. Although the vessels in malignancies often communicate

through shunts and do not have a muscular coat, the hard tumor consistency leads to a high flow resistance (**Fig. 19.2**). Even so, the flow velocities in most tumor vessels are increased but are highly variable. The same applies to the Doppler spectra that are sampled from the vessels.

In benign tumors, it is common to find an absence of vessels or a single vascular pedicle (**Table 19.2, Figs. 19.4, 19.5**). Nearby vessels often wind around the tumor instead of entering it. The flow velocities are usually low. However, proliferative fibrocystic

Table 19.1 Doppler criteria for malignant tumors

▸ Asymmetry relative to the opposite side
▸ Increased vascularity
▸ Radial pattern of converging vessels
▸ Branching vessels
▸ High flow velocities
▸ High total blood flow
▸ High flow resistance
▸ Variability of Doppler spectra

Table 19.2 Doppler criteria for benign masses

▸ Symmetric flow to opposite side
▸ Little or no vascularity
▸ Vessels run tangential to the mass
▸ Straight, solitary vessel
▸ Low flow velocities
▸ Low total blood flow
▸ Moderate flow resistance

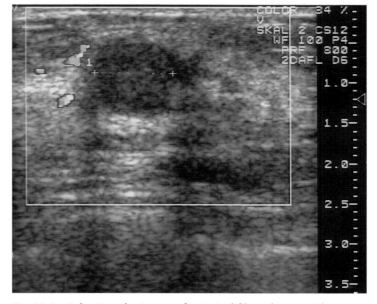

Fig. 19.4 Color Doppler image of a typical fibroadenoma. The tumor itself appears devoid of blood vessels, but a tangential vessel is seen in the adjacent tissue.

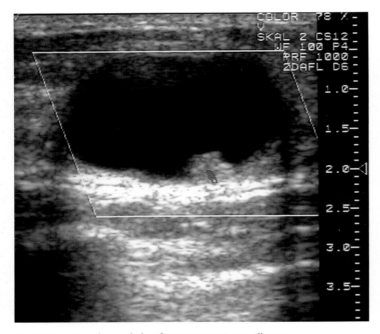

Fig. 19.5　Vascular pedicle of an intracystic papilloma.

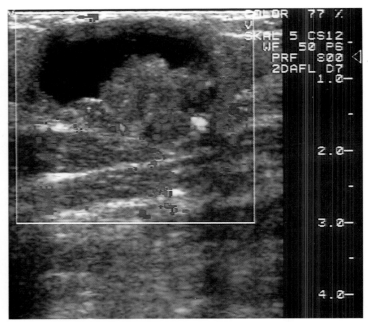

Fig. 19.6　Tumor vessels in an intracystic papilloma. The hypervascularity is due to the proliferative tendency of the neoplasm.

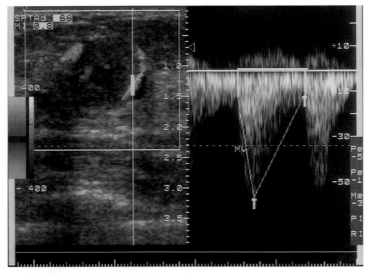

Fig. 19.7　Proliferative fibroadenoma with a rich blood supply. The vessels are numerous and the flow velocities are high (here 56.8 cm/s).

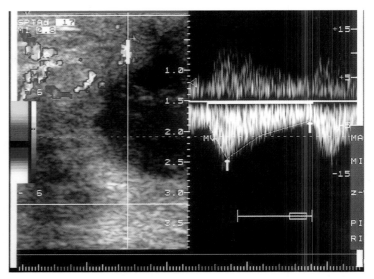

Fig. 19.8　Suppurative mastitis with increased peripheral vascularity.

> Inflammation is a frequent cause of increased vascular density. In most cases, however, the flow velocities are relatively low (here 11.9 cm/s).

changes, benign tumors with a proliferative tendency, and inflammatory processes are associated with an increase in blood flow (**Figs. 19.6, 19,7, 19.8**). Movements of the transducer or patient can generate spurious color signals. Frequency shifts caused by reflections from microcalcifications can also produce color signals (**Fig. 19.9**), and these should not be mistaken for increased blood flow. Nor should normal anatomic vessels in the breast be interpreted as tumor vessels if they happen to pass near a tumor. This particularly applies to the main branches of the axillary and internal thoracic arteries, which carry high-velocity flow.

Vascularity and Hemodynamic Parameters

The simplest quantifiable parameter is vascularity, or the number of blood vessels supplying a breast tumor. In our study population, benign tumors were associated with an average of 1.6 vessels while malignant tumors were associated with 11.3 vessels (**Table 19.3**). A cutoff value of > 3 vessels provides a sensitivity of 89 % and a specificity of 92 % in the diagnosis of malignancy (**Table 19.4**). Taking the difference in vascularity between the affected breast and the same quadrant of the contralateral breast, we find that a cutoff of > 2 vessels improves sensitivity to 90 % and specificity to

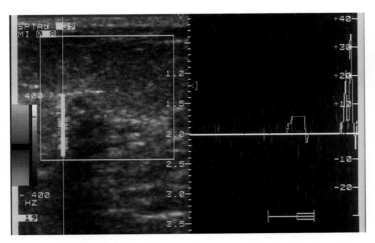

Fig. 19.9 Color Doppler artifact and corresponding frequency pattern associated with breast microcalcifications. The lesion was identified histologically as proliferative benign disease.

 Fluctuations of the color signals in the direction of the beam are an artifact commonly seen with microcalcifications and may be misinterpreted as blood flow. This artifact does not always occur, however, and therefore color Doppler is not useful in screening for microcalcifications.

93% (**Table 19.5**). Among the Doppler parameters, only the sum of the flow velocities (V_{sum}) yields a comparably good result (**Tables 19.3–19.5**). It is surprising that the Doppler spectra show such a high degree of overlap that the calculated indices are poor discriminators. For illustrative purposes, only the RI values are shown in the tables. The AB ratio and PI do not differ significantly. It is still noteworthy that all the parameters except the minimum RI show significant differences between benign and malignant tumors.

Table 19.3 Vascular and hemodynamic parameters measured for 325 benign and 133 malignant breast tumors

	Benign lesions		Malignant lesions	
	Mean	S.D.	Mean	S.D.
No. of vessels	1.63	1.46	11.27	9.66
V_{mean}	9.70	6.93	19.32	8.01
V_{max}	11.92	9.79	36.11	19.24
V_{sum}	22.24	27.95	253.48	307.52
RI_{mean}	0.69	0.11	0.74	0.10
RI_{max}	0.73	0.12	0.88	0.12
RI_{min}	0.64	0.12	0.61	0.12

V_{mean} = mean systolic flow velocity, V_{max} = maximum flow velocity, V_{sum} = sum of all flow velocities, RI = resistance index.

Despite the good discrimination achieved with optimum cutoff values, it is important to note that some carcinomas do not have a rich vascular supply (**Fig. 19.10**). Some are slow-growing neoplasms. Moreover, some vessels associated with heterogeneous malignancies or cancers with a large connective tissue component and intense posterior shadowing cannot be visualized. It is important, therefore, to evaluate all available diagnostic information. The data presented here were obtained under study conditions in a selected population using sophisticated technology. Thus, it is unreasonable to expect these results to be reproducible under routine diagnostic conditions using various types of equipment.

 Doppler sonography should never be used as an isolated study, but rather as an adjunct to supplement other findings.

Table 19.4 Correlation (%) of vascular and hemodynamic parameters with breast carcinoma

Cutoff value		Sensitivity	Specificity	PPV	NPV
Vessels	>2	97.7	81.5	68.4	98.9
Vessels	>3	88.7	92.3	79.7	95.2
V_{mean}	>10	91.7	49.2	42.5	93.6
V_{mean}	>20	42.1	93.2	71.8	79.7
V_{max}	>10	97	44	41.5	97.3
V_{max}	>20	81.2	83.4	66.7	91.6
V_{sum}	>40	91	85.5	72.5	95.9
V_{sum}	>50	86.5	90.8	79.3	94.3
V_{sum}	>60	84.2	93.8	84.9	93.6
RI_{mean}	>0.65	80.5	38.3	40.7	78.9
RI_{mean}	>0.75	46.6	78.3	53	74.4
RI_{max}	>0.75	79.7	65.6	54.9	86
RI_{max}	>0.85	60.2	83	65	79.9
RI_{min}	>0.6	53.4	36.4	30.6	59.7
RI_{min}	>0.7	22.6	77.9	34.9	65.7

PPV = positive predictive value. NPV = negative predictive value.

Table 19.5 Difference in vascular and hemodynamic parameters between affected/unaffected sides as a predictor of breast carcinoma (%)

Cutoff value		Sensitivity	Specificity	PPV	NPV
Vessels	>2	89.5	93.2	84.4	95.6
Vessels	>2	78.9	95.4	87.5	91.7
V_{mean}	>10	58.6	85.5	62.4	83.5
V_{mean}	>20	21.1	98.5	84.8	75.3
V_{max}	>10	82	80.3	63	91.6
V_{max}	>20	60.2	92.9	77.7	85.1
V_{sum}	>30	91	90.2	79.1	96.1
V_{sum}	>40	86.5	93.5	84.6	94.4
V_{sum}	>50	83.5	94.5	86	93.3
V_{sum}	>60	80.5	95.7	88.4	92.3
RI_{mean}	>0.05	46.1	77.3	48.2	75.8
RI_{mean}	>0.1	28.1	85.6	47.2	72.2
RI_{max}	>0.05	68.5	67.5	49.2	82.4
RI_{max}	>0.1	60.7	82	60.7	82
RI_{min}	>0.05	19.1	77.3	27.9	67.6
RI_{min}	>0.1	12.4	87.6	31.4	68.5

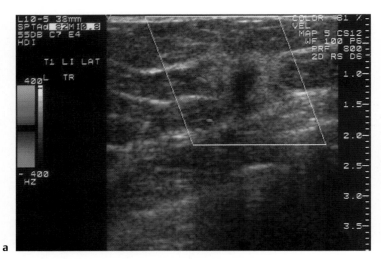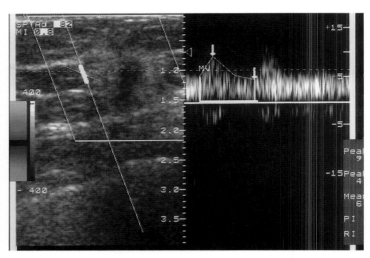

a   b

Fig. 19.10 a, b   Invasive ductal carcinoma with low blood flow.
a Color Doppler display of vessels.
b Duplex flow velocity measurement.

> If morphology shows a suspicious pattern, but the vascularity is sparse, one should not be dissuaded from a working diagnosis of carcinoma or from biopsy.

Possible Applications

Smoothly Marginated Carcinomas

The cases in **Figures 19.1–19.3** illustrate that cellular carcinomas, which may be mistaken for benign tumors in imaging studies, show conspicuous abnormalities on color Doppler images. Doppler ultrasound is particularly useful for confirming the suspicious nature of these tumors.

Proliferative Fibroadenomas

The proliferative activity of highly vascularized fibroadenomas can be predicted with Doppler ultrasound (**see Fig. 19.7**). Observations of these tumors following cytologic confirmation have confirmed their proliferative tendency. The histologic and cytologic analysis of these tumors consistently show proliferative changes, and therefore surgical excision can be recommended when a hypervascular fibroadenoma is found.

Multifocal and Multicentric Tumors

The detection of multifocality and multicentricity is an important part of preoperative diagnosis. Multifocal lesions can be difficult to identify mammographically, especially in women with dense breasts. If the decision between breast-conserving surgery and mastectomy must be based on ultrasound findings alone, it is very helpful if the diagnosis of multiple tumor masses is confirmed by demonstrating multiple vascularized lesions with color Doppler (**Fig. 19.11**).

Scars

In the follow-up of patients who have undergone breast-conserving surgery, major difficulties can arise in the exclusion of recurrent disease. It is advantageous in these cases to exclude a recurrence by noninvasive means (**Fig. 19.12**). Postsurgical scars generally have a low blood supply. Even so, much experience is required in differentiating a scar from a recurrence, because many recurrent tumors are hypovascular, especially after prior radiotherapy. If doubt exists concerning recurrence in a mature scar, contrast-enhanced breast MRI can be helpful in excluding recurrence. With an area of enhancement in or near the tumor, local recurrence is suspected, and image-guided percutaneous core biopsy should be directed to the area to confirm the diagnosis. Use of an

Fig. 19.11   **Multifocal breast cancer.** Color Doppler shows two small tumor masses, each of which is associated with a radial pattern of tumor vessels.

ultrasound contrast agent, not yet FDA-approved in the United States, may help accomplish this goal (see below).

Lymph Node Evaluation

The detection of nodal metastases plays an increasingly important role in preoperative planning. In metastatic lymph nodes that do not display some of the typical ultrasound findings, usually focal changes in the cortex of the node, color Doppler can advance the diagnosis by demonstrating a reactive pattern in enlarged lymph nodes. A concomitant increase in blood flow implies a higher index of suspicion for metastasis (**Fig. 19.13**). Inflammatory changes can also cause a slight increase in vascularization, but usually this is detectable in the hilar area of the node.

It is very important to detect metastatic involvement of the internal mammary nodes, because that region is not routinely included in lymphadenectomy. Color Doppler has a critical role in the surgical planning of these cases because of the proximity of these nodes to the pleura and internal thoracic vessels. Detecting or excluding direct vascular connections during the planning phase can reduce the subsequent risk of surgical complications (**Fig. 19.14**).

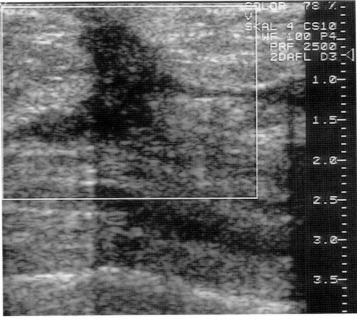

Fig. 19.12 Postsurgical scar following local excision of breast carcinoma. The scar appeared suspicious at ultrasound, but color Doppler shows no abnormal increase in vascularity, suggesting that the lesion is benign.

Prognostic Evaluation

Pathologic studies have shown that a correlation exists between tumor angiogenesis and disease prognosis. This type of study requires a large population to make a prognostic evaluation. The follow-up period in women examined by color Doppler ultrasound is not yet sufficient to make a definitive evaluation. We were able to make a tentative assessment, however, by comparing the numbers of tumor vessels and total blood flow (sum of flow velocities) in 51 patients with nodal metastases and 82 patients without

nodal metastases. We found a significant difference with regard to the number of tumor vessels ($p < 0.01$) in both groups. Measurements of total blood flow showed a tendency toward higher blood flow when metastases were present ($p < 0.062$). Thus, there is evidence that blood flow measurements can provide at least a crude prognostic assessment in that tumors with less blood flow correlate more frequently with an absence of metastases (**Fig. 19.15 a, b**).

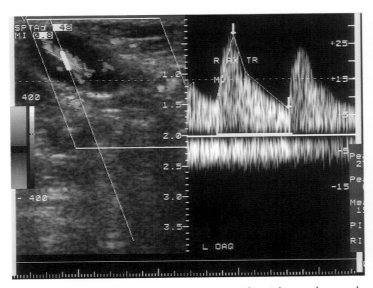

Fig. 19.13 Axillary lymph node metastasis with a rich vascular supply.

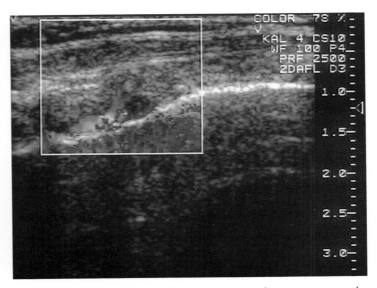

Fig. 19.14 Lymph node metastasis 3 × 4 mm in diameter next to the internal thoracic artery. A large, branched vascular pedicle runs directly from the artery into the lymph node. Parasternal transverse scan in the third intercostal space on the left side.

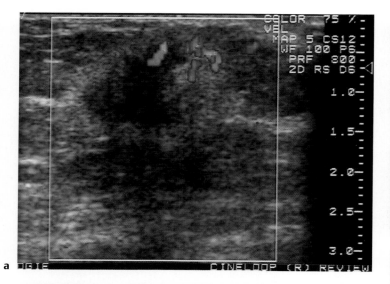

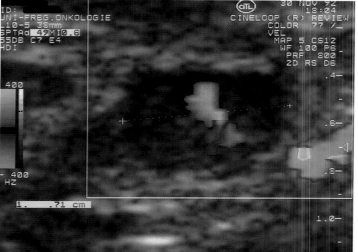

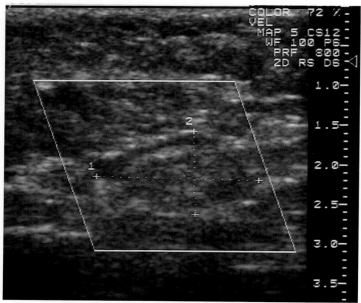

Fig. 19.16 a, b Lymph node metastasis 1 cm in diameter after earlier primary treatment.

a Initial image shows very high tumor blood flow. Chemotherapy with Taxol was initiated.

b The same lymph node 3 months after the start of treatment. The size of the node is unchanged, but the decrease in vascularity indicates significant tumor response.

Fig. 19.15 a, b Invasive ductal breast carcinoma.

a Hypovascular primary tumor.

b Enlarged reactive lymph node with no abnormal vascularity in color Doppler. Histology showed no metastatic involvement of the node.

Chemotherapy and Follow-Up

Malignant tumors vary greatly in their response to chemotherapy and often develop resistance during the course of treatment. It is very difficult to detect this clinically. We have already tested Doppler ultrasound in experimental animals and in various treatment modalities as a means of evaluating tumor response. Traditionally, tumor size measured clinically or by imaging has been the only parameter used to evaluate response. A constant tumor diameter is interpreted as "no change," and this may justify changing to a different therapy. But as **Figure 19.16 a, b** shows, a marked decrease in tumor blood flow may occur without an apparent change in tumor size. Thus, Doppler ultrasound provides a sensitive method for evaluating in vivo the chemotherapeutic response of tumors.

Use of Ultrasound Contrast Agents to Increase Doppler Signal

Ultrasound contrast agents are substances that increase the echogenicity of blood following intravenous injection. By improving the signal-to-noise ratio, these agents enhance the apparent echo contrast between hypervascular and hypovascular areas. Small vessels that were previously invisible can be detected following contrast administration. This technique can help differentiate a hypovascular carcinoma from scar tissue, whose morphology, for example, frequently mimics carcinoma at ultrasound.

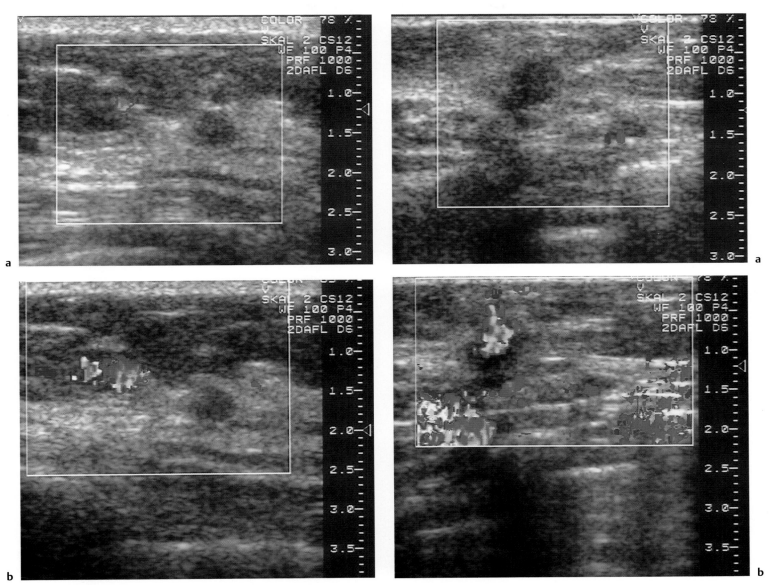

Fig. 19.17 a, b Scar granuloma 2 years after breast-conserving cancer surgery. Ultrasound showed a hypoechoic mass with ill-defined margins.
a Color Doppler prior to contrast administration shows a parenchymal vessel separate from the tumor.
b After the intravenous injection of 8 mL Levovist (400 mg/mL), the tumor still appears avascular but the parenchymal vessel is more clearly demonstrated.

Fig. 19.18 a, b Local recurrence 2 years after breast-conserving cancer surgery. Ultrasound showed a lesion similar to that in Fig. 19.17.
a The tumor itself is avascular, but a small parenchymal vessel is visible some distance away.
b Following contrast injection, the parenchymal vessel appears more prominent. But the major change is the increased signal intensity within the mass, indicating a high blood flow rate in the tumor.

Practical Application

Following intravenous injection of the echo-enhancing agent, it takes approximately 20–40 seconds for blood carrying the contrast material to reach the arterial bed. By increasing the echogenicity of the blood, the agent increases the amplitude of the Doppler signal while causing no significant increase in the frequency shift. Vessels that are faintly visualized in color Doppler become more conspicuous, and previously nonvisualized vessels can be seen. Vessels that were visible before contrast injection and are enhanced by the contrast agent should not be classified as suspicious (**Fig. 19.17 a, b**), but a focal increase of blood flow in an area that previously appeared avascular should raise suspicion of carcinoma (**Fig. 19.18 a, b**).

In our studies we employed the ultrasound contrast agent Levovist (Schering, Berlin), which is used primarily in cardiology, gastroenterology, and nephrology. The advantages of echo enhancement in breast tumors are currently being tested. The agent consists mainly of galactose granules that are stabilized with a special lipid-based preparation so that they will remain stable for a short time in the bloodstream. The particles are small enough to pass easily through the pulmonary capillary bed. We have observed no side effects other than an occasional warm or cold sensation at the injection site, and the agent may be administered repeatedly without concern. The injection solution is prepared by dissolving the dry mixture in water shortly before use. It is available in various dosages. We have obtained the best results by injecting 8 mL of a 400 mg/mL solution. Lower concentrations may not provide a sufficient degree of signal enhancement.

To facilitate image interpretation, it would be useful to record and document the degree of signal enhancement that is observed. Presumably the dynamic progression of contrast inflow and clearance would also be important. At present, however, no ultrasound imaging system is equipped with mechanisms for the rapid determination of Doppler signal intensity. This capability would be essential to define standard uptake curves and cutoff values like those used in radionuclide scanning and dynamic MRI. Nevertheless, from the examples presented here, we can appreciate the potential advantages of the routine use of ultrasound contrast agents in selected problem cases. Noncontrast Doppler studies, and outside of the United States, contrast-enhanced scans should be done by experienced examiners. Both methods are useful for the investigation of problem cases.

 For Doppler ultrasound to be used rationally and effectively, the examiner should be well trained. Ideally, careful B-mode imaging should be done first, with the Doppler study in a supportive role. The subjective interpretation of vascularity requires a particularly high degree of experience. Objective quantitative measurements would be preferable, but at present they are very difficult to do. Automated measuring programs can be of particular benefit in contrast-enhanced ultrasound examinations.

Breast Ultrasound Review Questions   20

Question	Find the answers in Chapter:
1. What are the physical principles on which ultrasound imaging is based? A. The measurement of: ▸ Transit time ▸ Echo amplitude ▸ Frequency shift B. The transmission of: ▸ A continuous wave ▸ Pulsed ultrasound	1
2. What physical principle is utilized in the evaluation of blood flow? What techniques do you know?	1
3. Please explain the basic principles of the following terms: ▸ A mode ▸ B mode ▸ M mode ▸ Duplex mode ▸ Color Doppler	1
4. What is a: ▸ Simple scan ▸ Compound scan ▸ Static scan ▸ Real-time scan ▸ Water-bath scan vs. contact scan	1, 18
5. Which examination techniques (see question 3) and which scanning techniques (see question 4) do you prefer? Why?	2
6. Name two different scanning techniques that are useful for examining the breast.	2
7. Explain the principles of these transducer types: ▸ Linear array ▸ Sector scanner ▸ Annular array ▸ Convex array	1
8. Name two different scanning techniques used in breast ultrasound examinations.	2
9. What is a simple scan? A compound scan?	1, 18

Question	Find the answers in Chapter:
10. What is meant by real-time scanning? Does it involve a water-bath technique or contact scanning?	1, 2
11. What is the advantage of a real-time scan over static scanning methods?	1, 18
12. What is a linear-array transducer? What is an annular-array transducer?	1
13. Is a sector transducer better than a linear-array transducer for breast imaging? If not, why?	1
14. What one or more of the following should be used for real-time breast ultrasound? An instrument with ▸ Long wavelength ▸ High frequency ▸ High resolution ▸ Short wavelength ▸ Low frequency	1
15. What ultrasound frequencies are suitable for breast ultrasound?	1
16. If a high frequency is used, should the power setting be increased or decreased, and should the TGC be increased or reduced?	1
17. How do the following parameters affect ultrasound resolution? ▸ Frequency ▸ Wavelength ▸ Pulse length ▸ Focusing	1
18. What are the advantages and disadvantages of different transducers? Which transducer types and frequency ranges are best for: ▸ Abdominal imaging ▸ Early pregnancy ▸ Late pregnancy ▸ Gynecologic imaging ▸ Breast imaging	1

Question	Find the answers in Chapter:	Question	Find the answers in Chapter:
19. Does real-time scanning involve a water-bath technique, static scanning, and/or contact scanning?	1, 2	28. Diagnostic criteria for carcinoma: *Margin* ▸ Circumscribed ▸ Indistinct *Echo pattern* ▸ Hyperechoic ▸ Anechoic *Posterior acoustic features* ▸ Enhancement ▸ Shadowing	3, 12
20. What one or more of the following causes acoustic enhancement deep to a mass? ▸ High sound velocity ▸ Low sound velocity ▸ High sound attenuation ▸ Low sound attenuation	1		
21. On which principle(s) of physics is ultrasound imaging based?	1	29. Diagnostic criteria for scars: *Margin* ▸ Circumscribed ▸ Indistinct *Echo pattern* ▸ Hyperechoic ▸ Anechoic *Posterior acoustic features* ▸ Enhancement ▸ Shadowing	3, 11
22. What principles or physics are utilized in the ultrasound evaluation of blood flow?	1,19		
23 Are there different Doppler techniques? What are they?	1, 19		
24. Describe a standard examination protocol for breast ultrasound.	2		
25 Please assign high or low echogenicity to each of the following (compared with the echogenicity of fat) ? ▸ Breast parenchyma ▸ Fat ▸ Carcinoma ▸ Skin ▸ Cooper ligaments ▸ Cysts	3, 4	30. What problems may arise with scars? How can these problems be solved? What are the advantages of ultrasound over mammography?	11
		31. What are the distinctive sonomorphologic features of proliferative fibroadenomas?	10
		32. What are the typical criteria for benign tumors? ▸ Acoustic shadowing ▸ Architectural distortion ▸ Indistinct margins ▸ Posterior acoustic enhancement	3, 10
26. Using BI-RADS,™ please select the diagnostic criteria for cysts by selecting one descriptor from each of the following feature categories: *Shape* ▸ Oval ▸ Irregular Margin ▸ Circumscribed ▸ Not circumscribed *Echo pattern* ▸ Hyperechoic ▸ Anechoic *Posterior Acoustic Features* ▸ Enhancement ▸ Shadowing	3,7	33. How would you proceed with a noncompressible, hypoechoic mass with indistinct margins and posterior acoustic shadow?	11, 12
		34. Which benign breast disease is associated with the highest risk of breast cancer? ▸ Papilloma ▸ Benign disease with atypical proliferation (grade III) ▸ Lipoma ▸ Fibroadenoma ▸ Abscess	6, 7
27. Diagnostic criteria for fibroadenoma: *Margin* ▸ Circumscribed ▸ Indistinct *Echo pattern* ▸ Hyperechoic ▸ Anechoic *Posterior acoustic features* ▸ Enhancement ▸ Shadowing	3, 10	35. Which three of the following are the most common ultrasound features applicable to diagnosis of carcinoma? ▸ Hyperechogenicity (compared with fat) ▸ Acoustic enhancement ▸ Indistinct margins ▸ Posterior acoustic shadowing ▸ Parallel orientation ▸ Poor compressibility	3, 12
		36. What nonsurgical options are available for the cytologic or histologic evaluation of indeterminate masses? Please explain the various techniques.	14

Question	Find the answers in Chapter:
37. What are the advantages and disadvantages of imaging-guided tissue sampling?	14
38. What methods are available for the preoperative localization of nonpalpable breast lesions?	14
39. When would you select ultrasound-guided pre-surgical localization, and for what types of findings might mammography be better?	14
40. What is the purpose of specimen mammography and specimen ultrasonography?	14
41. What are the advantages of ultrasound-guided needle procedures?	14
42. What is the purpose of fine-needle aspiration in breast diagnosis?	14
43. Does core biopsy have advantages over aspiration cytology?	14
44. Is fine-needle aspiration helpful in the differential diagnosis of focal lesions?	14
45. In what cases is aspiration cytology conclusive?	14
46. What are the potential pitfalls in aspiration cytology?	14
47. What are the advantages and disadvantages of mammographic stereotactic biopsy?	14
48. In what ways are mammography and ultrasound complementary?	3–19
49. Can breast ultrasound be used for screening? Why or why not?	16
50. What are the advantages of mammography over ultrasound?	16
51. Why is mammography useful for screening?	16
52. What are the advantages of ultrasound over mammography?	4, 5–8, 15, 16, 17, 19
53. What are the disadvantages of ultrasound?	16
54. Are mammography and ultrasound competitive or complementary modalities?	3–19
55. Name five important indications for breast ultrasound.	2–16
56. What points should be considered in acquiring an ultrasound imaging system?	1
57. Which one of the following is the purpose of duplex scan? ▸ Color imaging of large vessels ▸ Measurement of flow velocity ▸ Measurement of Doppler spectra ▸ Locating small vessels	19
58. What is color Doppler used for? ▸ Visualization of large vessels ▸ Measurement of flow velocity ▸ Visualization of small vessels ▸ Measurement of flow velocity	19

Question	Find the answers in Chapter:
59. The precise measurement of flow velocity in blood vessels requires: ▸ Color Doppler ▸ CW Doppler ▸ Pulsed Doppler ▸ Beam-vessel angle correction	19
60. Is Doppler ultrasound useful for routine examinations?	19
61. What is the advantage of color Doppler over CW Doppler?	19
62. What typical criteria would one expect to find in the color Doppler examination of breast cancer?	19
63. What filter and PRF settings should be used in tumor diagnosis?	19
64. What diagnostic criteria are relevant for Doppler examinations in breast diagnosis?	19
65. What indices are used in the evaluation of Doppler spectra?	19
66. What is the purpose of the filter setting in Doppler ultrasound?	19
67. Would it be more common to find high or low flow velocities in malignant tumors?	19
68. What filter setting should be used in the diagnosis of breast tumors? How would you decide?	19
69. The clinical examination is normal. Screening mammograms showed clustered, pleomorphic, suspicious-appearing microcalcifications. Ultrasound shows no abnormalities. You recommend: ▸ Follow-up mammograms in 6 months ▸ Fine-needle aspiration ▸ Stereotactically-guided vacuum-assisted large needle biopsy ▸ Mammographic localization and excisional biopsy	12, 14, 16
70. When you excise clustered microcalcifications, how do you confirm a successful operation? (More than one answer may be correct): ▸ Ultrasound at 6 months ▸ Mammography at 6 months ▸ Specimen ultrasonography ▸ Specimen mammography	14
71. At ultrasound you see a hypoechoic focal lesion with a posterior acoustic shadow. How would you further evaluate this lesion?	12, 14
72. At ultrasound you see a hypoechoic mass with indistinct margins and an acoustic shadow. When you press lightly over the mass with the transducer, both the mass and the shadow disappear. How do you interpret this?	11

Question	Find the answers in Chapter:	Question	Find the answers in Chapter:
73. The patient has a unilateral bloody nipple discharge. There are no palpable, mammographic, or sonographic abnormalities in the breast. How would you proceed?	6	77. You find a moderately compressible, hypoechoic focal lesion with indistinct margins and a posterior acoustic shadow. One year earlier, the patient underwent breast-conserving surgery in this region and postoperative radiotherapy. How do you interpret the finding? What are the differential diagnostic considerations?	11
74. You find an intracystic tumor at ultrasound. How would you further evaluate this lesion?	7	78. What is the best way to establish a diagnosis for the indeterminate lesion in question 77?	11, 14
75. What features distinguish malignant from benign tumors?	3, 7, 10, 12		
76. You see a solid, homogeneous mass with circumscribed margins. It correlates with a smooth, mobile mass on physical examination. How would you advise the patient?	10		

Appendix: IBUS Guidelines

The quality of ultrasound imaging depends on:
▸ Equipment
▸ Examination technique
▸ Interpretation

Equipment Requirements

Only high-resolution instrumentation producing high-quality images should be used. Important parameters include spatial, contrast, temporal, and vascular resolutions.

Linear-array or annular-array transducer configurations are suitable for high-quality images. The dominant transducer frequency should be 7.5 MHz or higher, preferably of a broad bandwidth construction. However, high frequency on its own is not a sufficient parameter to ensure quality.

A field of view greater than 4 cm is preferable for large area examinations, and smaller fields are suitable for detailed examination of specific findings.

A penetration depth of at least 4 cm with selectable focal regions is required.

The transducer dead zone should be minimal and limited to a distance of less than 2–3 mm to clearly display superficial structures.

When color Doppler imaging is included in the examination procedure, the color display only provides an estimate of vascularity. High sensitivity for low-amplitude and low-signal flow detection requires Doppler frequencies above 5 MHz. Low flow velocity detection requires wall filter settings in the range of 50–100 Hz and low pulse repetition frequency (PRF) around 1000 Hz.

Examination Technique

To evaluate breast anatomy and not to miss subtle pathology, the examination should be:
▸ Systematic
▸ Comprehensive
▸ Reproducible

Systematic

A planned approach for performance and documentation of the examination is required. When a specific lesion is examined, its precise position should be noted on the image and its correlation with the clinical and mammographic findings recorded. When the total breast volume needs to be assessed, overlapping scans will ensure complete examination.

Comprehensive

All breast structures must be completely displayed, and particular care taken in the area of interest to ensure that normal anatomical and/or pathological findings are recognized and recorded.

Reproducible

The imaging results must be readily reproducible, and ultrasound findings should be clearly identified on the stored images. It should be possible to confirm the same appearances on different types of high-resolution ultrasound scanning systems.

As the acquisition of ultrasound images is very operator dependent, a thorough understanding of the physical principles of ultrasound and of the normal anatomy are essential to achieve high-quality images.

A supine oblique or supine position is recommended to reduce breast thickness and to improve visualization of deeper tissues. The reduced thickness allows optimization of focusing.

One or both arms should be elevated behind the head or neck to stretch the pectoralis muscle for better fixation and immobilization of the breast.

When scanning, the transducer should always be perpendicular to the skin surface.

Transducer coupling to the surface of the skin should be gentle and should give complete contact.

Strong compression pushes lesions out of the scanning plane below the transducer and should be avoided as it deforms tissue structures, making interpretation more difficult.

Compression is useful to avoid refraction and scattering from normal anatomical structures when sound penetration is insufficient, and to examine tissue elasticity of benign and malignant findings.

The scanning procedure should involve overlapping scanning planes. These may be parasagittal, transverse, radial, or antiradial. Radial and antiradial scans follow normal anatomical patterns, assisting the recognition of abnormalities and better demonstrating ductal structure and changes.

Interpretation

Ultrasound examination of the breast is difficult and requires:
▸ Detailed knowledge of anatomy, physiological changes, and benign and malignant pathology.
▸ Correlation of findings with other imaging results, clinical information, and examination.

The minimum report should include:
▸ The indications for the examination.
▸ A description of any lesion(s) and adjacent features, including the size of the maximum diameter(s) or extent.
▸ The position of the lesion(s) as represented on a clock face, including distance from the nipple.
▸ Correlation with clinical and/or mammographic or other imaging findings.
▸ Opinion regarding provisional diagnosis(es) and significance of finding(s).

Continuous education and follow-up are essential to improve and maintain skills in technique and interpretation.

Recommendations by the IBUS to achieve accuracy and confidence:

▸ Performance of a minimum of 500 examinations in a multidisciplinary environment with at least 300 cytology or histology correlation cases.
▸ Performance of at least 50 interventional procedures with appropriate follow-up.

IBUS International Faculty

E Azavedo (Sweden), J C Bamber (United Kingdom), R Chersevani (Italy), Y-H Chou (Taiwan), F Degenhardt (Germany), E Durante (Italy), B B Goldberg (USA), B-J Hackelöer (Germany), W L Heindel (Germany), R Holland (Netherlands), J Jellins (Australia), Y X Jiang (China), W A Kaiser (Germany), T Kamio (Japan), F Kasumi (Japan), C K Kuhl (Germany), H Madjar (Germany), E B Mendelson (USA), V V Mitkov (Russia), W K Moon (Korea), A Mundinger (Germany), K K Oh (Korea), R Otto (Switzerland), S de Pace Bauab (Brazil), S Pankl (Austria), L E Philpotts (USA), Ch Rageth (Switzerland), M T Rickard (Australia), G Rizzatto (Italy), E Rubin (USA), R Schulz-Wendtland (Germany), E A Sickles (USA), L Steyaert (Belgium), G Svane (Sweden), W E Svensson (United Kingdom), K Szopinski (Poland), E Ueno (Japan), C F Weismann (Austria), R Wilson (United Kingdom), W T Yang (USA).

This information is correct at the time of publication. For further information, please visit:
http://www.ibus.org/

Further Reading

American College of Radiology. Standard for the performance of the breast ultrasound examination. Reston, VA: American College of Radiology; 2002

American College of Radiology. ACR-BI-RADS® - Ultrasound. In: ACR Breast Imaging Reporting and Data System. Breast Imaging Atlas. Reston VA: American College of Radiology; 2003

American College of Radiology. ACR Appropriateness Criteria. Imaging work-up of palpable breast masses. Reston, VA: American College of Radiology; 2003

American College of Radiology. ACR practice guideline for the performance of a breast ultrasound examination. Reston, VA: American College of Radiology; 2007

Azavedo E, Bone B. Imaging breasts with silicone implants. Eur Radiol 1999;9:349–355

Bäz E, Madjar H, Reuss Ch, Vetter M, Hackelöer B-J, Holz K. The role of enhanced Doppler Ultrasound in differentiation of benign versus malignant scar lesions after breast surgery for malignancy. Ultrasound Obstet Gynecol 2000;15(5):377–382

Baker JA, Kornguth PJ, Soo MS, Walsh R, Mengoni P. Sonography of solid breast lesions: observer variability of lesion description and assessment. AJR Am J Roentgenol 1999;172:1621–1625

Berg WA. Rationale for a trial of screening breast ultrasound: American College of Radiology Imaging Network (ACRIN) 6666. AJR Am J Roentgenol 2003;180:1225–1228

Berg WA, Gilbreath PL. Multicentric and multifocal cancer: whole-breast US in preoperative evaluation. Radiology 2000;214:59–66

Berg WA, Campassi CI, Ioffe OB. Cystic lesions of the breast; sonographic-pathologic correlation. Radiology 2003;227:183–191

Berg WA, Gutierrez L, NessAiver MS, et al. Diagnostic accuracy of Mammography, clinical examination, US, and MR imaging in preoperative assessment of breast cancer. Radiology 2004;233(3):830–849

Blood CH, Zetter BR. Tumor interactions with the vasculature: angiogenesis and tumor metastasis. Biochim Biophys Acta 1990;1032:89–118

Bosch AM, Kessels AG, Beets GL, et al. Interexamination variation of whole breast ultrasound. Br J Radiol 2003;76:328–331

Buchberger W, Niehoff A, Obrist P, et al. Clinically and mammographically occult breast lesions: detection and classification with high-resolution sonography. Semin Ultrasound CT MR 2000;21:325–336

Buchberger W, DeKoekkoek-Doll P, Springer P, Obrist P, Dünser M. Incidental Findings on Sonography of the Breast: Clinical Significance and Diagnostic Workup. AJR Am J Roentgenol 1999;173:921–927

Cole-Beuglet C, Soriano RZ, Kurtz AB, et al. Ultrasound analysis of 104 primary breast carcinomas classified according to histopathologic type. Radiology 1983;147:191–196

Cosgrove DO, Bamber JC, Davey JB, McKinna JA, Sinnet HD. Color doppler signals from breast tumors. Radiology 1990;176:175–180

D'Orsi CJ, Bassett LW, Berg WA, et al. BI-RADS, Breast Imaging Reporting and Data System. 4th ed. Reston, VA: American College of Radiology; 2003

DeBruhl ND, Gorczyca DP, Ahn CY, Shaw WW, Bassett LW. Silicone breast implants: US evaluation. Radiology 1993;189:95–98

Dennis MA, Parker SH, Klaus AJ. Breast biopsy avoidance—value of normal mammograms and normal sonograms in the setting of a palpable lump. Radiology 2001;219:186–191

Deurloo EE, Tanis PJ, Gilhuijs KG, et al. Reduction in the number of sentinel lymph node procedures by preoperative ultrasonography of the axilla in breast cancer. Eur J Cancer 2003;39:1068–1073

Dodd GD, Wallace JD, Freundlich IM, Marsh L, Zermino A. Thermography and cancer of the breast. Cancer 1969;23(4):797–802

Drevs J, Hofmann I, Hugenschmidt H, et al. Effects of PTK787/ZK 222584, a specific inhibitor of vascular endothelial growth factor receptor tyrosine kinases, on primary tumor, metastasis, vessel density, and blood flow in a murine renal cell carcinoma modell. Cancer Res 2000;60(17):4819–4824

Entrekin RR, Porter BA, Sillesen HH, et al. Real-time spatial compound imaging: application to breast, vascular, and musculoskeletal ultrasound. Semin Ultrasound CT MR 2001;22:50–64

Feldman F. Angiography of cancer of the breast. Cancer 1969;23:803–810

Feu J, Tresserra F, Fabregas R. Metastatic breast carcinoma in axillary lymph nodes: In vitro US detection. Radiology 1997;205:831–835

Fischer U, Zachariae O, Baum F, von Heyden D, Funke M, Liersch T. The influence of preoperative MRI of the breast on recurrence rate in patients with breast cancer. Eur Radiol 2004;14:1725–1731

Flobbe K, Bosch AM, Kessels AG, et al. The additional diagnostic value of ultrasonography in the diagnosis of breast cancer. Arch Intern Med 2003;163:1194–1199

Folkman J, Watson K, Ingber D, Hanahan D. Induction of angiogenesis during the transition from hyperplasia to neoplasia. Nature 1989;339:58–61

Fornage BD, Toubas O, Morel M. Clinical, mammographic and sonographic determination of preoperative breast cancer size. Cancer 1987;60:765–771

Fornage BD, Sneige N, Faroux MJ, Andry E. Sonographic appearance and ultrasound-guided fine-needle aspiration biopsy of breast carcinomas smaller than 1 cm^3. J Ultrasound Med 1990;9:559–568

Fung HM, Jackson FI. Clinically and mammographically occult breast lesions demonstrated by ultrasound. J R Soc Med 1990;83:696–701

Garra BS, Cespedes EI, Ophir J, et al. Elastography of breast lesions: initial clinical results. Radiology 1997;202(1):79–86

Gautherie M, Haehnel P, Walter JP, Keith LG. Thermovascular changes associated with in situ and minimal breast cancers. J Reprod Med 1987;32:833–841

Georgian-Smith D, Taylor KJW, Madjar H, et al. Sonography of palpable breast cancer. J Clin Ultrasound 2000;28(5):211–216

Gordon PB, Goldenberg SL. Malignant breast masses detected only by ultrasound: a retrospective review. Cancer 1995;76:626–630

Gordon PB, Goldenberg SL, Chan NH. Solid breast lesions: Diagnosis with US-guided fine-needle aspiration biopsy. Radiology 1993;189:573–580

Gøtzsche PC, Olsen O. Is screening for breast cancer with mammography justifiable? Lancet 2000;355:129–134

Guyer PB, Dewbury KC. Ultrasound of the breast in the symptomatic and x-ray dense breast. Clin Radiol 1985;36:69–76

Harris KM, Ganott MA, Shestak KC, et al. Detection of silicone leaks: a new sonographic sign. Radiology 1991;181:134

Harris KM, Ganott MA, Shestak KC, et al. Silicone implant rupture: detection with US. Radiology 1993;187:761–768

Hergan K. Sonography of the axilla and supraclavicular region. Eur J Ultrasound 1996;3:113–124

Hernan I, Vargas HI, Masood S. Implementation of a Minimally Invasive Breast Biopsy Program in Countries with Limited Resources. Breast J 2003;9:S 81–S 85

Hernandez A, Bassest O, Bremond A, Magnin IE. Stereoscopic visualization of three-dimensional ultrasonic data applied to breast tumor. Eur J Ultrasound 1998;8:51–65

Hilton SV, Leopold GR, Olson LK, et al. Real-time breast sonography; application in 300 consecutive patients. AJR Am J Roentgenol 1986;147:479–486

Hlawatsch A, Teifke A, Schmidt M, Thelen M. Preoperative assessment of breast cancer: sonography versus MR imaging. AJR Am J Roentgenol 2002;179:1493–1501

Hou MF, Chuang HY, Ou-Yang F, et al. Comparison of breast mammography, sonography and physical examination for screening women at high risk of breast cancer in Taiwan. Ultrasound Med Biol 2001;28:641–649

Hughes LE, Mansel RE, Webster DJT. Benign disorders and diseases of the breast. 2nd ed., London: WB Saunders; 2000

Itoh A, Ueno E, Tohno E, et al. Breast disease: clinical application of US elastography for diagnosis. Radiology 2006;239(2):341–350

Jellins J. Combining imaging and vascularity assessment of breast lesions. Ultrasound Med Biol 1988;14(Suppl. 1):121–130

Kallinowski F, Moehle R, Schaefer C, Vaupel P. Effects of tumor necrosis factor a on tumor blood flow and hyperthermic treatment. Onkologie 1989;12:131–135

Kamio T, Kameoka S, Muraki H, et al. Significance of ductal findings in ultrasonic examination of the breast: Diagnosis of intraductal tumor and intraductal spreading of breast cancer. In: Kasumi F, Ueno E. Topics in Breast Ultrasound. Tokyo: Shinohara; 1991 (pp. 200–205)

Kaplan SS. Clinical utility of bilateral whole-breast US in the evaluation of women with dense breast tissue. Radiology 2001;221:641–649

Kolb TM, Lichy J, Newhouse JH. Occult cancer in women with dense breasts: detection with screening US–diagnostic yield and tumor characteristics. Radiology 1998;207:191–199

Kolb TM, Lichy J, Newhouse JH. Comparison of the performance of screening mammography, physical examination, and breast US and evaluation of factors that influence them: an analysis pf 27,825 patient evaluations. Radiology 2002;225:165–175

Kopans DB. Breast imaging. 3rd ed. Philadelphia: Lippincott Williams and Wilkins; 2007:555–605

Kossoff G, Jellins J, Reeve TS. Potential solutions to the limitations of the sonographic examination of the breast. In: Jellins T, Kobayashi T. Ultrasonic Examination of the Breast. New York: Wiley; 1983 (pp. 229–231)

Kremkau FW. Diagnostic ultrasound. Physical principles and exercises. New York: Grune & Stratton; 1981

Kriege M, Brekelmans C, Boetes C, et al. Efficacy of MRI and mammography for breast cancer screening in women with a familial or genetic predisposition. N Engl J Med 2004;351:427–429

Kwak JY, Kim EK, Keun KJ. Variable breast conditions-comparison of conventional and real-time compound ultrasonography. J Ultrasound Med 2004;23:85–96

Laine HR, Tukeva T, Mikkola P, Holström PT. Assessment of mammography and ultrasound examination in the diagnosis of breast cancer. Eur J Ultrasound 1996;3:9–14

Leonard C, Harlow CL, Coffin C. Use of US to guide radiation boost planning following lumpectomy for carcinoma of the breast. Int J Radiat Oncol Biol Phys 1993;27:1193–1197

Leung JW, Sickles EA. Multiple bilateral masses detected on screening mammography: assessment of need for recall imaging. AJR Am J Roentgenol 2000;175:23–29

Madjar H. Breast examination with continuous wave and color Doppler. Ultrasound Obstet Gynecol 1992;2:215–220

Madjar H. Echo-enhanced ultrasound – clinical and technical aspects. Ultrasound Obstet Gynecol 2000;16:111–114

Madjar H, Jellins J. Role of echo enhanced ultrasound in breast mass investigations. Eur J Ultrasound 1997;5:65–75

Madjar H, Sauerbrei W, Münch S, Schillinger H. Continuous-wave and pulsed doppler studies of the breast: Clinical results and effect of transducer frequency. Ultrasound Med Biol 1991;17:31–39

Madjar H, Du Bois A, Kommoss F, Meerpohl HG, Pfleiderer A. Implementation of Doppler ultrasound for therapy control of breast malignancies treated with chemotherapy. Onkologie 1993;16:183–188

Madjar H, Ladner HA, Sauerbrei W, Oberstein A, Prömpeler H, Pfleiderer A. Preoperative staging of breast cancer by palpation, mammography and high-resolution ultrasound. Ultrasound Obstet Gynecol 1993;3:185–190

Madjar H, Vetter M, Prömpeler H, Breckwoldt M, Pfleiderer A. Doppler measurement of breast vascularity in women under pharmacologic treatment of benign breast disease. J Reprod Med 1993;38:935–940

Madjar H, Prömpeler HJ, Sauerbrei W, Wolfarth R, Pfleiderer A. Color doppler flow criteria of breast lesions. Ultrasound Med Biol 1994;20:849–858

Madjar H, Teubner J, Hackelöer B-J. Breast Ultrasound Update. Karger, Basel 1994

Madjar H, Prömpeler HJ, Sauerbrei W, Mundinger A, Pfleiderer A. Differential diagnosis of breast lesions by color doppler. Ultrasound Obstet Gynecol 1995;6:199–204

Madjar H, Sauerbrei W, Prömpeler HJ, Wolfarth R, Gufler H. Color doppler and duplex flow analysis for classification of breast lesions. Gynecol Oncol 1997;64:392–403

Madjar H, Rickard M, Jellins J, Otto R. IBUS guidelines for the ultrasonic examination of the breast. Eur J Ultrasound 1999;9:99–102

Madjar H, Prömpeler HJ, Del Favero C, Hackelöer BJ, Llull JB. A new Doppler signal enhancing agent for flow assessment in breast lesions. Eur J Ultrasound 2000;12:123–130

Mainiero MB, Goldkamo A, Lazarus E. Characterization of breast masses with sonography—can biopsy of some solid masses be deferred? J Ultrasound Med 2005;24:161–167

McNicholas MMJ, Mercer PM, Miller JC, McDermott EWM, O'Higgins NJ, MacErlean DP. Color Doppler sonography in the evaluation of palpable breast masses. AJR Am J Roentgenol 1993;161:765–771

Memis A, Ustun EE, Orguc S. Mammographic and ultrasonographic evaluation of breast after excisional biopsy. Eur J Ultrasound 1997;5:47–51

Mendelson EB. Evaluation of the postoperative breast. Radiol Clin North Am 1992;30:107–138

Mendelson EB. Radiation changes in the breast. Semin Roentgenol 1993;28:344–362

Mendelson EB. The development and meaning of appropriateness guidelines. Radiol Clin North Am 1995;33:1081–1084

Mendelson EB. Ultrasonography of the Breast. In: Callen, PW. Ultrasonography in Obstetrics and Gynecology, 5th ed. Amsterdam: Elsevier; 2008;1077–1097

Mendelson EB, Berg WA, Merritt CR. Toward a standardized breast ultrasound lexicon, BI-RADS: ultrasound. Semin Roentgenol 2001;36:217–225

Mendelson EB, Baum J, Berg WA, Merritt CRB, Rubin E. American College of Radiology, Breast Imaging Reporting and Data System (BI-RADS®): Ultrasound, Reston, VA, 2003

Merritt CRB. Future directions in breast ultrasonography. Seminars in Breast Disease 1999;2(1):89–96

Merritt CRB. Physics of Ultrasound. In: Rumack CM, Wilson SR, Charboneau JW. Diagnostic Ultrasound. 3rd ed., St. Louis, MO: Elsevier Mosby; 2005: pp. 3–34

Miller AB, Baines CJ, Wall C. Canadian National Breast Screening Study-2: 13-year results of a randomised trial in women aged 50–59 years. J Natl Cancer Inst 2000;92:1490–1499

Mitchell DG, Merton DA, Liu JB, Goldberg B. Superficial masses with color Doppler imaging. J Clin Ultrasound 1991;19:555–560

Moon WK, Noh D-Y, Im J-G. Multifocal, multicentric, and contralateral breast cancers: bilateral whole-breast US in the preoperative evaluation of patients. Radiology 2002;224(2):569–576

Mund DF, Farria DM, Gorczyca DP, et al. MR imaging of the breast in patients with silicone-gel implants: spectrum of findings. AJR Am J Roentgenol 1993;161:773–778

Natsuki S, Yamazaki K. A study on the vascular proliferation in tissues around the tumor in breast cancer. Jpn J Surg 1988;18:235–242

Nyström L, Andersson I, Bjurstam N, Frisell J, Nordenskjöld B, Rutqvist LE. Long-term effects of mammography screening: updated overview of the Swedish randomised trials. Lancet 2002;359:909–919

Olsen O, Gøtzsche PC. Cochrane review on screening for breast cancer with mammography. Lancet 2001;358:1340–1342

Ophir J, Alam SK, Garra B, et al. Elastography: ultrasonic estimation and imaging of the elastic properties of tissues. Proc Inst Mech Eng [H] 1999;213(3):203–233

Ophir J, Cespedes I, Garra B, Ponnekanti H, Huang Y, Maklad N. Elastography: ultrasound imaging of tissue strain and elastic modulus in vivo. Eur J Ultrasound 1996;3:49–70

Parker SH, Jobe WE, Dennis MA, et al. US-guided automated large-core breast biopsy. Radiology 1993;187:507–511

Peer PG, Holland R, Hendriks JHCL, Mravunac M, Verbeek ALM. Age-Specific Effectiveness of the Nijmegen Population-Based Breast Cancer-Screening Program: Assessment of Early Indicators of Screening Effectiveness. J Natl Cancer Inst 1994;86(6):436–441

Plate KH, Breier G, Weich HA, Risau W. Vascular endothelial growth factor is a potential tumour angiogenesis factor in human gliomas in vivo. Nature 1992;359:845–848

Powell DE, Stelling CB. Magnetic resonance imaging of the human female breast. Current status and pathologic correlations. Pathol Annu 1988;23:159–194

Rahbar G, Sie AC, Hansen GC, et al. Benign versus malignant solid breast masses: US differentiation. Radiology 1999;213:889–894

Richter K, Heywang-Köbrunner SH. Sonographic Differentiation of benign from malignant breast lesions: Value of indirect measurement of ultrasound velocity. AJR Am J Roentgenol 1995;165:825–831

Rizzatto G, Chersevani R, Guiseppetti GM, Baldassarre S, Bonifacino A, Ranieri E. Breast Ultrasound. Bologna: Grasso; 1993

Rosen EL, Soo MS. Tissue harmonic imaging sonography of breast leasions. Clin Imaging 2001;25:379–384

Rosen PP. Rosen's Breast Pathology. 2nd ed. Philadelphia: Lippincott Williams and Wilkins; 2001:164

Rubin E. Cutting-edge sonography obviates breast biopsy. Diagn Imag Suppl 1996;9:

Rubin E, Miller VE, Berland LL, Han SY, Koehler RE, Stanley RJ. Hand-held real-time breast sonography. AJR Am J Roentgenol 1985;144(3):623–627

Saarela AO, Rissanen TJ, Kiviniemi HO, Paloneva TK. Mammographic and ultrasonographic findings in bilateral breast chemotherapy of breast cancer. Eur Radiol 1998;8(4):634–638

Satake H, Shimamoti K, Endo T, Ishigaki T, Funahashi H. Value of sonography and galactography in dilated ducts or cysts of the breast. Eur J Ultrasound 1997;6:127–130

Sauerbrei W, Madjar H, Prömpeler HJ. Differentiation of benign and malignant breast tumors by logistic regression and a classification tree using Doppler flow signals. Methods Inf Med 1998;37(3):226–234

Schlief R. Diagostic potential of intravenous contrast enhancement in various areas of cardiovascular Doppler ultrasound: Efficacy results of a multinational clinical trial with the galactose-based agent SHU 508 A. Echocardiography 1993;10:665–682

Schneider B, Laubenberger J, Kommoss F, Madjar H, Gröne K, Langer M. Multiple giant fibroadenomas: clinical presentation and radiologic findings. Gynecol Obstet Invest 1997;43(4):278–280

Seymour MT, Moskovic EC, Walsh G, Trott P, Smith IE. Ultrasound assessment of residual abnormalities following primary chemotherapy of breast cancer. Br J Cancer 1997;76(3):371–376

Shetty MK, Shah YP, Sharman RS. Prospective evaluation of combined mammographic and sonographic assessment in patients with palpable abnormalities of the breast. J Ultrasound Med 2003;22:263–270

Sickles EA. Periodic mammographic follow-up of probably benign lesions: results in 3,184 consecutive cases. Radiology 1991;179:463–468

Sickles EA. Probably benign breast lesions: when should follow-up be recommended and what is the optimal follow-up protocol? Radiology 1999;213:11–14

Skaane P, Engedal K, Skjennald A. Interobserver variation in the interpretation of breast imaging: comparison of mammography, ultrasonography, and both combined in the interpretation of palpable noncalcified breast masses. Acta Radiol 1997;38:497–502

Smitt MC, Birdwell RL, Goffinet DR. Breast electron boost planning: comparison of CT and US. Radiology 2001;219:203–206

Snider HC, Rubin E, Henson R. Axillary ultrasonography to detect recurrence after sentinel node biopsy in breast cancer. Ann Surg Oncol 2006;13(4):501–507

Soo MS, Rosen EL, Baker JA, et al. Negative predictive value of sonography with mammography in patients with palpable breast lesions. AJR Am J Roentgenol 2001;177:1167–1170

Stack JP, Redmond OM, Codd MB, Dervan PA, Ennis JT. Breast disease: Tissue characterization with Gd-DTPA enhancement profiles. Radiology 1990;174:491–494

Stavros AT, Thickman D, Rapp CL, Dennis MA, Parker SH, Sisney GA. Solid breast nodules: use of sonography to distinguish between benign and malignant lesions. Radiology 1995;196:123–134

Sterns EE, Zee B. Thermography as a predictor of prognosis in cancer of the breast. Cancer 1991;67:1678–1680

Svensson WE. A review of the current status of breast ultrasound. Eur J Ultrasound 1997;6:77–101

Szopinski KT, Pajk AM, Wysocki M, et al. Tissue harmonic imaging: utility in breast sonography. J Ultrasound Med 2003;22:479–487

Tabar L, Dean PB, Tot T. Teaching atlas of mammography. 3rd ed. Stuttgart: Thieme; 2001

Tabar L, Yen MF, Vitak B, Chen HHT, Smith RA, Duffy SW. Mammography service screening and mortality in breast cancer patients: 20 year follow-up before and after introduction of screening. Lancet 2003; 361:1405–1410

Teboul M, Halliwell M. Atlas of Ultrasound and Ductal Echography of the Breast. Oxford: Blackwell; 1995

Tohno E, Cosgrove DO, Sloane JP. Ultrasound diagosis of breast disease. Edinburgh: Churchill Livingstone; 1994

Ueno E, Tsunodo-Shimizu H, Nakamura N, Hirano M, Imanura A. Colour Doppler imaging for the diagnosis of solid breast masses. In: Kasumi F, Uenu E. Topics in Breast Ultrasound. Seventh International Congress on the Ultrasonic Examination of the Breast, Tokyo 1991, Shinohara

Weidner R, Semple JP, Welch WR. Tumor angiogenesis and metastasis-correlation in invasive breast carcinoma. N Engl J Med 1991;324:1–8

Weissmann CF. Breast ultrasound: new frontiers in imaging? Ultrasound Obstet Gynecol 2000;15:279–282

Wells PT, Halliwell M, Skidmore R, Webb AJ, Woodcock JP. Tumour detection by ultrasonic Doppler blood-flow signals. Ultrasonics 1977;15:231–232

White DN, Cledgett PR. Breast carcinoma detection by ultrasonic Doppler signals. Ultrasound Med Biol 1978;4:329–335

Williams KL, Phillips BH, Jones PA, Beaman SA, Fleming PJ. Thermography in screening for breast cancer. J Epidemiol Community Health 1990;44:112–113

Winehouse J, Douek M, Holz K, et al. Contrast-enhanced colour Doppler ultrasonography in suspected breast cancer recurrence. Br J Surg 1999;86(9):1198–1201

Index

Page numbers in *italics* refer to illustrations

A

A-mode (amplitude modulation) imaging 6, *6*
abscesses 131–139, *133*, *134*
  calcified *136*
  diagnostic criteria 132–138
    edema 132
    excluding malignancy 135–136
    long-standing lesions 136
    mass 132–134
    peri-implant inflammatory processes 137
    skin thickening 137
  documentation 139
  imaging role 138–139
  lactational 131
  management 138
  nonpuerperal 131–132
  see also mastitis
acoustic enhancement 4–5, *5*, *52*
acoustic impedance 3
acoustic shadow 3, 4, 52
  carcinoma *4*, *25–27*, *53*, *169–171*, 171
  scars *4*, 159, 160
adenofibroma 141, *148*
adenomyoepithelioma *148*
adenosis tumor 141
adolescent breast 25, 63, *63*, *64*, *66*
American College of Radiology accreditation 59
American Institute of Ultrasound in Medicine accreditation 59
anechoic pattern 50, *50*
angular margin 48, *48*
annular-array sector transducer 9, *10*
antiradial scans 39
apocrine metaplasia *206*
architectural distortion 55, *55*
areola *64*, *65*
aspiration
  abscesses 138
  benign tumors 153
  breast implants and 127, 128, *128*, 207, *208*
  carcinoma 188, *188*, *206*
  cysts *103*, 108–109, *109*, 114, 138, *139*, *206*, 207
  fibrocystic tissue 97, *97*
  fine-needle aspiration cytology 205–208, *206*, *242*
    fluid-filled lesions 207, *207*, 208
    instruments 205
    solid lesions 205–207, *206*, *207*
  lymph node 197
  needle insertion technique 201–205, *202–204*
attenuation 3–4
atypical ductal hyperplasia *52*
axilla 62, *62*, 67, *68–69*
  metastases *231*, *232*, *240*, *241*, *251*
  see also lymph nodes
axillary artery *68*
axillary vein *68*, *69*
  thrombosis *231*

B

B-cell lymphoma *177*
B-mode (brightness modulation) imaging 6, 7, 12
background echotexture 44, *44*
benign solid tumors 141
  diagnostic criteria 141–149
  differential diagnosis 150–151
  documentation 156
  mammography 153
  MRI 153–155
  ultrasound 153
  see also specific tumors
BI-RADS-US system 43–60
  assessment categories 59, 75–76
  classification categories 44–58
    background echotexture 44, *44*
    calcifications 55–56, *55–56*
    masses 45–55, *45–55*
    special cases 56–58
    vascularity 58, 59
  development of 43
  feature analysis 43–44
  quality assurance 59–60
biopsy 208–210
  see also core biopsy
blood flow measurement 245–246, *246*
  see also Doppler ultrasound
breast
  anatomy 61–62, *61*, 72–73, *72*
  sonographic morphology 62–67, *63–66*
breast augmentation *117*, *118*, *121*
  carcinoma and 126
  see also breast implants
breast carcinoma 32, *34*, 167–190, *247*
  acoustic shadow *4*, *25–27*, *53*, *169–171*, 171
  aspiration 188, *188*, 207
  clinical significance 167–168
  core biopsy 188, *188*, 221, *239*
  cystic disease and *185*, *186*, *187*
  diagnostic criteria 168–176
    echogenicity 169, *170*
    effect on surrounding tissue *173*, *174*
    hyperechogenicity 175–176, *175*
    margins 168–169, *169*, *170*
    orientation 171–173, *172–174*
    posterior features 171, *172*
    shape 168–169
  differential diagnosis 92, *165*, *168*, 180, *181*
  documentation 190
  Doppler ultrasound applications 250
  heterogenous *4*
  implants and 126–127, *127*, *128*
  infiltrating
    ductal 47–49, 53, 56, 112, 175, 217–218
    lobular 47, 175, 218
  inflammatory 55, *59*, 137, 138
  intracystic *48*, *51*, *107*, *110*, *112*, *185*, *186*
  intraductal *35*, 56, 216–218, *216–218*
  invasive *11*, *26*, *31*, *75*, *95*, *111*, *113*, *168*, 216
    ductal 56, 59, 138, 189–190, 250, 252
      diagnosis 47–48, 94, 95, 112, 151, 168–174, 178, 181–184, 186
      imaging 26, 33, 38, 236–238, *239–242*, 245
      screening 226
      staging 215–217, 220
    lobular 53, 54, 177, 178
    squamous cell 179
  male *49*
  medullary *179*
  metaplastic *55*
  mucinous *150*, 179
  multicentric 167, *186*, *187*, 190, 218–219, 220, 221, 224, 227, 250
  multifocal *34*, *113*, 167, *177*, *182*, *213*, 216, 218–219, *219*, *225*, *237*, *240*, 250, *250*
  necrotic *187*
  papillary *48*, *178*
  recurrence 229, *230*, *233*, *234*, *253*
    after mastectomy 126–127, *127*, 128
    detection of locoregional recurrences 229–233
    ultrasound role 234
  sites of occurrence 167
  surgical planning 220–222
  tubular *179*
  types of 167

ultrasound role 189
vascularity 248–249
see also preoperative staging; screening
breast implants 117–129, *117*
  aspiration and 127, 128, *128*, 207, *208*
  clinical significance 117–119
  differential diagnosis 128
  documentation 129
  implant abnormalities 122, 123
    capsular contraction 122, 123
    fibrous encapsulation 122
    rupture 123–126, *124*, *125*, *126*
    tumors 126–127, *127*, 128
  indications for 117
  inflammatory processes and 137, *137*
  sites of 117
  sonographic findings 119–127
    different types of implants 118–123, *120*, *121*
  types of 117
  ultrasound role 128–129
brightness settings 12, *12*

C

calcifications 55–56
  abscess *136*
  ductal carcinoma in situ 54, *56*
  fibroadenoma *146*
  macrocalcifications 55, *55*
  microcalcifications *54*, 56, *56*, 98, 105, *112*, 215, *248*, *249*
    fibrocystic change 88–89, *89*, *90*, *95*
    invasive ductal carcinoma 94
  milk of calcium 88, *104*, 146
  "popcorn" *53*
  secretory *85*
  "teacup" 88, 146
carcinoma *see* breast carcinoma
chemotherapy 252, *252*
circumscribed margin 48, *48*
clinical examination 71–72
color-flow Doppler imaging 10, *11*, 245, *246*
  carcinoma *245*
  fibrocystic change 96
  see also Doppler ultrasound
comedocarcinoma *176*, *219*
complex echo pattern 50, *51*
compounding 9, 241, *241–242*
  see also real-time compound scan
compression 40, *40*, *41*, 62, 63, *64*, 72, 83
  carcinoma and *25*, *27*, *170*
  fibrocystic change and 86, *87*
  scars and *160*, *161*, *162*
continuous-wave Doppler (CW Doppler) 10, *11*
contrast agents 252–254
contrast settings 12, *12*, 16
Cooper ligament changes 54, *54*, *174*, *175*
core biopsy 208, *209*
  abscess *138*
  benign tumors 153–155
    fibroadenoma 155
  carcinoma 188, *188*, 221, *239*
  fibrocystic tissue 97
  lymph node 197
cysts 10, 32, 33, 75, 84, 88, 93, 99–115, *100*, *147*
  acoustic enhancement *5*, *6*, *52*
  aspiration *103*, 108–109, *109*, 114, 138, *139*, *206*, 207
  carcinoma and cystic disease *185*, *186*, *187*
  causes 99
  clinical significance 99
  complicated *51*, 56, *56*, 100–108
    fluid levels 105, *105*, 108–109, *108*
  diagnostic criteria 99–108
  differential diagnosis 108–114, *146*
  documentation 115
  echo pattern *50*, *51*
  functional resolution 16
  hemosiderin-containing *104*

image quality 18, *20*
inclusion *57*, *165*
infected 132, *139*
interventional procedures 114–115
intracystic carcinoma 48, *51*, *107*, *110*, *112*, *185*, *186*
intracystic papilloma 105–106, *106*, *107*, 109, *248*
intracystic reverberations 100, *102*, *103*, 109
intracystic thrombus *46*
juvenile 106, *107*, *108*, *114*
  infected 132
macrocysts 99, *101*
microcysts *83*, *84*, 88–89, *93*, 99, *100*, *102*
  clustered 56, *56*, 105
multiple septations *101*
oil 105, *105*
orientation *47*
sebaceous *57*
silicone 126, *127*
treatment 99
ultrasound role 115
wall proliferation 105–106
water-path scanning techniques *23*, *24*
see also fibrocystic change

D

demographic documentation 13
desmoplasia 171
diabetic mastopathy/fibrosis 86, *88*
discharge, nipple 89–91, *92*
display modes 6, *6*
documentation 77
  abscesses 139
  benign tumors 156
  breast implants 129
  carcinoma 190
  cysts 115
  demographic 13
  fibrocystic change 98
  lymph nodes 198
  scars 166
documentation unit 12
Doppler ultrasound 9–11, 245–254
  applications 250–252
    carcinomas 250, *250*
    chemotherapy and follow-up 252, *252*
    fibroadenomas 250
    lymph node evaluation 251, *251*
    multifocal and multicentric tumors 250, *250*
    prognostic evaluation 252
    scars 250–251, *251*
  clinical principles 245
  continuous-wave Doppler (CW Doppler) 10, *11*
  contrast agent use 252–254
  duplex scanning 10, *11*
  examination technique 246
  historical development 245–246
  interpretive criteria 247–249
    vascularity 248–249
  power Doppler 10
  scars 166
  see also color-flow Doppler imaging
ductal carcinoma in situ 49, 54, *56*, *112*, 175, 217–218
ductal ectasia 38, 54, 84, *85*, 86
ductography 97
ducts 63, *74*
  dilated *85*, *93*, *95*, 96
  in fibrocystic change 82–85, 86, *89*
  proliferative expansion 217, *217*
  see also ductal ectasia
duplex scanning 10, *11*
dynamic examination 39–40
  compression 40, *40*, *41*
  evaluating spatial extent 39, *39*, *40*
dynamic range 16

E

echogenic halo 50, *50*
ectatic veins *96*
edema 55, *55*
    mastitis 132, *132*
    postirradiation *162*
electronic convex-array transducer 8
electronic linear-array transducer 7–8, *8, 9, 241*
electronic sector transducer 9
enhancement 4–5, *5*, 52, *52*
European Group for Breast Cancer Screening 60
examination 71–72
extended field-of-view ultrasound 235, 243
    sample applications 239–241, *239*
    technical principles 236–237

F

fat 62, *63, 64, 65, 66*, 72
    lobules 44, *44, 45*, 150
    necrosis 151, *152*, 164, *164*
fatty breast *25, 39*, 73, *73, 151*
fibroadenolipoma 143, 146–149
fibroadenoma 40, 52, *53, 75*, 141, *142–144, 152, 238, 247*
    acoustic enhancement *5*
    aspiration 206, *206*
    bilateral *144*
    calcified *146*
    core biopsy *155*
    diagnostic criteria 141–145
    differential diagnosis 150–151, *168, 181*
    echo pattern *51*
    lesion boundary *50*
    lobulated *143*
    multiple *154*
    proliferative 145, *145, 146*
        Doppler ultrasound application 248, 250
    resection *209*
    shape *45, 46*
    see also benign solid tumors
fibrocystic change *38, 52*, 63, 73, 81–98, *93, 102, 242*
    aspiration 97
    causes 81
    clinical significance 81
    color Doppler 96
    core biopsy 97
    diagnostic criteria 82, 86
    differential diagnosis *181*
    documentation 98
    ductography 97–98
    MRI 96
    proliferative 89, *94*, 97
    symptoms 81
    treatment options 81
    ultrasound diagnosis 82–92
        pitfalls 92
        role of 98
    see also cysts; fibrotic change
fibrocystic nodules 88, 145–146, *147*
fibroglandular tissue *25*, 44, *44*
fibrolipoma 146, *148*, 207
fibroma 142
fibrotic change 66, 73, 82–83
    diabetic fibrosis 86, *88*
    postirradiation fibrosis *162*
    see also fibrocystic change
final evaluation 76
fine-needle aspiration 205–208, *206, 242*
    fluid-filled lesions 207, *207, 208*
    instruments *205*
    solid lesions 205–207, *206, 207*
    see also aspiration
fluid levels 105, *105*, 108–109, *108*
foam cells *206*
focusing 6–7, *9*, 13

follow-up
    clinical significance 229
    detection of locoregional recurrences 229–233
    Doppler ultrasound application 252, *252*
    postoperative 159–164
    ultrasound role 234
foreign bodies 57, *57*
foreign body granuloma *50*
    silicone 126, *127*
Freiburg Screening Study 226–227
    conclusions 227

G

gain settings 12–13, *13*
galactocele *54*, 153, *154*
gel pads 31
granular cell tumor *49, 147*
granuloma
    foreign body *50*
        silicone 126, 127
    scar 164, *165, 253*
granulomatous inflammation *135, 136*
granulomatous tumor *155*
gray-level reproduction 16

H

hamartoma 146–149, *149*
hemangioma 149
hematoma, postoperative 162–164, *163, 166, 180, 183*
hemodynamic parameters 248–249
hemosiderin *93, 104*
heterogeneous background 44, *44*
history 71
homogeneous background echotexture 44, *44*
hyperechoic pattern 50, *51*
    carcinoma 175–176, *175*
hypoechoic pattern 50, *51*

I

image field 16
image labeling 13
image scale 13
immersion scanning 24–25, *24–27, 62, 63, 64*
impedance, acoustic 3
implants *see* breast implants
inclusion cyst *57, 165*
indistinct margin 48, *48*
inflammation
    granulomatous *135, 136*
    inflammatory carcinoma 55, *59, 138*
    lymph nodes 58, *58*
    peri-implant inflammatory processes 137
internal thoracic artery 62, *62*, 67, *67*
International Breast Ultrasound School 60
interventional ultrasound 201–213
    clinical significance 201
    core biopsy 208, *209*
    fine-needle aspiration cytology 205–208, *206*
        fluid-filled lesions 207, 207, 208
        instruments 205
        solid lesions 205–207, *206, 207*
    indications for 201
    large needle biopsy 208
    methods 201
    needle insertion technique 201–205, *202–204*
    specimen ultrasonography 212, *212, 213*
    ultrasound-guided localization 210, *211, 212*
    vacuum-assisted devices 208, *209, 210*
involuted breast *63, 64, 65, 66*, 85
isoechoic pattern 50, *51*

J

juvenile cyst 106, *107, 108, 114*
  infected 132

K

keloid formation 162, *163*

L

lactational abscesses 131
Levovist 253–254
lipoma *51*, 146, *152*
lobular carcinoma in situ (LCIS) *218*
lymph nodes 62, *62*, 67, *67*, 191–198
  aspiration 197
  axillary 58, *58*, 68, *69*
  clinical significance 191
  core biopsy 197
  diagnostic criteria 191–196
  differential diagnosis 196
  documentation 198
  Doppler ultrasound applications 251, *251*
  intramammary 58, *58*, 153, *155*
  metastases 67, *69*, 191, 192–196, *192–196*, 197, 230, 232, 251, 252
    hilar 194, *194*, 195
    peripheral 194
  reactive 191–192, *192, 237*
  ultrasound role 197
lymphadenopathy 139
lymphatic drainage *62*
lymphoma, B-cell *177*

M

M-mode (motion mode) imaging 6, *7*
macrocalcifications 55, *55*
macrocysts 99, *101*
magnetic resonance imaging (MRI)
  benign tumors 153–155
  breast implants 118, *118*, 128, 129
  fibrocystic change 96
  mastitis 139
  scars 164–166
mammography
  advantages of 76
  benign tumors 153
  breast carcinoma *169*
  disadvantages of 76
  mastitis 138
  prior mammograms 72
  role in follow-up 234
  scars 164
  see also screening
Mammotome *209, 210*
masses 45–55, *45*
  boundary 50, *50*
  echo pattern 50, *51, 52*
  in or on the skin 57, *57*
  margin 48, *48, 49*
  orientation 46, *47*
  posterior acoustic features 52, *52, 53*
  shape 45–46, *45, 46, 47*
  surrounding tissue 54–55, *54, 55*
  see also specific masses
mastitis *55*, 131–132
  edema 132, *132*
  following implant insertion *137*
  forms of 131
  imaging role 138–139
  lymphoplasmacytic periductal *135*
  plasma cell 85

suppurative *132, 248*
treatment 131
see also abscesses
mechanical sector transducer 7, *8*
metastases 67, *69, 137*, 150, *230, 231*, 233, *251, 252*
  axillary *231, 232, 240, 241, 251*
  clinical significance 191
  diagnostic criteria 191–196, *192–196*
  differential diagnosis 196
  see also lymph nodes
microcalcifications *54*, 56, *56*, 98, 105, *112, 248, 249*
  fibrocystic change 88–89, *89, 90, 95*
  invasive ductal carcinoma *94*
microcysts *83, 84*, 88–89, *93*, 99, *100, 102*
  clustered 56, *56*, 105
microlobulated margin 48, *49*
milk of calcium 88, *104*, 146
monitor settings 12, *12*
multicentricity 167, *186, 187, 190*, 218–219, *220, 221, 224, 227*, 250
multifocality *34, 113*, 167, *177, 182*, 213, 216, 218–219, *219*, 225, *237, 240*, 250, *250*
myoepithelioma 149

N

necrosis
  fat 151, *152*, 164, *164*
  necrotic carcinoma *187*
neurofibroma 149
nipple *64, 65*
  discharge 89–91, 92
nonpuerperal abscesses 131–132

O

oil cysts 105, *105*

P

Paget disease 217, *219*
palpation 71
papilloma
  intracystic 105–106, *106, 107*, 109, *248*
  intraductal 89, *91, 240*
    localization 92
parasternal region 62, 67, *67*
parenchyma 62, 63, *63, 66*, 73
  patterns 62, *74*
patient history 71
patient positioning 28–29, *29*
phyllodes tumor 149, *149, 150*
plasma cell mastitis 85
pleural effusion 233, *233*
pneumocystography 114–115
"popcorn" calcifications 53
postirradiation changes *162*
postmastectomy reconstruction *117, 120, 121, 123*
  carcinoma and 126–127, *127, 128*
  see also breast implants
postmastectomy seroma 128, *129*
postoperative follow-up 159–164
power Doppler 10
pregnancy 153
preoperative staging 215–222
  clinical significance 215
  intraductal carcinomas and components 216–218, *216–218*
  multicentricity 218–219, *220, 221*
  multifocality 218–219, *219*
  tumor size 215–216
prognostic evaluation 251
pseudomass *39, 40*
pulsatility index (PI) 246
pulsed sound waves 6

Q

quality control 15
   quality assurance programs 59–60
   see also test phantoms

R

radial scans 37, *38*
real-time compound scan 235, *241*, 243
   sample applications 241, *241–242*
   technical principles 237–238
real-time examination 28–39, *28*, 62–67, *64–66*
   patient positioning 28–29, *29*
   scanning technique 32–39
      antiradial or tangential scans 39, *39*
      radial scans 37, *38*
      sagittal scans 32–35, *35*, *36–37*, *38*
      target ultrasound assessment of palpable masses 39
      transverse scans 35–37, *37*
   transducer coupling 31–32, *32*
   transducer handling 29–31, *30*
   transducer selection 31, *31*
   see also real-time compound scan
resistance index (RI) 246
retroareolar region *242*
reverberations
   breast implants *119*, *122*, *123*, *125*
   intracystic 100, *102*, *103*, 109
ribs *45*, 65, *66*, *67*, 151, *152*

S

sagittal scans 32–35, *35*, *36–37*, *38*
sarcoidosis *58*, *135*, *155*
scars *4*, *5*, *55*, 151, 157–166, *160*, *161*
   acoustic shadowing *4*, 159, *160*
   clinical significance 157
   diagnostic criteria 159–164
   diagnostic problems 157–159, *157*, *158*, *159*
   diagnostic procedures 164–166
   differential diagnosis 164, *180*, *181*
   documentation 166
   Doppler ultrasound applications 250–251, *251*
   granuloma 164, *165*, 253
   hypertrophic scar formation 160–162, *162*
   ultrasound role 166
sclerosing adenosis 86, *87*, 98
screening 223–227
   clinical significance 223
   prerequisites 223–224
   studies on 226–227
   target group 223
sebaceous cyst 57
sentinel node imaging 191
   see also lymph nodes
seroma, postoperative 128, *129*, 162, *163*, 164, *166*, *234*, *240*
shadowing *see* acoustic shadow
silicone 57
   cyst 126, *127*
   granuloma 126, *127*
   see also breast implants
sinus histiocytosis 191
skin retraction/irregularity 55, *55*
skin thickening 55, *55*, 137
sound
   acoustic enhancement 4–5, *5*
   acoustic impedance 3

   attenuation 3–4
   pulsed sound waves 6
   speed of 3
   wavelength 3
spatial resolution 16
specimen ultrasonography 212, *212*, *213*
spiculated margin 48, *49*
staging *see* preoperative staging
standoff pads 31, *31*
stromal fibrosis *52*
surgical planning 220–222

T

tangential scans 39, *39*
target ultrasound assessment of palpable masses 39
"teacup" calcifications 88, 146
test phantoms 15–21
   characteristics 15–16, *16*
   test protocol 16–17
   test results 17–21, *17–20*
thoracodorsal artery *68*, 231
thoracodorsal vein *68*
three-dimensional ultrasound 235, 243
   sample applications 238, *239*
   technical principles 235–236, *236–238*
thrombus *46*
   axillary vein *231*
time gain compensation (TGC) 5, 12, *14*
tissue harmonic imaging 9
transducers 7–9
   electronic convex-array transducer *8*
   electronic linear-array transducer 7–8, *8*, *9*, *241*
   electronic sector transducer 9
   mechanical sector transducer 7, *8*
   selection of 14–15
      field of view 14–15
      transducer frequencies 14
   two-dimensional annular-array sector transducer 9, *10*
transverse scans 35–37, *37*

U

ultrasound
   advantages of 76
   disadvantages of 77
   see also Doppler ultrasound; extended field-of-view ultrasound; interventional ultrasound; *specific applications*; three-dimensional ultrasound
ultrasound-guided localization 210, *211*, *212*

V

VacuFlash system *210*
vacuum-assisted devices 208, *209*, *210*
vascularity *58*, *59*, 248–249

W

water-path scanning 23–27, *28*
   immersion technique 24–25, *24–27*, *28*, 62, *63*, *64*
   water-bag technique 23, *23*
wavelength 3
wide field-of-view imaging *see* extended field-of-view ultrasound